T0182142

Contemporary Endocrinology

Series Editor

Leonid Poretsky
Division of Endocrinology
Lenox Hill Hospital
New York, NY, USA

More information about this series at http://www.springer.com/series/7680

Lewis Landsberg
Editor

Pheochromocytomas, Paragangliomas and Disorders of the Sympathoadrenal System

Clinical Features, Diagnosis and Management

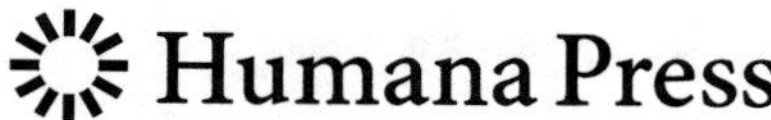

Editor
Lewis Landsberg
Northwestern University
Feinberg School of Medicine
Chicago, IL, USA

ISSN 2523-3785 ISSN 2523-3793 (electronic)
Contemporary Endocrinology
ISBN 978-3-030-08357-1 ISBN 978-3-319-77048-2 (eBook)
https://doi.org/10.1007/978-3-319-77048-2

Printed on acid-free paper

This Humana Press imprint is published by the registered company Springer International Publishing AG part of Springer Nature.
The registered company address is: Gewerbestrasse 11, 6330 Cham, Switzerland

Series Editor Foreword

Although it is my privilege as a Series Editor to write a foreword for every volume, sometimes this privilege proves to be truly special, as is the case with the current volume – *Pheochromocytomas, Paragangliomas and Disorders of the Sympathoadrenal System: Clinical Features, Diagnosis and Management.* The volume is edited by Dr. Lewis Landsberg, who was my mentor during the fellowship training at Boston's Beth Israel Hospital (now Beth Israel Deaconess) and Harvard Medical School more than three decades ago. At the time, Lew was already a giant in the field, having authored the chapters on pheochromocytoma in major textbooks, including our specialty's "bible" – *The Williams Textbook of Endocrinology.* It is extraordinarily rewarding to see Dr. Landsberg continuing to advance our fund of knowledge in truly remarkable ways, as he has done with this volume.

As noticed in one of the chapters in the current volume, pheochromocytomas are rare but their symptoms are common. Indeed, we think of a possibility of pheochromocytoma in our patients and undertake the diagnostic work-up frequently, while we do not find the disease very often. Pheochromocytomas and paragangliomas, therefore, continue to present diagnostic and therapeutic challenges for practicing endocrinologists.

The current volume addresses its subject using a "classical" approach, starting with etiology (including genetics), continuing to pathogenesis, clinical presentation, diagnostic work-up, and management (both medical and surgical) with chapters written in a clear but comprehensive style by international authorities in the field. As expected from this group of authors, the book does not limit itself to pheochromocytomas and paragangliomas but also addresses disorders of the sympathoadrenal system, including, for example, such a common condition as hypertension.

Without a doubt, *Pheochromocytomas, Paragangliomas and Disorders of the Sympathoadrenal System: Clinical Features, Diagnosis and Management* will prove to be extremely useful and enjoyable reading to those interested in this fascinating and challenging subject.

New York, NY, USA Leonid Poretsky

Preface

Pheochromocytomas, catecholamine-producing tumors derived from chromaffin cells, have intrigued and perplexed clinicians for over 100 years. Although relatively uncommon, pheochromocytoma is an important tumor for the following reasons: Correctly diagnosed and properly treated, it is almost always curable; misdiagnosed or improperly treated, it is usually lethal. Unselected autopsy series demonstrate that more than 50% of pheochromocytomas are not recognized during life; postmortem review of these cases indicates that death was usually attributable to the tumor. Pheochromocytomas are dangerous by virtue of the secretion of their stored, biologically active compounds, principally catecholamines; as a result, truly spectacular and alarming clinical manifestations commonly occur. Although malignancy does occur in a minority of cases, the principal threat to life is the unrestrained and unregulated release of catecholamines.

The first description of pheochromocytoma is attributed to Felix Frankel (Freiburg, Switzerland) in 1886, who reported a young woman who had suffered from headaches and palpitations and who was found to have bilateral adrenal medullary tumors at postmortem examination. The term *pheochromocytoma* was coined in 1912 by Ludvig Pick, the renowned German pathologist, who noted the marked darkening of adrenal medullary tumors when exposed to chromium salts. The term *chromaffin* is a portmanteau word designating an affinity for chromium salts; the cut surface of pheochromocytomas darken on exposure to potassium dichromate, which oxidizes the catecholamines to highly polymerized, darkly pigmented compounds.

The first successful surgical removal of a pheochromocytoma was performed in 1926 by Cesar Roux in Switzerland and Charles Mayo in the United States. Progressive advances in the diagnosis and treatment of pheochromocytoma over the ensuing decades, as well as the delineation of genetic pheochromocytoma syndromes, make this a propitious time for a thorough review of the subject. It is the aim of this book to provide just such a review. Other chapters considering disease states that may mimic some of the manifestations of chromaffin cell tumors are included as well.

This volume should be of interest to general internists, endocrinologists, endocrine fellows, endocrine surgeons, anesthesiologists, and intensivists as well as medical students and graduate students in the biological sciences.

For the sake of brevity, pheochromocytomas are frequently referred to as "pheos." Extra-adrenal pheos are commonly known as "paragangliomas."

Chicago, IL, USA Lewis Landsberg

Contents

Contributors

Ana Maria Arbelaez, MD Washington University School of Medicine, St. Louis, MO, USA

Monica Bianco, MD Department of Pediatrics, Northwestern University Feinberg School of Medicine, Chicago, IL, USA

Division of Endocrinology, Ann and Robert H. Lurie Children's Hospital of Chicago, Chicago, IL, USA

Kenneth K. Chen, MD Division & Fellowship Director, Obstetric & Consultative Medicine Staff Endocrinologist, Women & Infants' Hospital of Rhode Island, Alpert Medical School of Brown University, Providence, RI, USA

Philip E. Cryer, MD Washington University School of Medicine, St. Louis, MO, USA

Elizabeth Dabrowski, MD Department of Pediatrics, Northwestern University Feinberg School of Medicine, Chicago, IL, USA

Division of Endocrinology, Ann and Robert H. Lurie Children's Hospital of Chicago, Chicago, IL, USA

Benjamin Deschner, MD Department of Surgery, Northwestern University Feinberg School of Medicine, Chicago, IL, USA

Dina Elaraj, MD, FACS Department of Surgery, Northwestern University Feinberg School of Medicine, Chicago, IL, USA

Section of Endocrine Surgery, Northwestern University Feinberg School of Medicine, Chicago, IL, USA

Roy Freeman, MD Autonomic and Peripheral Nerve Laboratory, Department of Neurology, Beth Israel Deaconess Medical Center, Boston, MA, USA

Anthony J. Gill, MD, FRCPA University of Sydney and Cancer Diagnosis and Pathology Group, Kolling Institute of Medical Research, Royal North Shore Hospital, St Leonards, NSW, Australia

Guido Grassi, MD Clinica Medica, Università Milano-Bicocca, Monza, and IRCCS Multimedica, Sesto San Giovanni/Milan, Italy

Clinica Medica, Ospedale S. Gerardo dei Tintori, Monza, Italy

Carla B. Harmath, MD Department of Radiology, Section of Abdominal Imaging, The University of Chicago Medicine, Chicago, IL, USA

Pearl K. Jones, MD Lotus Spine and Pain, San Antonio, TX, USA

Rachel Kadakia, MD Department of Pediatrics, Northwestern University Feinberg School of Medicine, Chicago, IL, USA

Division of Endocrinology, Ann and Robert H. Lurie Children's Hospital of Chicago, Chicago, IL, USA

Peter Kopp, MD Division of Endocrinology, Metabolism and Molecular Medicine and Center for Genetic Medicine, Feinberg School of Medicine, Northwestern University, Chicago, IL, USA

Lewis Landsberg, MD Northwestern University, Feinberg School of Medicine, Chicago, IL, USA

Giuseppe Mancia, MD Università Milano Bicocca, Monza, Italy

Mark E. Molitch, MD Division of Endocrinology, Metabolism and Molecular Medicine, Northwestern University Feinberg School of Medicine, Chicago, IL, USA

Hatice Savas, MD University of Chicago Medicine, Chicago, IL, USA

Gino Seravalle, MD Cardiologia, Ospedale San Luca, IRCCS Istituto Auxologico Italiano, Milan, Italy

Ljuba Stojiljkovic, MD, PhD Department of Anesthesiology, Northwestern University, Feinberg School of Medicine, Northwestern Medical Group, Chicago, IL, USA

Arthur S. Tischler, MD Department of Pathology and Laboratory Medicine, Tufts Medical Center, Boston, MA, USA

Daniel J. Toft, MD, PhD Division of Endocrinology, Metabolism and Molecular Medicine, Northwestern University Feinberg School of Medicine, Chicago, IL, USA

John Turchini, MD University of Sydney and Cancer Diagnosis and Pathology Group, Kolling Institute of Medical Research, Royal North Shore Hospital, St Leonards, NSW, Australia

William F. Young, MD, MSc Division of Endocrinology, Diabetes, Metabolism, and Nutrition, Mayo Clinic, Rochester, MN, USA

Donald Zimmerman, MD Department of Pediatrics, Northwestern University Feinberg School of Medicine, Chicago, IL, USA

Division of Endocrinology, Ann and Robert H. Lurie Children's Hospital of Chicago, Chicago, IL, USA

Chapter 1
Catecholamines

Lewis Landsberg

The naturally occurring, biologically important catecholamines are *epinephrine* (adrenaline in the UK), *norepinephrine* (noradrenaline in the UK), and *dopamine*. These compounds are synthesized in vivo from tyrosine which is sequentially hydroxylated to form dihydroxyphenylalanine (DOPA), decarboxylated to form dopamine (DA), β-hydroxylated to form norepinephrine (NE), and N-methylated to form epinephrine (E) (Fig. 1.1). The initial step, the hydroxylation of tyrosine by tyrosine hydroxylase, is rate limiting for the entire pathway. N-methylation of NE to E occurs only in the adrenal medulla and in those central neurons that utilize E as a neurotransmitter [1].

E is a circulating hormone, synthesized and stored in the adrenal medulla and secreted from that gland in response to acetylcholine released from the preganglionic splanchnic nerves. The latter originate in the intermediolateral column of the thoracic spinal cord (Fig. 1.2). E also serves as a neurotransmitter in the central nervous system (CNS) [2].

NE is the neurotransmitter at all sympathetic nerve endings (SNE) except those innervating the sweat glands which utilize acetylcholine as a neurotransmitter. The peripheral sympathetic nerves originate in the paravertebral sympathetic ganglia. Like the adrenal medulla, they are innervated by preganglionic nerves originating in the intermediolateral column of the spinal cord [1]. Although NE is also stored and released from the adrenal medulla, it does not function as a circulating hormone unless the levels are very high, as may occur from intense adrenal medullary stimulation or secretion from a pheochromocytoma. NE is also a neurotransmitter in the CNS.

DA is an important neurotransmitter in the CNS; in the periphery DA appears to generate its physiologic effects from the decarboxylation of its circulating precursor (DOPA) in effector tissues such as the kidneys and the gut. The origin of circulating

L. Landsberg (✉)
Northwestern University, Feinberg School of Medicine, Chicago, IL, USA
e-mail: l-landsberg@northwestern.edu

L. Landsberg (ed.), *Pheochromocytomas, Paragangliomas and Disorders of the Sympathoadrenal System*, Contemporary Endocrinology,
https://doi.org/10.1007/978-3-319-77048-2_1

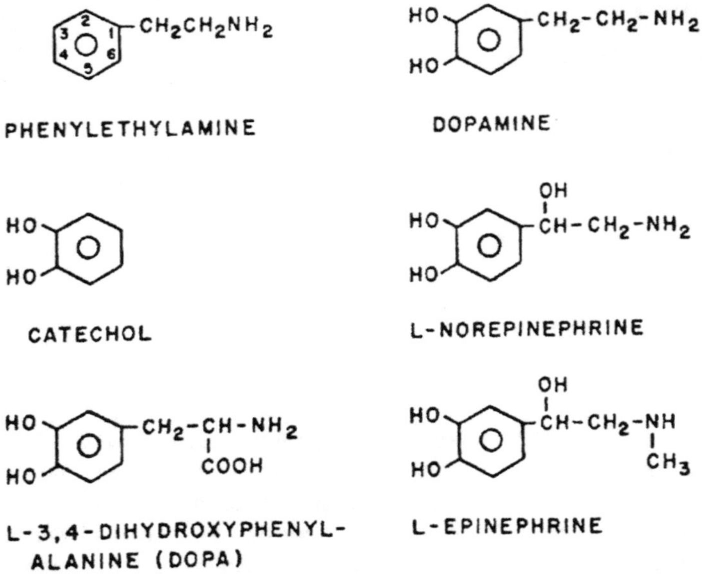

Fig. 1.1 Structures of naturally occurring catecholamines and related compounds. The conventional numbering system for ring and side chain substituents is shown for phenylethylamine, which may be considered the parent compound of many sympathomimetic amines. Catecholamines are hydroxylated at positions 3 and 4 on the ring (From Landsberg and Young [17], with permission)

DOPA is obscure, but a reasonable hypothesis localizes DOPA formation to the small intensely fluorescent (SIF) cells of the sympathetic ganglia [1, 3, 4].

Storage and Release of Catecholamines from Adrenal Medulla and Sympathetic Nerve Endings

Both the SNEs and the adrenal medulla contain large stores of catecholamines within discrete subcellular organelles known as chromaffin granules in the adrenal medulla and dense core vesicles in the nerve endings (Fig. 1.3). Storage within these structures provides a large functional reserve of catecholamines which are protected from enzymatic degradation by intracellular monoamine oxidase (MAO) [2, 5]. Catecholamine release is by exocytosis: fusion of the granule membrane with the cell wall and extrusion of the entire soluble contents of the granule or vesicle [1]. Exocytosis is triggered by the release of acetylcholine from the splanchnic preganglionic nerves that innervate the adrenal medulla and by depolarizing impulse traffic in the postganglionic sympathetic nerves (Fig. 1.4).

In the normal adrenal E constitutes about 75–80% of the total catecholamine content. In pheochromocytomas the relative concentration of NE is often increased.

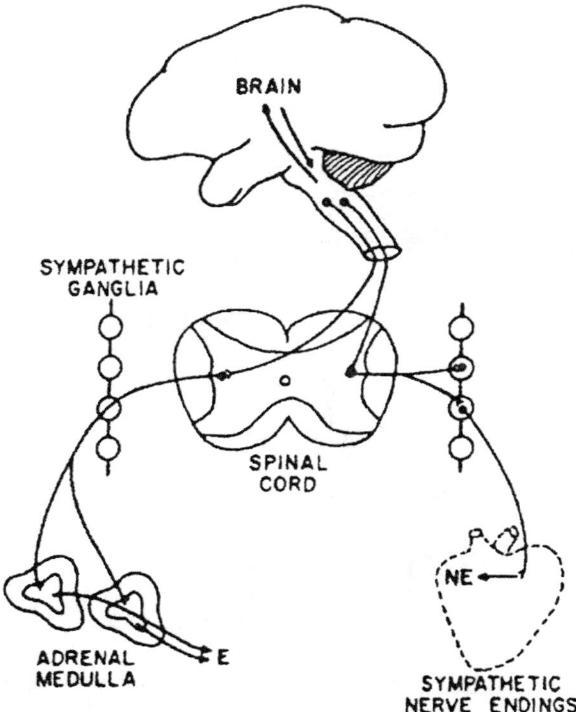

Fig. 1.2 Organization of the sympathoadrenal system. Descending tracts from the medulla, pons, and hypothalamus synapse with preganglionic sympathetic neurons in the spinal cord, which in turn innervate the adrenal medulla directly or synapse in paravertebral ganglia with postganglionic sympathetic neurons. The latter gives rise to sympathetic nerves, which are distributed widely to viscera and blood vessels. Release of epinephrine (E) or norepinephrine (NE) at the adrenal medulla or at sympathetic nerve endings occurs in response to a downward flow of nerve impulses from regulatory centers in the brain (From Landsberg and Young [17], with permission)

Fig. 1.3 Electron photomicrograph of human adrenal medulla. Cells at the lower left containing small, electro-dense particles are adrenomedullary chromaffin cells with chromaffin granules; those above are adrenocortical cells. Magnification ×7250. Inset (upper right) shows chromaffin granules with clearly defined limiting membranes under higher magnification (×50,000) (Courtesy of Dr. James Connolly)

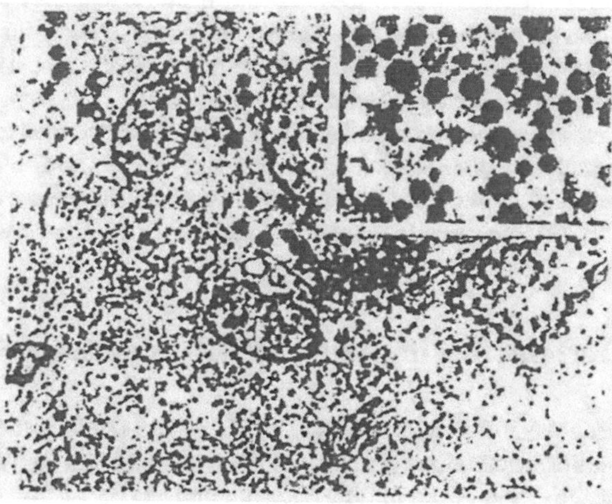

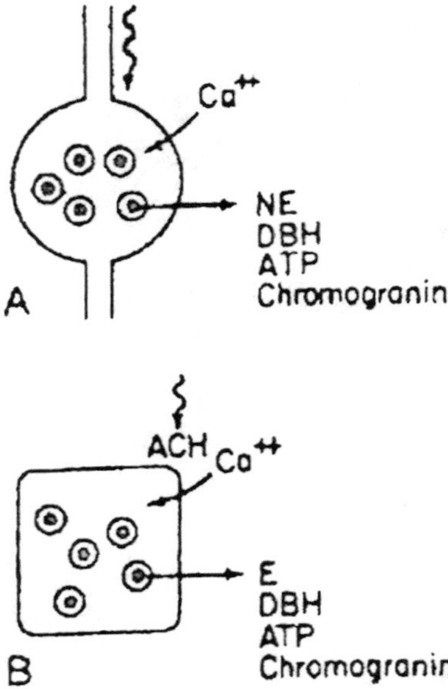

Fig. 1.4 Schematic representation of catecholamine release from a sympathetic nerve ending (**a**) and from an adrenomedullary chromaffin cell (**b**). Catecholamines, DBH, ATP, and chromogranin, as well as enkephalins (not shown), are released in stoichiometric amounts from the storage granule in response to nerve impulses. E, epinephrine; NE, norepinephrine (From Landsberg [18], with permission)

Central Regulation of Catecholamine Release

Descending tracts from the brainstem and the hypothalamus synapse with the preganglionic neurons in the intermediolateral cell column of the spinal cord (Fig. 1.2). Impulse traffic generated from these central neurons regulates the release of catecholamines from the adrenal medulla and SNS, thereby providing the CNS with control of the autonomic functions which maintain homeostasis and which react to external threats to the internal environment (fight or flight) [2, 6, 7]. The sympathoadrenal outflow is responsive to changes in arterial and venous pressure and to changes in the constituents of the circulating plasma such as oxygen and carbon dioxide tension, tonicity, pH, and the levels of hormones and substrates. In contrast the release of catecholamines from pheochromocytomas is unregulated since pheos are not innervated.

Termination of Action and Metabolism of Catecholamines

Reuptake of locally released NE from the SNEs is the major mechanism of transmitter inactivation; uptake into the nerve endings also plays an important role in the inactivation of circulating catecholamines (Fig. 1.5).

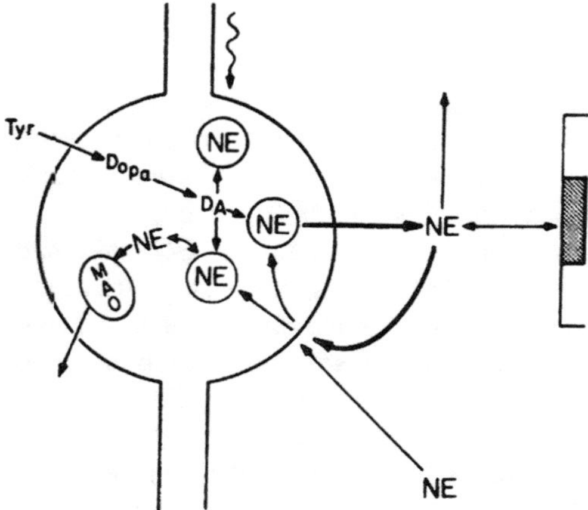

Fig. 1.5 Schematic representation of a sympathetic nerve ending. Tyrosine (Tyr) is taken up by the neuron and is sequentially converted to dopa and dopamine (DA); after uptake into the granule, DA is converted to norepinephrine (NE). In response to nerve impulses, NE is released into the synaptic cleft, where it may diffuse into circulation or be recaptured by a nerve. Accumulation of extragranular NE and DA is prevented by monoamine oxidase (MAO). NE within the synaptic cleft also interacts with presynaptic (or prejunctional) α- and β-adrenergic receptors on the axonal membrane that modulate NE release (not shown). A variety of other mediators also affect the presynaptic membrane and modulate NE release (From Landsberg and Young [17], with permission)

Table 1.1 Average[a] 24-h excretion of catecholamines and metabolites

Compound	μg/day	Major source(s)
Epinephrine (E)	5	Adrenal medulla
Norepinephrine (NE)	30	SNS
Conjugated NE + E	100	Dietary catechols
Metanephrine	65	Adrenal medulla
Normetanephrine	100	SNS
3-methoxy-4-hydroxy mandelic acid (VMA)	4000	SNS, adrenal, CNS
3-methoxy-4-hydroxyphenylglycol (MHPG)	2000	SNS, adrenal, CNS
Dopamine	225	Kidney
Homovanillic acid (HVA)	6900	CNS

[a]Not upper limit

Both E and NE are metabolized by catechol-O-methyltransferase (COMT) and monoamine oxidase (MAO), enzymes with high concentration in the liver and kidney. The action of COMT produces normetanephrine (NMN) from NE and metanephrine (MN) from E. Both of these metabolites are important in the diagnosis of pheochromocytoma. The product of both enzymes, 3-methoxy-4-hydroxy mandelic acid (VMA), is no longer used in the diagnosis of pheos. Both DA and homovanillic acid (HVA) (the end product of DA metabolism) are useful in the diagnosis of neuroblastoma. Average normal values (not upper limits) for the excretion of catecholamines and metabolites are shown in Table 1.1 [1, 2].

Adrenergic Receptors

Catecholamines influence the function of every organ system. The effects are mediated by cell surface receptors. Stimulation of these receptors by the excessive amounts of catecholamines released from pheochromocytomas accounts for many of the clinical manifestations noted in this disease.

Differential responses to catecholamines and SNS stimulation had been noted, respectively, by Sir Henry Dale and Professor Walter Cannon in the early years of the twentieth century. It was, however, Professor Raymond Ahlquist, in 1948, who postulated the existence of two types of adrenergic receptors, based on the differential potency of sympathomimetic amines on a variety of physiologic responses. He designated these α and β adrenergic receptors. Over the ensuing decades, the structure and function of adrenergic receptors have been established and the intracellular cascades responsible for tissue-specific responses identified [8]. To summarize briefly, adrenergic receptors are cell membrane proteins with seven-membrane-spanning domains, an extracellular amino terminus, intracellular carboxy terminus, and three intracellular loops; the third intracellular loop and the carboxy terminus have regulatory phosphorylation sites that influence receptor function. Receptor occupancy triggers adrenergic responses that depend, in turn, upon regulatory G proteins that associate with the receptors and initiate the intracellular cascades that result in responses characteristic of the receptor stimulated and the effector tissue. The calcium ion is involved as a second messenger in these intracellular cascades [9–11].

Specific agonists and antagonists have been developed for each receptor type and have wide applicability in medical practice and in the treatment of patients with pheochromocytoma. Subsequent work has identified major subtypes of the α and β receptors (designated α1 and α2 and β1, β2, and β3) with clinically useful selective agonists and antagonists available for many of these subtypes [12].

Some classic physiologic effects of α receptor stimulation are vasoconstriction (arteries and veins), intestinal relaxation, and pupillary dilatation; activation of the β receptor results in cardiac stimulation, lipolysis, bronchodilation, vasodilation, and glycogenolysis. These receptor actions are summarized in Table 1.2 along with the relevant receptor subtypes.

Table 1.2 Adrenergic receptors and major catecholamine responses

	α1	**α2**	
Potency	**E = NE**	**E = NE**	
Effects	Vasoconstriction Smooth muscle relaxation Pupillary dilation	Vasoconstriction ↓ Prejunctional NE release ↓ Insulin secretion ↑ Platelet aggregation	
	β1	**β2**	**β3**
Potency	**E = NE**	**E >>> NE**	**NE >>> E**
Effects	Cardiac stimulation ↑ Lipolysis ↑ Renin secretion	Vasodilation Bronchodilation ↑Hepatic glucose output	↑ Lipolysis ↑ BAT heat production

Physiologic Effects of Catecholamines

The regulatory role of catecholamines in controlling organ function may be grouped into three major categories: circulatory, metabolic, and visceral. The manifestations of pheochromocytoma reflect the impact of excessive catecholamine stimulation in these three categories.

Circulatory effects Catecholamines cause vasoconstriction and cardiac stimulation resulting in high blood pressure and tachycardia, thereby accounting for two of the most common manifestations of pheochromocytoma: hypertension and palpitations. The vasoconstrictive effects involve the venous (capacitance) as well as the arterial (resistance) portions of the circulation and are mediated by the α1 and α2 receptors. Cardiac stimulation is mediated by the β1 receptor [12]. The multiple effects of catecholamines on the circulation are shown graphically in Fig. 1.6.

The effects of catecholamines to diminish plasma volume are particularly important. Contraction of the great veins increases venous pressure which stimulates the low pressure baroreceptors; this increase in pressure is read in the CNS as volume expansion, and a diuresis is initiated, thereby diminishing plasma volume. This mechanism reflects the fact that the body cannot assess volume status directly; it senses volume by changes in pressure in the capacitance (low pressure) portion of the circulation.

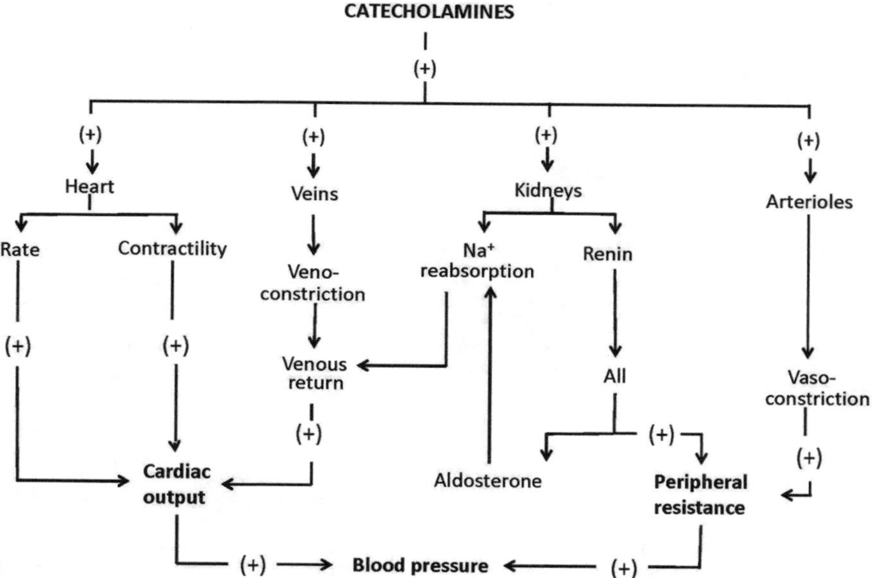

Fig. 1.6 Catecholamine effects on blood pressure. Sympathetic stimulation (+) increases blood pressure by effects on the heart, the veins, the kidneys, and the arterioles. The net result of sympathetic stimulation is an increase in both cardiac output and peripheral resistance. *AII* angiotensin II (Modified from Young and Landsberg [19])

The venoconstriction thus explains several important features of pheochromocytoma such as orthostatic hypotension and large swings in blood pressure: low volume reserve impairs the capacity to compensate for a fall in cardiac output by increasing venous return from the reservoir in the great veins. The diminished plasma volume also explains the high hematocrit occasionally noted (the so-called stress polycythemia) [2].

Metabolic effects Catecholamines have two major effects on metabolism: they cause substrate mobilization (lipolysis, glycogenolysis, and gluconeogenesis) [2, 13] and an increase in metabolic rate [1, 14–16]. The direct stimulatory effects on stored fuel are amplified by catecholamine induced suppression of insulin release, since substrate mobilization depends on a balance between catecholamines and insulin. Suppression of insulin (mediated by the $\alpha2$ receptor) and stimulation of hepatic glucose output ($\beta2$ receptor) account for the carbohydrate intolerance frequently noted in pheochromocytoma patients. Lipolysis in white adipose tissue stores is mediated by the $\beta1$ and $\beta3$ receptor.

The increase in metabolic rate is secondary to catecholamine stimulation of brown adipose tissue (BAT). The latter has been noted for decades to be hypertrophied and activated in patients with pheochromocytoma. BAT is a heat generating organ that operates via a unique mechanism that uncouples fatty acid oxidation from ATP synthesis (Fig. 1.7). The generation of heat from BAT may be briefly summarized as follows:

1. When stimulated by catecholamines, hormone-sensitive lipase in BAT generates free fatty acids which activates uncoupling protein (UCP 1).
2. The latter, a mitochondrial carrier protein, is uniquely localized to BAT.

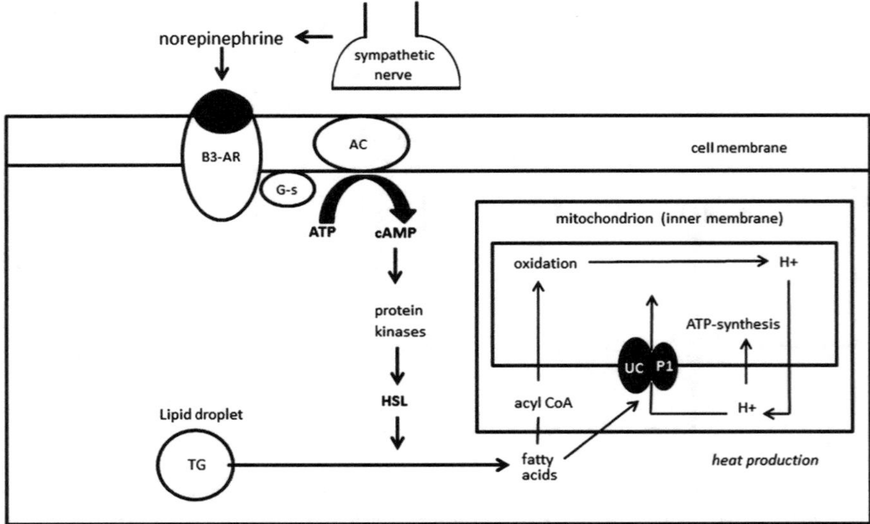

Fig. 1.7 BAT stimulation (see text for details)

3. UCP 1 permits hydrogen ions, formed from the action of the respiratory chain enzymes and excluded from the inner mitochondrial matrix during substrate oxidation, to reenter the inner mitochondrial matrix along its electromotive gradient without the synthesis of ATP.
4. In the normal coupled state reentry is tightly coupled to ATP synthesis which stores the energy released from the exothermic oxidative reactions.
5. When UCP1 is activated, ATP synthesis is bypassed, and the heat generated from the exothermic reactions increases the local temperature of BAT.
6. This heat is then exported to organs throughout the body via the vascular system [1].

During cold exposure this mechanism helps homoeothermic animals to maintain body temperature. Note that in patients with pheochromocytoma, this does not result in fever since the central set point for temperature regulation is not altered. The excess heat is dissipated by sweating, thereby accounting for a major symptom of pheochromocytoma.

Visceral effects Catecholamines relax visceral smooth muscle in the bronchial tree, the intestines, and the urinary bladder while stimulating the corresponding sphincters. The implications of these effects for patients with pheochromocytoma are less clear than the cardiovascular or metabolic effects described above, although alterations in GI motility are occasionally noted in pheochromocytoma patients. Both direct and indirect effects of catecholamines on the kidneys result in enhanced renal sodium reabsorption. The indirect effects are from stimulation of renin release and activation of the angiotensin-aldosterone system (Fig. 1.6). These effects might contribute to the hypertension in patients with a pheochromocytoma.

Pharmacology

The identification of adrenergic receptors was an important prelude to the development of agonists and antagonists to the classic α and β receptors and to several of their subtypes.

Adrenergic Agonists

The naturally occurring catecholamines, E and NE, stimulate α and β receptors and have limited but important therapeutic uses [8]. E is critical in the treatment of anaphylactic reactions, and its appropriate use is frequently lifesaving. E is also used as a cardiac stimulant in cardiac arrests. NE is a potent pressor agent used in the treatment of severe hypotension or shock. DA, administered intravenously, has a complex pharmacology that is dose dependent: at low doses it stimulates DA receptors and increases renal and mesenteric blood flow; at intermediate doses it stimulates, in addition, β receptors, while at high dose it activates α receptors which overrides the other effects.

Direct and Indirect Acting Sympathomimetic Amines

Sympathomimetic amines are congeners of the naturally occurring catecholamines that have been structurally modified to enhance one or more biologic properties [12]. These modifications influence, singly or in concert, various properties including reduction in metabolism and prolongation of action, increase in bioavailability via the oral route, effect specifically α or β receptors or their subtypes, and diminished or enhanced CNS penetration. Sympathomimetic amines are said to have direct effects when they interact with adrenergic receptors directly and indirect effects when they release the neurotransmitter, NE, from the SNEs. Some sympathomimetic amines have both direct and indirect effects; some are selective for the α1 receptor subtype. Some commonly utilized sympathomimetic amines, and their properties and indications are shown in Table 1.3. These drugs are useful in treating hypotension; they have also been used with limited success in patients with hepatorenal syndrome and pure autonomic neuropathy.

In pheochromocytoma patients, the catecholamine stores in the SNEs are increased due to the higher levels of circulating catecholamines; this results in an enhanced response to indirect acting sympathomimetic amines.

Adrenergic Prodrugs

Midodrine, droxidopa, α-methyldopa, and L-DOPA are prodrugs that are metabolized to active moieties in vivo. Midodrine is deglycinated to desglymidodrine, an α1 selective agonist used, with limited efficacy, in patients with hepatorenal syndrome

Table 1.3 Sympathomimetic amines

Agent	Action	Receptor	Therapeutic use
Phenylephrine	Direct	α1	Hypotension
Midodrine	Direct	α1	Orthostatic ↓ BP
Clonidine	Direct	α2	Hypertension
Isoproterenol	Direct	β1, β2	Bradycardia
Albuterol	Direct	β2	Bronchospasm
Terbutaline	Direct	β2	Bronchospasm
Formoterol	Direct	β2	Asthma (long acting)
Salmeterol	Direct	β2	Asthma (long acting)
Dobutamine	Direct	β1, β2, α1	CHF
Pseudoephedrine	Direct	α1, α2, β2	Decongestant
Ephedrine	Direct/indirect	α, β	Bronchospasm
Amphetamine	Indirect	α, β	Narcolepsy
Methylphenidate	Indirect	α, β	ADHD

CHF Congestive heart failure, *ADHD* Attention deficit hyperactivity disorder and orthostatic hypotension. Droxidopa (L-dihydroxyphenylserine, L-DOPS), a synthetic amino acid that forms NE when decarboxylated by aromatic amino acid decarboxylase (DOPA decarboxylase), is an enzyme widely distributed throughout the body. The NE so formed functions as a circulating pressor rather than as a neurotransmitter. It is used with limited success in the treatment of orthostatic hypotension. α-methyldopa (Aldomet), an antihypertensive medication rarely used today except in pregnancy induced hypertension, is decarboxylated and β-hydroxylated to α-methyl NE, a centrally active α2 agonist that lowers BP. L-DOPA, when given orally, is decarboxylated by the same decarboxylase and forms DA in vivo. It is used in the treatment of Parkinson's disease with some success. It is given in combination with carbidopa, a decarboxylase inhibitor that does not cross the blood brain barrier, thereby allowing increased concentrations of L-DOPA to enter the CNS where it is converted to DA and partially restores DA mediated neurotransmission in the basal ganglia [12].

Adrenergic Antagonists (α- and β-Blockers)

Blocking the action of the excessive amounts of catecholamines in patients with pheochromocytoma is the goal of medical management. The judicious use of adrenergic blocking agents will almost always reverse the symptoms of catecholamine excess and permit safe surgical removal of the tumor [1].

α-Blocking Agents

Two *nonspecific α-blockers* are useful in the treatment of pheochromocytoma although their availability may be limited due to short supply and expense [12]. *Phentolamine* has been used intravenously to provide a short-acting competitive blockade in the treatment of pheochromocytoma paroxysms. Its use has been largely replaced by other short-acting specific α1-blockers as described below. *Phenoxybenzamine* provides long-acting, noncompetitive blockade of both the α1 and α2 receptors, features that make it the drug of choice for the treatment of pheochromocytoma patients prior to surgery. Disadvantages of phenoxybenzamine include hypotension after surgical removal of the tumor because of the long duration of action and accentuation of the tachycardia that occurs in pheochromocytoma patients after α2 blockade which antagonizes the presynaptic inhibition of NE release at adrenergic synapses. These adverse effects can be effectively managed by fluid administration on the one hand and β blockade on the other.

Selective α1-blockers with differing duration of action are available and have proved useful in the treatment of pheochromocytoma (Table 1.4). *Doxazosin* produces a

Table 1.4 Adrenergic blocking agents

Agent	Receptor	Major therapeutic uses
Phentolamine (iv)	α1, α2	Pressor crises (pheochromocytoma, cocaine, MAOI)
Phenoxybenzamine	α1, α2	Pheochromocytoma
Prazosin	α1	Pressor crises
Terazosin	α1	Hypertension, BPH
Doxazosin	α1	Pheochromocytoma, hypertension, BPH
Tamsulosin	α1	BPH
Propranolol	β1, β2	Pheochromocytoma, hyperthyroidism, tachycardia
Metoprolol	β1	CAD, CHF, tachycardia
Atenolol	β1	Hypertension, HCM, hyperthyroidism
Esmolol (iv)	β1	OR, ICU: Tachycardia, aortic dissection
Carvedilol	β1, β2, α1	Hypertension, CHF, CAD
Labetalol	β1, β2, α1	Hypertension

MAOI Monoamine oxidase inhibition reactions, *BPH* Benign prostatic hypertrophy, *CAD* Coronary artery disease, *HCM* Hypertrophic cardiomyopathy

long-acting competitive blockade making it a reasonable alternative to phenoxybenzamine for the medical management and preoperative preparation of pheochromocytoma patients. Postoperative hypotension may be less with doxazosin than with phenoxybenzamine, and the α1 selectivity may result in less tachycardia. Although the competitive nature of the blockade means that catecholamine surges from the tumor could overcome the blockade, doxazosin has been quite successful when used in the treatment of pheochromocytoma. *Prazosin* is a selective α1-blocker with a very short duration of action. It has established usefulness in the treatment of individual paroxysms in patients with pheochromocytoma. *Tamsulosin* is a selective α1-blocker with specificity for the prostate gland and is used to treat lower urinary tract symptoms related to prostatic hypertrophy and outflow tract obstruction.

β-Blocking Agents

β-blockers are among the most widely prescribed drugs with a variety of indications involving cardiovascular and non-cardiovascular diseases, as outlined in Table 1.4 [1, 12]. The so-called first-generation β-blockers nonselectively block β1 and β2 receptors. *Propranolol* is the prototypic agent in this class and is the drug used most frequently in the management of patients with pheochromocytoma. It should be administered to all pheochromocytoma patients but only after α blockade has been introduced to avoid unopposed α-mediated vasoconstriction. In addition to slowing the heart rate, β-blockers antagonize anesthesia-related arrhythmias.

Second-generation β-blockers are selective for the β1 receptor although this selectivity is only relative and less than that noted for the α1-selective agents. These are also referred to as cardioselective β-blockers and include *metoprolol*, *atenolol*, and *esmolol*. Esmolol is a very short-acting agent used intravenously in the intensive care unit and the operating room where rapid onset and offset are important.

Third-generation β-blockers have a vasodilating moiety which is applied in addition to blockade of the β receptor. *Carvedilol* and *labetalol* are the two commonly used agents in this class; they block the β1, β2, and the α1 adrenergic receptors. Carvedilol is used in the treatment of CHF and hypertension; the vasodilating moiety lessens the unfavorable metabolic effects of β blockade. Labetalol is available in intravenous as well as oral formulation and finds its greatest use in the treatment of severe hypertension. Of note, it may interfere with catecholamine measurements in the diagnosis of pheochromocytoma. The potency of the effects on the β receptor is much greater than the effects on the α receptor.

References

1. Landsberg L. Catecholamines; Philadelphia: Wolters-Kluwer; 2017.
2. Young JB, Landsberg L. Chapter 13. Physiology of the sympathoadrenal system. In: Williams textbook. Philadelphia: 9th ed. Saunders; 1998.
3. Hall AK, Principal Neurons LSC. Small intensely fluorescent (SIF) cells in the rat superior cervical ganglion have distinct developmental histories. J Neurosci. 1991;11:472–84.
4. Carey RM. Chapter 45. Dopamine mechanisms in the kidney. In: Primer on the autonomic nervous system. Amsterdam: Elsevier Inc; 2012. p. 221–3.
5. Winkler H. The adrenal chromaffin granule: a model for large dense core vesicles of endocrine and nervous tissue. J Anat. 1993;183:237–52.
6. Benarroch EE. Chapter 2. Central autonomic control. In: Primer on the autonomic nervous system; Amsterdam: Acdamic press (Elsevier) 2012. p. 9–12.
7. Morrison SF. Differential control of sympathetic outflow. Am J Physiol Regulatory Integrative Comp Physiol. 2001;281:R683–98.
8. Westfall TC, Westfall DP. Neurotransmission: the autonomic and somatic motor nervous systems. In: Goodman & Gilman's the pharmacological basis of therapeutics. New York: McGraw Hill; 2011.
9. Gilman AG. G proteins: transducers of receptor-generated signals. Annu Rev Biochem. 1987;56:615–49.
10. Tobin AB. G-protein-coupled receptor phosphorylation: where, when and by whom. Br J Pharmacol. 2008;153(suppl 1):S167–S176.
11. Kohout TA, Lefkowitz RJ. Regulation of G protein-coupled receptor kinases and Arrestins during receptor desensitization. Mol Pharmacol. 2003;63:9–18.
12. Westfall TC, Westfall DP. Adrenergic agonists and antagonists. In: Goodman & Gilman's the pharmacological basis of therapeutics. 12th ed. New York: McGraw-Hill; 2011.
13. Coppack SW, Jensen MD, Miles JM. In vivo regulation of lipolysis in humans. J Lipid Res. 1994;35:177–86.
14. Enerbäck S. Brown adipose tissue in humans. Int J Obes. 2010;34:S43–6.

15. Morrison SF, Madden CJ, Tupone D. Central control of brown adipose tissue thermogenesis. Front Endocrinol. 2012;3:1–19.
16. Ricquier D. Uncoupling protein 1 of brown adipocytes, the only uncoupler: a historical perspective. Front Endocrinol. 2011;2:1–7.
17. Landsberg L, Young JB. Catecholamines and the adrenal medulla. In: Bondy PK, Rosenberg LE, et al., editors. Metabolic control and disease. 8th ed. Philadelphia: W.B. Saunders; 1980. p. 1621–93.
18. Landsberg L. Catecholamines and the sympathoadrenal system. In: Ingbar SH, editor. The year in endocrinology. New York: Plenum; 1976. p. 177–231.
19. Young JB, Landsberg L. Obesity and circulation. In: Sleight P, et al., editors. Scientific foundations of cardiology. London: Heineman; 1983.

Chapter 2
Pathology of Pheochromocytoma and Paraganglioma

John Turchini, Anthony J. Gill, and Arthur S. Tischler

Introduction

Pheochromocytomas and paragangliomas are tumors that arise from related neural crest-derived cells of the autonomic nervous system. The World Health Organization classification of endocrine tumors arbitrarily reserves the name pheochromocytoma for tumors that arise from the chromaffin cells of the adrenal medulla. Paragangliomas [1] are similar tumors that occur throughout the distribution of sympathetic nerves and ganglia and along branches of the glossopharyngeal and vagus nerves in the head and neck. Pheochromocytomas and paragangliomas may be morphologically and functionally identical or may show functional differences associated with different anatomic sites. Recent molecular and genetic advances have led to greatly increased understanding of these tumors. It is now known that as many as 30% are hereditary [2]. While some of the hereditary disorders, including von Hippel-Lindau syndrome (VHL), MEN2, and neurofibromatosis type 1 (NF1), have been well recognized for decades, recent discoveries have put a new focus on enzymes within the Krebs cycle, especially the *succinate dehydrogenase* (SDH) genes [3, 4]. Pathogenic germline mutations in the genes encoding subunits of SDH, collectively known as *SDHx* genes, now account for the largest share of hereditary pheochromocytoma and paraganglioma. Moreover, SDH deficiencies have also been identified in gastrointestinal stromal tumor, renal cell carcinoma [5, 6], and pituitary adenoma [9] – summarized in Table 2.1. Isocitrate dehydrogenase has also been implicated in a small number of cases [7]. Germline mutations in at least 19 genes have now been identified, and

J. Turchini · A. J. Gill
University of Sydney and Cancer Diagnosis and Pathology Group, Kolling Institute of Medical Research, Royal North Shore Hospital, St Leonards, NSW, Australia

A. S. Tischler (✉)
Department of Pathology and Laboratory Medicine, Tufts Medical Center, Boston, MA, USA
e-mail: atischler@tuftsmedicalcenter.org

L. Landsberg (ed.), *Pheochromocytomas, Paragangliomas and Disorders of the Sympathoadrenal System*, Contemporary Endocrinology,
https://doi.org/10.1007/978-3-319-77048-2_2

Table 2.1 SDH abnormalities in pheochromocytoma and paraganglioma

Syndrome	Gene	Chromo-some	Inheritance	Fre-quency (%)[a]	Age at primary diagnosis (yrs)	Sex	Adrenal PCC	PGL abdo-minal	PGL tho-racic	PGL head and neck	Metas-tatic rate[a]	SDH-deficient GIST	SDH-deficient RCC	SDH-deficient PA	Pulmo-nary chondroma
PGL1/CSS	*SDHD*	11q23	Ad;PT	~5	30s	M = F	+	+	++	+++	<5%	+	+/–	+	–
PGL2/CSS	*SDHAF2*	11q12.2	Ad;PT	<1	30s	M = F	+/–	+/–	+/–	+	Low	–+/–	+/–	+/–	–
PGL3/CSS	*SDHC*	1q23.3	AD	~1	40s	M = F	+/–	+/–	+	+ + (esp carotid body)	Low	+	++	+	–
PGL4/CSS	*SDHB*	1p36.1-p35	AD	~5	30s	M = F	+	++++	++	++	31–71%	+	+++	+	–
PGL5/CSS	*SDHA*	5p15	AD	<1	27–77	M = F	+	++	+/–	+	?	+++ (30% of SDH-deficient GISTs)	+	++	–
Carney triad	*SDHC promoter hyper-methylation*	1q23.3	Not hereditary	<1	10s–20s	F >> M		+		+	?	++++ (50% of SDH-deficient GIST)	–	–	++

Abbreviations: *AD* autosomal dominant, *AD;PT* autosomal dominant with paternal transmission (maternally imprinted, disease is inherited only from paternal carrier), *CSS* Carney-Stratakis syndrome, *GIST* gastrointestinal stromal tumor, *PCC* pheochromocytoma, *RCC* renal cell carcinoma, *PGL* paraganglioma, *PA* pituitary adenoma, *PGL1–5* paraganglioma syndrome types 1–5, ? not known (insufficient data)

[a]Combined data for PCC and PGL

many of these have also been reported to occur as somatic-only mutations in genuinely sporadic tumors [2, 3, 8–11]. Given the newly recognized importance of heredity, prospective recognition, and accurate pathological diagnosis of pheochromocytoma, paraganglioma, and their syndromically associated tumors is now essential for patient care.

Pheochromocytoma

The World Health Organization classification of endocrine tumors arbitrarily reserves the name pheochromocytoma for tumors that arise from the chromaffin cells of the adrenal medulla, while their extra-adrenal counterparts are called paragangliomas [1] . The name pheochromocytoma translates to *dusky-colored tumor* and is derived from a pigment produced when catecholamines within the tumor react with oxidizing agents causing the cut surface to turn brown. The color change was discovered in the mid-nineteenth century by anatomists employing solutions of chromate salts to study the normal adrenal gland and was consequently named, somewhat incorrectly, the chromaffin reaction [12]. It was used in diagnosing pheochromocytomas roughly from 1912 [13] until immunohistochemistry became widely available in the 1980s.

Pheochromocytomas are rare, with a reported annual incidence of 0.4–9.1 cases per 1 million [14–16]. In some series as many as 61% are found incidentally [17, 18]. They usually present in the 4th to 5th decades of life but can arise at any age [19]. Hereditary disease is more likely to present in younger patients [19]. In children presenting with apparently sporadic pheochromocytoma, hereditary disease is proven in up to 70% of cases [20]. However older age at presentation and absence of a family history do not exclude a pathogenic germline mutation [19]. Males and females are affected equally.

Most symptoms of pheochromocytoma are related to catecholamine synthesis, as the majority of tumors are functional. The classic triad includes headache, tachycardia/palpitations, and sweating. Although 25% or fewer patients experience the classic triad, about half have at least one of the symptoms [17]. Sustained hypertension or paroxysmal hypertension are the most common findings. About 6% of patients present with constipation [21]. Additional paraneoplastic syndromes can also occur, the most common of which is Cushing's syndrome caused by ectopic production of ACTH [22]. Less often, ectopic VIP can be produced, leading to diarrhea and hypokalemia (Verner-Morrison syndrome) [23]. This is especially but not exclusively associated with composite tumors consisting of pheochromocytoma and ganglioneuroma. Polycythemia has been reported due to overproduction of, or oversensitization to, erythropoietin and is particularly associated with pheochromocytomas arising in the setting of *EPAS1* or *EGLN1*/2 mutations [24]. Other presenting complaints can include orthostatic hypotension and pallor, anxiety, panic attacks, and tremor. Typically symptoms occur simultaneously in a "spell." However this is a non-specific finding raising multiple diagnostic possibilities [25]. Some patients are asymptomatic, particularly those who have a small tumor or one that secretes methylated catecholamine metabolites. It is important to remember that hereditary pheochromocytomas are often found during evaluation of patients who present with a syndromically associated tumor such as a gastrointestinal stromal tumor, medullary thyroid carcinoma, or renal cell carcinoma.

Biochemical testing is mandatory for diagnosis if pheochromocytoma is suspected and can be of assistance in determining the genotype of a hereditary pheochromocytoma. Tumors typically associated with MEN2 or NF1 secrete predominantly epinephrine, whereas those associated with VHL produce norepinephrine. Biochemical testing also discriminates pheochromocytomas from paragangliomas, which may synthesize norepinephrine or dopamine or be nonfunctional but only extremely rarely produce epinephrine. Levels of plasma-free metanephrines or fractionated urine metanephrines are sensitive test parameters because tumor-derived catecholamines are metabolized by intratumoral catechol-O-methyltransferase. Metanephrine and normetanephrine therefore reflect the presence of pheochromocytoma better than catecholamines themselves, which are produced throughout the normal sympathetic nervous system [26, 27]. High levels of the dopamine metabolite 3-methoxytyramine are highly suggestive of an SDH-deficient pheochromocytoma or paraganglioma [28, 29] and can be a useful guide to preoperative staging as these tumors are more likely to be metastatic or multifocal.

Imaging is always warranted when there is biochemical evidence of pheochromocytoma. Anatomic imaging modalities include CT and MRI, whereby the latter produces the characteristic ring-enhancing lesional mass or lightbulb sign. Other features which may be seen include calcification, hemorrhage, necrosis, and cystic change. Functional imaging including ^{123}I-MIBG scintigraphy is also a valuable tool that can be used to detect metastases and is preferable to CT for that purpose [30]. Somatostatin receptor imaging, especially by PET/CT using ^{68}Ga-DOTATATE or other new somatostatin analogs, is by far the most sensitive and specific modality for detecting metastases or second primaries [31, 32] but is not yet widely available.

The risk of metastasis for pheochromocytoma remains approximately 10% [33], and there can be a delay between the primary and metastatic disease of years to decades [34, 35]. Frequent sites of metastasis include regional lymph nodes, lung, liver, and bone. A staging system for pheochromocytoma and abdominal paragangliomas was introduced in the 8th edition of the American Joint Committee on Cancer staging manual published in 2017 [36].

Pheochromocytomas usually range in size from 30 to 50 mm but can be over 100 mm or less than 10 mm. Using an arbitrary cutoff, tumors smaller than 10 mm have often been categorized as hyperplastic medullary nodules, but recent molecular studies do not support that distinction [37]. Grossly, pheochromocytoma is usually well circumscribed and unencapsulated. The cut surface is pink, gray, or tan and can be easily distinguished from the bright yellow of adrenal cortical tumors (Fig. 2.1). Fibrosis, hemorrhage, central degeneration, and cystic change are common [38]. Large tumors typically compress or obliterate the surrounding adrenal cortex and may show extensive cystic change.

Microscopically, pheochromocytoma may be well delineated, or there may be intermingling of tumor cells with the adrenal cortex [38]. Varied architectural patterns and cytological features may be seen, sometimes within an individual tumor.

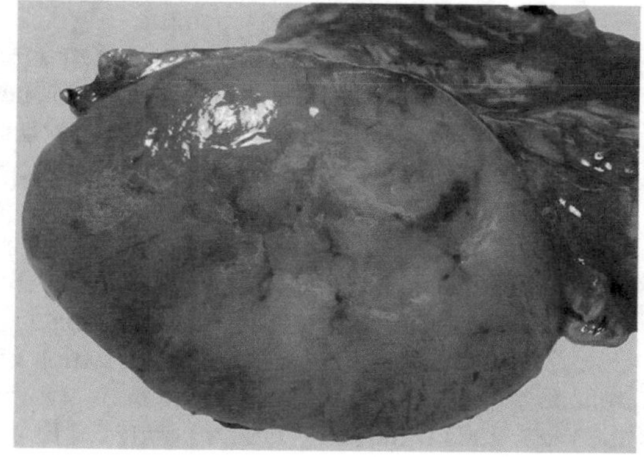

Fig. 2.1 Fresh gross specimen of a pheochromocytoma. The pink-tan cut surface contrasts with the distinct golden yellow of residual adrenal cortex

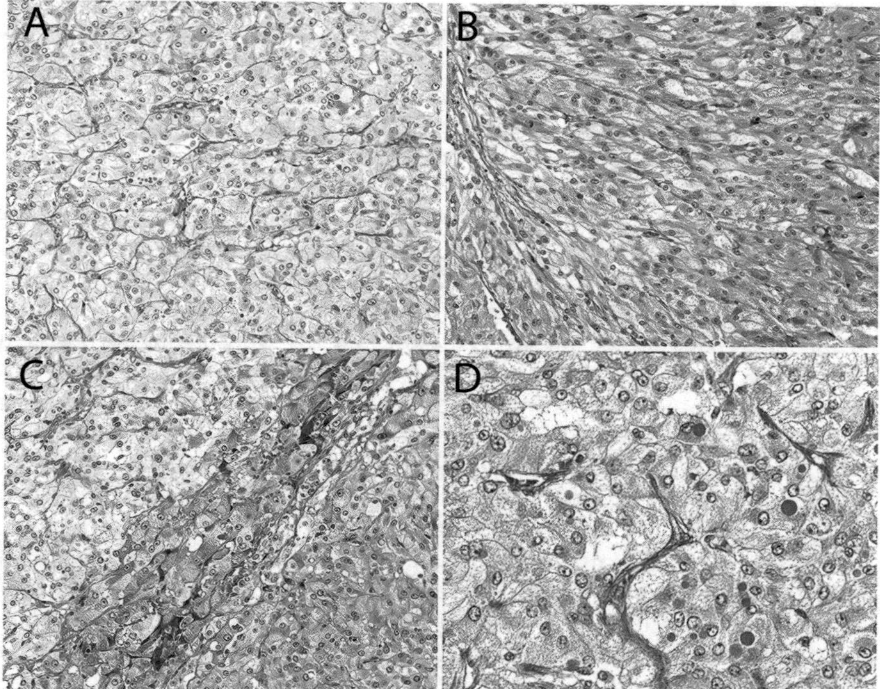

Fig. 2.2 Varied appearances of pheochromocytoma in single adrenal from a patient with MEN2A. (**a**) Classic "Zellballen" pattern, with polygonal tumor cells in discrete nests with intervening capillaries. (**b**) Diffuse spindle cell growth. (**c**) Three architecturally and cytologically distinct cell populations side-by-side. (**d**) High magnification of nested cells containing numerous eosinophilic hyaline globules (original magnification **a**–**c** 200×)

The most typical pattern is the alveolar "Zellballen" (German for "cell balls") architecture characterized by nests of polygonal tumor cells with peripheral sustentacular cells, surrounded by capillaries (Fig. 2.2). Other patterns include trabecular growth or diffuse "sheet-like" growth. Vascular spaces may be prominent, giving rise to a pseudoangiomatous pattern (Fig. 2.2) [39]. The cytoplasm is usually amphophilic or basophilic and granular. Intracytoplasmic hyaline globules may be present. These are diastase resistant and can be highlighted with a periodic acid Schiff stain. The tumor cells may closely resemble normal chromaffin cells in size or may be larger or smaller. Nuclei range from round to oval with fine chromatin and inconspicuous nucleoli to vesicular with prominent nucleoli. There can be prominent intranuclear pseudoinclusions. Cells may be conspicuously pleomorphic, commonly with "endocrine-type" atypia characterized by nuclear enlargement and pleomorphism but with relatively preserved nuclear to cytoplasmic ratios (Fig. 2.2). Other cytological variations, which may be present focally or diffusely, include spindle cells [40], oncocytic cells with prominent eosinophilic cytoplasm, and clear cells mimicking adrenal cortex. Mitoses are rare [41]. With the possible exception of spindle cells [42], none of the cytological variations appears to have clinical significance. A distinct type of tumor is composite pheochromocytoma, defined as pheochromocytoma intimately associated with a nonpheochromocytoma tumor, including ganglioneuroblastoma, ganglioneuroma, or schwannoma. To diagnose a composite pheochromocytoma, the complete architecture of the second component must be present. Scattered neurons ("ganglion cells") occasionally present in a pheochromocytoma do not change the diagnosis to composite pheochromocytoma-ganglioneuroma [38].

The most frequent differential diagnosis of pheochromocytoma is adrenal cortical neoplasia, especially for oncocytic tumors [43]. Others include renal cell carcinoma, hepatocellular carcinoma, and metastases. In contrast to most tumors in the differential diagnoses, essentially all pheochromocytomas show diffuse immunohistochemical staining for chromogranin A [38]. Staining for tyrosine hydroxylase, which is required for catecholamine synthesis [44], can usually differentiate pheochromocytoma from metastases of other neuroendocrine tumors. Cytokeratin expression is typically absent, although it has been reported very focally. Adrenal cortical markers SF1, MelanA, and inhibin are also negative [45]. S100 staining frequently highlights sustentacular cells, but these are not always present [46]. Immunohistochemistry for peptides that may be secreted by the tumor, such as ACTH, is usually not required for diagnosis but may be helpful to localize the source of a peptide known to be in excess [47]. Immunohistochemistry for succinate dehydrogenase B (SDHB) is very useful in determining the presence of any *SDH*x mutation, with associated higher risk of metastasis and likely inheritance (Fig. 2.4) [48–50]. Several notes of caution pertain to differentiation of pheochromocytoma from adrenal cortical tumors. Both tumor types stain for synaptophysin, which therefore should not be used to make the distinction. Both also may contain hyaline globules and intranuclear pseudoinclusions. Immunohistochemical staining of oncocytic tumors requires particular caution because of non-specific "stickiness" for some antibodies that may cause artefactual staining [51].

A long-standing conundrum for pathologists has been whether a primary pheochromocytoma can be diagnosed as benign or malignant. Because of the difficulties in making this distinction, the 2004 World Health Organization classification of endocrine tumors defined malignancy by the development of metastases, specified as the occurrence of pheochromocytoma at a site where chromaffin tissue is not present in order to rule out second primary tumors. While implicitly maintaining this concept, the 2017 WHO classification considers that all pheochromocytomas have some metastatic potential, and dichotomous classification has been superseded by a risk stratification approach [1]. While there is widespread agreement with a risk-based approach, and several risk stratification schemes have been proposed, there is no universally accepted system in widespread clinical use. However, several features are recognized to occur more frequently in pheochromocytomas that metastasize than in those cured by surgery alone. These include invasion, variably defined as into vessels, the adrenal capsule, or periadrenal soft tissue; certain architectural patterns including large, irregular, and confluent nests; necrosis, including spotty, infarct-like, or comedo necrosis; and small cells, spindle cells, and increased proliferative activity indicated by increased mitoses or a high Ki-67 proliferative index [52, 53]. Other features reported to be associated with increased risk but not as widely accepted include coarse nodularity, absence of hyaline globules, decreased sustentacular cells, and tumor size greater than 50 mm [33, 54–56].

Several multiparameter scoring systems based on these and other features have been developed; however, no system is universally accepted or endorsed. These include the Pheochromocytoma of the Adrenal Gland Scaled Score (PASS), the modified PASS, and the grading system for the Adrenal Pheochromocytoma and Paraganglioma (GAPP). PASS has been proposed to provide a threshold for identifying tumors that may metastasize, whereas GAPP has been proposed as an assessment for risk of metastasis and patient survival [52, 57]. Both these systems require further validation in independent cohorts before they can be considered as routine in clinical practice, and new ways of scoring putative adverse features shared by PASS and GAPP [42] might still be developed. At present the greatest risk for metastasis is the presence of *SDHB* mutations.

Histology can sometimes play a role in identifying patients with genetic mutations. Multiple pheochromocytomas with adrenal medullary hyperplasia are suggestive of MEN2 and can also be indicative of nonheritable germline mutations in the *TMEM127* gene [58]. Medullary tissue is usually confined to the head and body of the adrenal. Extension into the tail and alae is highly suggestive of hyperplasia [38] and should be carefully sought in adrenalectomy specimens [59]. In addition, the tumor should be confirmed to be originating from within the adrenal gland and not adjacent to it. This can be confirmed by searching for residual cortex at the periphery of the tumor. Other features such as small tumor cells, vascular pseudocapsule, and myxoid change can suggest von Hippel-Lindau disease (Fig. 2.3) [60]. However these features may be affected by multiple factors including interobserver disagreement and specimen processing [42]. Therefore, while they may help to link particular tumors with a higher probability of specific mutations, they cannot replace molecular testing. A valuable and now widely employed adjunct to molecular testing is immunohistochemical staining for SDHB protein, which becomes negative when *SDHA*, *SDHB*, *SDHC*, or *SDHD* are mutated (Fig. 2.4) [48–50].

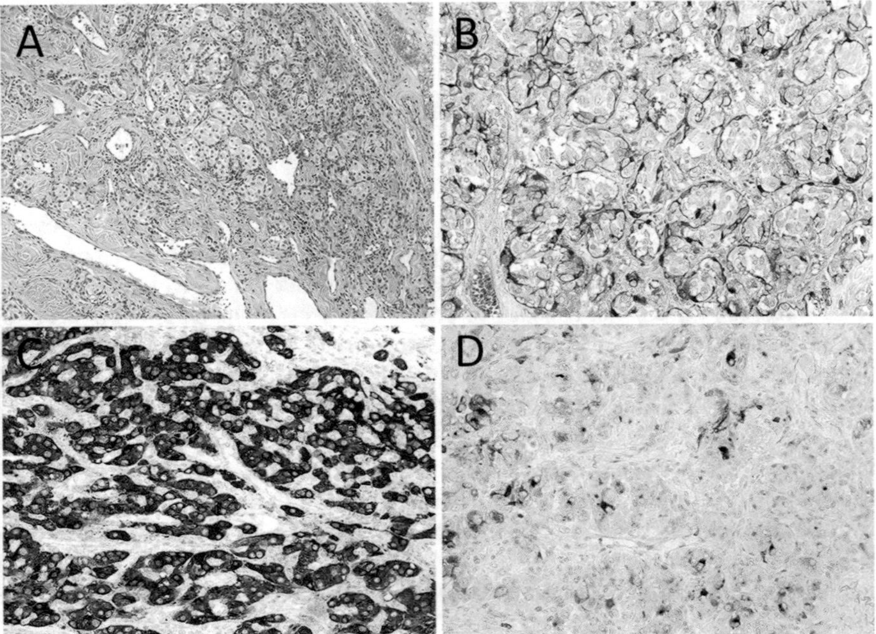

Fig. 2.3 Carotid body paraganglioma. (**a**) Low magnification showing Zellballen more sharply defined than in the pheochromocytoma in Fig. 2.2, relatively clear cytoplasm, and cavernous blood vessels. (**b**) Immunohistochemical stain for S100 showing numerous sustentacular cells highlighting the Zellballen pattern. (**c**) Immunohistochemical stain for synaptophysin, showing immunoreactivity in essentially all neuroendocrine cells ("chief cells"). (**d**) Immunohistochemical stain for chromogranin A, showing immunoreactivity in scattered cells, often only in a dot-like pattern corresponding to the Golgi apparatus. Synaptophysin, which is a constituent of secretory granule membrane, is typically a more sensitive but less specific neuroendocrine marker than granins, which are in the granule matrix. This tumor was negative for tyrosine hydroxylase and somatostatin receptor 2A

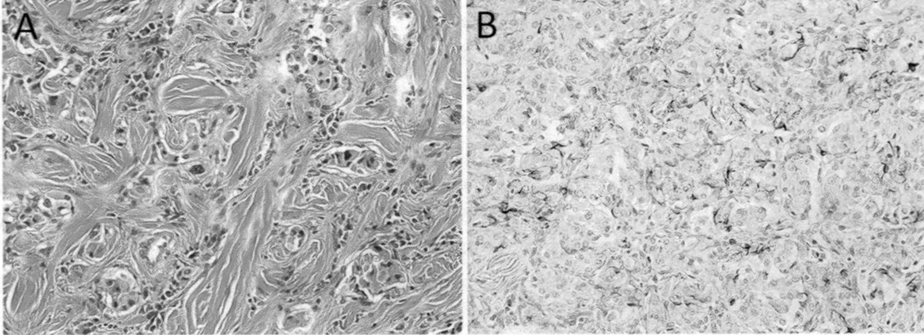

Fig. 2.4 Unusual features in a carotid body paraganglioma. (**a**) Sclerosis and cellular pleomorphism and nuclear atypia, mimicking invasive carcinoma. (**b**) Focal immunostaining for keratins, with pankeratin antibody. Paragangliomas are usually negative for keratins. In this case the antibody reacts focally with a subset of sustentacular cells

In view of the very strong association with hereditary disease, it is recommended that all patients with pheochromocytoma or paraganglioma be offered genetic testing, with the depth of testing depending on clinical risk factors and local resources [30]. Approximately 30–40% of these tumors are associated with an hereditary susceptibility gene, and 11–24% of patients with a solitary apparently sporadic tumor actually harbor an occult germline mutation [61–63]. To date, at least 19 separate susceptibility genes have been identified [64]. Many of these are tumor suppressor genes, and the mutation causes loss or inactivation of the wild-type allele. *RET* proto-oncogene and *HIF2A* (*EPAS1*) are genes that have gain of function mutations for which a second hit is not required, although allelic imbalance can occur [65]. Inheritance is typically autosomal dominant. However, mutations in *SDHD*, *SDHAF2*, and *MAX* demonstrate a parent of origin effect, whereby the mutated gene may be inherited from either parent, but only paternal transmission produces phenotypic expression [66, 67]. This parent of origin effect can mask family histories by causing skipped generations [66, 67].

In hereditary pheochromocytomas, mutations are usually mutually exclusive. Although some double mutations involving hereditary susceptibility genes and somatic mutations of other genes have been reported [68], the latter usually prove to involve variants of uncertain significance (VUS) with no effect on the structure of the encoded protein. The genetics of truly sporadic pheochromocytomas that occur in patients without germline mutations have become increasingly interesting with the recognition that they harbor a somatic mutation in one of the hereditary susceptibility genes, usually *NF1* [4, 69, 70], in up to 20% of cases. A distinguishing feature of the *NF1*-associated cases is that it is rare for patients with germline *NF1* mutations to present with pheochromocytoma before cutaneous manifestations are apparent. *HRAS* and *BRAF* mutations have been reported to occur as somatic-only events in 8.9% of pheochromocytomas and appear to be mutually exclusive with known pathogenic germline mutations [71].

In the absence of germline mutation, somatic-only mutations in the succinate dehydrogenase genes are extremely rare [69, 70, 72]. Therefore, the demonstration of somatic dysfunction in the succinate dehydrogenase genes by negative immunohistochemistry for SDHB is usually taken as prima facie evidence of germline mutation in one of the genes encoding SDH subunits (Fig. 2.4) [48–50].

Gene mutations are necessary but do not appear to be sufficient for tumorigenesis. The remaining factors that contribute remain unclear, but several genetic alterations in the form of gains and losses are associated with certain mutations. Most commonly these are loss of tumor suppressor genes on chromosomes 1p and 3q, 11p, 11q, 6q, 17p, 9q, 17q, 19p13.3, and 20q [71], with a range of effects on downstream pathways. SDH mutations are most commonly associated with hypermethylation [73, 74].

Prognosis for patients with pheochromocytomas is mostly predicted by resectability, as complete surgical resection is considered the only cure. The genetic mutations harbored by the tumor also have a bearing on prognosis, with *SDHB* mutations being associated with both a particularly high risk of metastasis and the shortest survival [61, 75, 76]. Soft tissue invasion alone appears to have little or no adverse effect on survival [77], but local recurrence is common if the tumor is not completely resected. Five-year survival after metastasis has been reported to range from 34% to 60%. If the liver or lungs are involved, then the survival is typically less than 5 years. When bone involvement occurs alone, survival tends to be longer [78]. Early identification of hereditary mutations can identify patients requiring additional surveillance for synchronous or metachronous disease tumors including paraganglioma, renal carcinoma, GIST, pituitary adenoma, or pancreatic tumors.

Paraganglioma

The autonomic nervous system consists of the parasympathetic system and the sympathetic system. The parasympathetic system arises both from the brain stem extending branches into the head, neck, and thorax and from the sacral spinal cord extending branches into the pelvis. In contrast, the sympathetic system arises from the spinal cord and traverses bilaterally along the entire length of the vertebral column, extending branches into nearby organs from the neck to the pelvis. During development, predominantly microscopic groupings of chromaffin cells or chromaffin-like cells are present in or near the sympathetic ganglia, along sympathetic nerve branches and along mostly proximal regions of the vagus and glossopharyngeal nerves. These microscopic groupings are highly variable in size, location, and anatomic organization, and in some locations they either involute or become almost impossible to find in adults [79] . In addition to microscopic structures, the sympathetic nervous system has two macroscopic organs containing chromaffin cells, the organ(s) of Zuckerkandl at the origin of the inferior mesenteric artery in fetuses and neonates, and the adrenal medulla in adults. Similarly, the parasympathetic nervous system has the carotid bodies, at the bifurcations of the carotid arteries. The functions of these anatomically diverse structures vary and in most locations are poorly understood. All were demonstrated to be capable of producing catecholamines by early anatomists using the chromaffin reaction, though the reaction in the head and neck was weaker and sometimes absent. Because they were *analogous* to sympathetic ganglia in development and biochemical function but were not ganglia, they were called *paraganglia* [80].

Paragangliomas occur in any location where normal paraganglionic cells are present during development or in adult life, most frequently where the cells are most numerous: the adrenal medulla (a pheochromocytoma is an intra-adrenal paraganglioma); the retroperitoneum, especially near the root of the inferior mesenteric artery; the carotid bodies, the jugulotympanic paraganglia in the floor and wall of the middle ear; and the vagus nerve near the nodose ganglion. Familiarity with these distributions is essential in formulating a differential diagnosis that includes paraganglioma for tumors in these locations.

The biochemical function of paragangliomas mirrors their developmental forebears. Sympathetic (also known as sympathoadrenal) paragangliomas are usually clinically or at least biochemically functional, producing norepinephrine and/or dopamine. Parasympathetic (also known as head and neck) paragangliomas are usually clinically silent mass lesions, but a substantial minority can be shown to produce norepinephrine or dopamine biochemically, and rare cases are clinically symptomatic. In some cases parasympathetic paragangliomas do not express tyrosine hydroxylase and only focally express chromogranin A, complicating the differential diagnosis.

Paragangliomas in any site can be morphologically identical to pheochromocytomas [38]. They demonstrate the same range of appearances, frequently with a "Zellballen" architecture comprised of chief cells and sustentacular cells. Sclerosing, angiomatous, trabecular, and spindle cell forms may be seen. Mitoses are usually rare. Despite these morphological overlaps, some histological features in individual tumors can suggest particular anatomic sites. Paragangliomas of the parasympathetic system are often composed of smaller cells than their sympathetic counterparts, have higher cellularity, and have more sharply defined Zellballen. In addition, they often have cavernous blood vessels.

Somewhat clear cells can be prominent in both sympathetic and parasympathetic paragangliomas. Caution should be used in assessing bladder biopsies as sympathetic paraganglioma can be misdiagnosed as urothelial carcinoma [81].

Head and Neck Paragangliomas

Head and neck tumors comprise approximately 20% of all paragangliomas and 0.6% of head and neck neoplasms [82, 83]. The reported incidence ranges from 1 in 30,000 to 1 in 100,000.

Paragangliomas can arise in any age from as young at 13 to the elderly [84, 85]. The mean age is 41–47 years with a female-to-male ratio of up to 8:1 [86, 87]. The vast majority of head and neck paragangliomas, around 60%, arise from the carotid body. The next most common location is at the jugular bulb (23%) and within or adjacent to the vagus nerve near the ganglion nodosum (13%). Middle ear, or tympanic, paragangliomas arising from the medial promontory wall account for 6% [88, 89]. Paragangliomas arising in the larynx are exceptionally rare and may present as thyroid masses. Head and neck paragangliomas are often incidentalomas detected during imaging of the thyroid or neck or may be found secondarily to nerve compression.

Hereditary paragangliomas tend to arise in a younger population, about 10 years earlier than sporadic forms [90]. They may occur in conjunction with sympathetic paragangliomas or pheochromocytomas. Head and neck paragangliomas can be bilateral (up to 25%) or multiple (up to 37%), and this is common in hereditary cases (up to 80%) [85, 89, 91]. Metastasis is uncommon overall, being reported in 4–6% of cases, and appears to be more frequent in younger patients with multifocal tumors, perhaps because of association with germline *SDHB* mutations. Metastatic paragangliomas are more frequently functional (only 3% of paragangliomas are secretory), and the gender distribution is equal [86, 88, 92]. The most common secondary sites are cervical lymph nodes (in two thirds of cases) followed by the lung, bone, and liver. The 5-year survival for metastatic tumors is 60–80% [86, 92]. Distant metastases presenting in a patient over 50 years of age are associated with shorter survival. Patients with *SDHB* mutations have the greatest risk of metastasis, up to one third by the age of 70 years.

Risk factors for head and neck paragangliomas include chronic hypoxic conditions and familial inheritance [90, 93–96]. Germline mutations occur in up to 18% of cases, mostly in the genes coding for succinate dehydrogenase (*SDHD* in 80%, *SDHB* in 8%, *SDHAF2* in 6%). *VHL* accounts for 6% of mutations, while *RET*, *NF1*, and *TMEM127* are rare [97, 98]. Again it is recommended that screening for at least the most common hereditary mutations be offered to all patients [1–11].

By immunohistochemistry, head and neck paragangliomas usually express chromogranin A, synaptophysin, CD56, and somatostatin receptor type 2A (SSTR2A) [97, 99]. Cytokeratin, carcinoembryonic antigen (CEA), and calcitonin are usually negative. Tyrosine hydroxylase is expressed in 30% and dopamine beta-hydroxylase in 11% [100, 101]. S100 and glial fibrillary acid protein (GFAP) are expressed by the sustentacular cells, which are usually present. The Ki-67 proliferation labeling is typically less than 1%. Mutations in any of the SDH complex genes will result in a loss of expression of SDHB. In addition, paragangliomas associated with *SDHA* mutation will also lose expression of SDHA (Figs. 2.4 and 2.5) [49, 50, 102].

Recurrence can occur in about less than 10% of cases. However, local recurrence does not equate to malignancy. Surgery, fractionated radiotherapy, or stereotactic

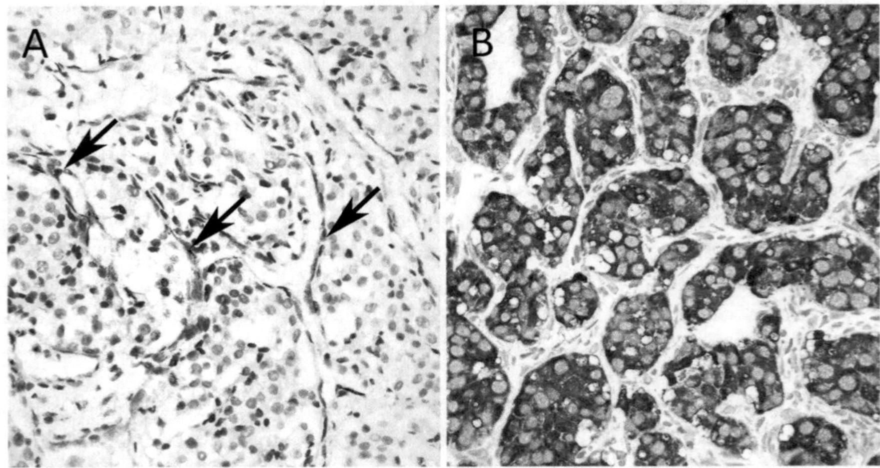

Fig. 2.5 Immunohistochemistry from serial sections from a paraganglioma stained for both SDHB (panel **a**) and SDHA (panel **b**). (**a**) In this case the neoplastic cells show completely absent staining for SDHB, denoting mutation of one of the SDH subunits (*SDHA*, *SDHB*, *SDHC*, or *SDHD*). In contrast, the endothelial and stromal cells (arrows) demonstrate preserved cytoplasmic granular staining for SDHB. This serves as an internal positive control and indicates that the loss of staining is genuine. (**b**) The neoplastic cells show diffuse strong positive staining for SDHA in the typical granular cytoplasmic (mitochondrial) pattern. The positive staining for SDHA excludes *SDHA* mutation [102]

radiosurgery are valid treatment options. However, because the tumors are usually slow-growing, active surveillance is often the best option to avoid the severe complications associated with interventions [103–105]. An exception is for tumors with *SDHB* mutations where early intervention may be preferred [106].

Sympathetic Paragangliomas

Sympathetic paragangliomas develop at all ages and have an equal sex distribution. The highest incidence is between 40 and 50 years of age. Pediatric paragangliomas are more likely to be bilateral, multifocal, and familial [107]. The reported incidence of metastasis ranges from 2.5% to 50% and is higher in the pediatric population [108–110]. About one third are hereditary, and, as for head and neck paraganglioma and pheochromocytoma, genetic testing should be offered for all patients.

Most sympathetic paragangliomas arise below the diaphragm, particularly near the adrenal gland (42%), the organ of Zuckerkandl (28%), and the urinary bladder (10%). About 12% arise in the thorax, with the heart constituting about 2% [111–115]. Hematuria may be the presenting symptom in 40–50% of tumors involving the urinary bladder. Unlike most head and neck paragangliomas, sympathetic paragangliomas usually are capable of catecholamine synthesis, and their signs and symptoms may be similar to those of pheochromocytoma. However, they do not usually secrete epinephrine because phenylethanolamine N-methyltransferase, the enzyme required for conversion of norepinephrine to epinephrine, is absent in normal extra-adrenal paraganglia. High levels of normetanephrine and/or methoxytyramine without elevated metanephrine therefore usually point to an extra-adrenal source. An important exception is pheochromocytoma in VHL syndrome [121]. From 17 to 43% of sympathetic paragangliomas are clinically nonsecretory [53, 116, 117]. Invasion into adjacent organs is rare. If metastases occur, lymph nodes, lung, liver, and bone are most common sites. Metastases to the pleura, ovary, testis, and peritoneum can also occur [117, 118].

Immunohistochemical findings are similar to those in head and neck paragangliomas, with the exception that tyrosine hydroxylase and dopamine beta-hydroxylase are more often expressed. Reportedly, dopamine beta-hydroxylase is always expressed, even in nonfunctional tumors, distinguishing them from parasympathetic paragangliomas [118].

Similarly to pheochromocytoma, the concept of benign and malignant paraganglioma has been replaced by an approach based on risk stratification. As discussed above, various grading systems, most recently the GAPP system [53], have been proposed to stratify risk. These systems are based on invasion, proliferative activity, necrosis, and growth patterns but need further validation before they are adopted for widespread clinical use. Other factors contributing to prognosis are older age, tumor size, high Ki-67 proliferative index, and biochemical phenotype [119–122].

Composite Pheochromocytoma and Composite Paraganglioma

Composite pheochromocytomas are tumors with two components: a pheochromocytoma or paraganglioma and a related neurogenic tumor. They comprise approximately 3–9% of all pheochromocytomas and less than 1% of paragangliomas. The second component is usually ganglioneuroma but in up to 20% of cases can be a ganglioneuroblastoma or, extremely rarely, malignant peripheral nerve sheath tumor [123–127]. Macroscopically they may appear heterogeneous, but most are only recognized microscopically. The diagnosis requires the presence of a pheochromocytoma or paraganglioma with a second tumor that has sufficient features to also be regarded as a tumor in its own right. The presence of occasional ganglion cells in an otherwise ordinary pheochromocytoma or paraganglioma is insufficient for the diagnosis.

Immunohistochemical findings should also be appropriate to the two source tumors. The second population of cells is usually associated with Schwann cell-containing stroma that can be stained for S100 and Sox10 as an aid to diagnosis [128].

Composite pheochromocytomas arise in the adrenal medulla and can be bilateral in up to 7% of cases [125]. They are most frequent in adults but can occur in children as young as 5 and in the elderly. Median age of diagnosis is 40–50 years. Male-to-female ratio is equal [123, 125]. Signs and symptoms are identical to those of conventional pheochromocytoma; however, the Verner-Morrison syndrome due to overproduction of VIP is more frequent [123, 125, 129]. Expression of RET protein and VIP are often associated with neuronal differentiation [130, 131].

NF1 is the most common mutation associated with composite pheochromocytoma, being present in 17% of cases, of which up to 50% are bilateral [125]. Two composite pheochromocytomas associated with MEN2A have been reported [132, 133]. There have also been reported associations with hemangiomas and renal angiomyolipoma [134, 135].

Metastatic risk is low, and the reported sites of metastasis are the same as for conventional pheochromocytoma. Metastasis is more common in tumors containing ganglioneuroblastoma and malignant peripheral nerve sheath tumor [125]. Metastatic deposits may harbor one or both components of a composite tumor [127]. It has also been reported that some primary conventional pheochromocytomas have the potential to metastasize as composite tumors [127, 136], but this is clearly a rare event and could potentially be attributable to undersampling of the primary tumor. Similarly to pheochromocytomas, composite pheochromocytomas that are completely surgically excised usually do not metastasize or recur. However, long-term follow-up remains important as the clinical course can be unpredictable [137].

Composite paragangliomas can arise at any age and have been reported in patients as young as 15 months, females slightly more often than males. Morphologically they are identical to composite pheochromocytomas [138, 139]. Almost all composite paragangliomas reported to date have consisted of paraganglioma with ganglioneuroma or, extremely rarely, ganglioneuroblastoma. No malignant peripheral nerve sheath tumors have been reported in composite paraganglioma.

Composite paragangliomas most commonly occur in the urinary bladder and the retroperitoneum, filum terminale, and mediastinum. Most are clinically silent. One case has been reported with local lymph node invasion [140] and none with metastases. It is of interest that no composite paragangliomas have been reported in the head and neck [123, 140–143], probably reflecting developmental differences between normal sympathetic and parasympathetic paraganglia.

References

1. Kloeppel G, Lloyd RV, Osamura R, Rosai J, editors. Pathology and genetics of tumors of endocrine organs. 4th ed. Lyon: IARC Press; 2017.
2. Boedeker CC, Hensen EF, Neumann HP, Maier W, van Nederveen FH, Suárez C, Kunst HP, Rodrigo JP, Takes RP, Pellitteri PK, Rinaldo A, Ferlito A. Genetics of hereditary head and neck paragangliomas. Head Neck. 2014;36(6):907–16.
3. Giubellino A, Lara K, Martucci V, Huynh T, Agarwal P, Pacak K, Merino MJ. Urinary bladder paragangliomas: how immunohistochemistry can assist to identify patients with SDHB germline and somatic mutations. Am J Surg Pathol. 2015;39(11):1488–92.
4. Pasini B, Stratakis CA. SDH mutations in tumorigenesis and inherited endocrine tumors: lesson from the pheochromocytoma-paraganglioma syndromes. J Intern Med. 2009;266(1):19–42.
5. Gill AJ, Chou A, Vilain R, Clarkson A, Lui M, Jin R, Tobias V, Samra J, Goldstein D, Smith C, Sioson L, Parker N, Smith RC, Sywak M, Sidhu SB, Wyatt JM, Robinson BG, Eckstein RP, Benn DE, Clifton-Bligh RJ. Immunohistochemistry for SDHB divides gastrointestinal stromal tumors (GISTs) into 2 distinct types. Am J Surg Pathol. 2010;34(5):63644.
6. Gill AJ, Pachter NS, Chou A, Young B, Clarkson A, Tucker KM, Winship IM, Earls P, Benn DE, Robinson BG, Fleming S, Clifton-Bligh RJ. Renal tumors associated with germline SDHB mutation show distinctive morphology. Am J Surg Pathol. 2011;35(10):1578–85.
7. Gaal J, Burnichon N, Korpershoek E, Roncelin I, Bertherat J, Plouin PF, de Krijger RR, GimenezRoqueplo AP, Dinjens WN. Isocitrate dehydrogenase mutations are rare in pheochromocytomas and paragangliomas. J Clin Endocrinol Metab. 2010;95(3):1274–8.
8. Dahia PL. Pheochromocytoma and paraganglioma pathogenesis: learning from genetic heterogeneity. Nat Rev Cancer. 2014;14(2):108–19.
9. Dénes J, Swords F, Rattenberry E, Stals K, Owens M, Cranston T, Xekouki P, Moran L, Kumar A, Wassif C, Fersht N, Baldeweg SE, Morris D, Lightman S, Agha A, Rees A, Grieve J, Powell M, Boguszewski CL, Dutta P, Thakker RV, Srirangalingam U, Thompson CJ, Druce M, Higham C, Davis J, Eeles R, Stevenson M, O'Sullivan B, Taniere P, Skordilis K, Gabrovska P, Barlier A, Webb SM, Aulinas A, Drake WM, Bevan JS, Preda C, Dalantaeva N, Ribeiro-Oliveira A, Garcia IT, Yordanova G, Iotova V, Evanson J, Grossman AB, Trouillas J, Ellard S, Stratakis CA, Maher ER, Roncaroli F, Korbonits M. Heterogeneous genetic background of the association of pheochromocytoma/paraganglioma and pituitary adenoma: results from a large patient cohort. J Clin Endocrinol Metab. 2015;100(3):E531–41.
10. Currás-Freixes M, Inglada-Pérez L, Mancikova V, Montero-Conde C, Letón R, Comino-Méndez I, Apellániz-Ruiz M, Sánchez-Barroso L, Aguirre Sánchez-Covisa M, Alcázar V, Aller J, Álvarez-Escolá C, Andía-Melero VM, Azriel-Mira S, Calatayud-Gutiérrez M, Díaz JÁ, Díez-Hernández A, Lamas-Oliveira C, Marazuela M, Matias-Guiu X, Meoro-Avilés A, Patiño-García A, Pedrinaci S, Riesco-Eizaguirre G, Sábado-Álvarez C, Sáez-Villaverde R, Sainz de Los Terreros A, Sanz Guadarrama Ó, Sastre-Marcos J, Scolá-Yurrita B, Segura-Huerta Á, Serrano-Corredor Mde L, Villar-Vicente MR, Rodríguez-Antona C, Korpershoek E, Cascón A, Robledo M. Recommendations for somatic and germline genetic testing of single pheochromocytoma and paraganglioma based on findings from a series of 329 patients. Journal of Medical Genetics. 2015;52(10):647–56.

11. Burnichon N, Vescovo L, Amar L, Libé R, de Reynies A, Venisse A, Jouanno E, Laurendeau I, Parfait B, Bertherat J, Plouin PF, Jeunemaitre X, Favier J, Gimenez-Roqueplo AP. Integrative genomic analysis reveals somatic mutations in pheochromocytoma and paraganglioma. Hum Mol Genet. 2011;20(20):3974–85.
12. Carmichael SW. The history of the adrenal medulla. Rev Neurosci. 1989;2:83–100.
13. Pick L. Das Ganglioma embryonale sympathicum (Sympathoma embryonale), eine typische bösartige Geschwulstform des sympathischen Nervensystems. Berlin Klin Wochenschr. 1912;49:16–22.
14. Andersen GS, Toftdahl DB, Lund JO, Strandgaard S, Nielsen PE. The incidence rate of pheochromocytoma and Conn's syndrome in Denmark, 1977—1981. Journal of Human Hypertension. 1988;2(3):187–9.
15. Fernández-Calvet L, García-Mayor RV. Incidence of pheochromocytoma in South Galicia, Spain. J Intern Med. 1994;236(6):675–7.
16. Holland J, Chandurkar V. A retrospective study of surgically excised pheochromocytomas in Newfoundland, Canada. Indian J Endocrinol Metab. 2014;18(4):542–5.
17. Baguet JP, Hammer L, Mazzuco TL, Chabre O, Mallion JM, Sturm N, Chaffanjon P. Circumstances of discovery of pheochromocytoma: a retrospective study of 41 consecutive patients. Eur J Endocrinol Eur Fed Endocr Soc. 2004;150(5):681–6.
18. Oshmyansky AR, Mahammedi A, Dackiw A, Ball DW, Schulick RD, Zeiger MA, Siegelman SS. Serendipity in the diagnosis of pheochromocytoma. J Comput Assist Tomogr. 2013;37(5):820–3.
19. Weinhäusel A, Behmel A, Ponder BA, Haas OA, Niederle B, Gessl A, Vierhapper H, Pfragner R. Long-term follow up of a "sporadic" unilateral pheochromocytoma revealing multiple endocrine neoplasia MEN2A-2 in an elderly woman. Endocr Pathol. 2003;14(4):37582.
20. Waguespack SG, Rich T, Grubbs E, Ying AK, Perrier ND, Ayala-Ramirez M, Jimenez C. A current review of the etiology, diagnosis, and treatment of pediatric pheochromocytoma and paraganglioma. J Clin Endocrinol Metab. 2010;95(5):2023–37.
21. Thosani S, Ayala-Ramirez M, Román-González A, Zhou S, Thosani N, Bisanz A, Jimenez C. Constipation: an overlooked, unmanaged symptom of patients with pheochromocytoma and sympathetic paraganglioma. Eur J Endocrinol Eur Fed Endocr Soc. 2015;173(3):377–87.
22. Nijhoff MF, Dekkers OM, Vleming LJ, Smit JW, Romijn JA, Pereira AM. ACTHproducing pheochromocytoma: clinical considerations and concise review of the literature. Eur J Intern Med. 2009;20(7):682–5.
23. Loehry CA, Kingham JG, Whorwell PJ. Watery diarrhoea and hypokalaemia associated with a pheochromocytoma. Postgrad Med J. 1975;51(596):416–9.
24. Yang C, Zhuang Z. Fliedner SMet al. Germ-line PHD1 and PHD2 mutations detected in patients with pheochromocytoma/paraganglioma-polycythemia. J Mol Med (Berl). 2015;93:93104.
25. Young WF, Maddox DE. Spells: in search of a cause. Mayo Clin Proc. 1995;70(8):757–65.
26. Lenders JW, Duh QY, Eisenhofer G, Gimenez-Roqueplo AP, Grebe SK, Murad MH, Naruse M, Pacak K, Young WF. Pheochromocytoma and paraganglioma: an endocrine society clinical practice guideline. J Clin Endocrinol Metab. 2014;99(6):191542.
27. Eisenhofer G, Peitzsch M. Laboratory evaluation of pheochromocytoma and paraganglioma. Clin Chem. 2014;60:1486–99.
28. Eisenhofer G, Lenders JW, Timmers H, Mannelli M, Grebe SK, Hofbauer LC, Bornstein SR, Tiebel O, Adams K, Bratslavsky G, Linehan WM, Pacak K. Measurements of plasma methoxytyramine, normetanephrine, and metanephrine as discriminators of different hereditary forms of pheochromocytoma. Clin Chem. 2011;57(3):411–20.
29. Eisenhofer G, Peitzsch M. Laboratory evaluation of pheochromocytoma and paraganglioma. Clin Chem. 2014;60(12):1486–99.
30. Lenders JW, Duh QY, Eisenhofer G, Gimenez-Roqueplo AP, Grebe SK, Murad MH, Naruse M, Pacak K, Young WF. Pheochromocytoma and paraganglioma: an endocrine society clinical practice guideline. J Clin Endocrinol Metab. 2014;99(6):191542.

31. Castinetti F, Kroiss A, Kumar R, Pacak K, Taieb D. 15 years of paraganglioma: imaging and imaging-based treatment of pheochromocytoma and paraganglioma. Endocr Relat Cancer. 2015;22(4):T135–45.
32. Janssen I, Blanchet EM, Adams K, Chen CC, Millo CM, Herscovitch P, Taieb D, Kebebew E, Lehnert H, Fojo AT, Pacak K. Superiority of [68Ga]-DOTATATE PET/CT to other functional imaging modalities in the localization of SDHB-associated metastatic pheochromocytoma and paraganglioma. Clin Cancer Res Off J Am Assoc Cancer Res. 2015;21(17):3888–95.
33. Eisenhofer G, Tischler AS, de Krijger RR. Diagnostic tests and biomarkers for pheochromocytoma and extra-adrenal paraganglioma: from routine laboratory methods to disease stratification. Endocr Pathol. 2012;23(1):4–14.
34. Scopsi L, Castellani MR, Gullo M, Cusumano F, Camerini E, Pasini B, Orefice S. Malignant pheochromocytoma in multiple endocrine neoplasia type 2B syndrome. Case report and review of the literature. Tumori. 1996;82(5):480–4.
35. Zhu D, Kumar A, Weintraub WS, Rahman E. A large pheochromocytoma with invasion of multiple local organs. J Clin Hypertens (Greenwich, Conn.). 2011;13(1):60–4.
36. Amin MB, Edge S, Greene F, Byrd DR, Brookland RK, Washington MK, Gershenwald JE, Compton CC, Hess KR, Sullivan DC, Jessup JM, Brierley JD, Gaspar LE, Schilsky RL, Balch CM, Winchester DP, Asare EA, Madera M, Gress DM, Meyer LR, editors. AJCC cancer staging manual. 8th ed. New York: Springer; 2017.
37. Korpershoek E, Petri BJ, Post E, van Eijck CH, Oldenburg RA, Belt EJ, de Herder WW, de Krijger RR, Dinjens WN. Adrenal medullary hyperplasia is a precursor lesion for pheochromocytoma in MEN2 syndrome. Neoplasia (New York, N.Y.). 2014;16(10):868–73.
38. Lack EE. Tumors of the adrenal glands and extraadrenal paraganglia, armed forces. Series 4, vol. 8. Washington, D.C.: Institute of Pathology Atlas of Tumor Pathology; 2000. ISBN-13: 978-1881041016.
39. Shin WY, Groman GS, Berkman JI. Pheochromocytoma with angiomatous features. A case report and ultrastructural study. Cancer. 1977;40(1):275–83.
40. Kasem K, Lam AK. Adrenal oncocytic pheochromocytoma with putative adverse histologic features: a unique case report and review of the literature. Endocr Pathol. 2014;25(4):416–21.
41. Strong VE, Kennedy T, Al-Ahmadie H, Tang L, Coleman J, Fong Y, Brennan M, Ghossein RA. Prognostic indicators of malignancy in adrenal pheochromocytomas: clinical, histopathologic, and cell cycle/apoptosis gene expression analysis. Surgery. 2008;143(6):759–68.
42. Tischler AS, deKrijger RR. 15 years of paraganglioma: pathology of pheochromocytoma and paraganglioma. Endocr Relat Cancer. 2015;22(4):T123–33.
43. Duregon E, Volante M, Bollito E, Goia M, Buttigliero C, Zaggia B, Berruti A, Scagliotti GV, Papotti M. Pitfalls in the diagnosis of adrenocortical tumors: a lesson from 300 consultation cases. Hum Pathol. 2015;46(12):1799–807.
44. Tischler AS. Pheochromocytoma and extra-adrenal paraganglioma: updates. Arch Pathol Lab Med. 2008;132(8):1272–84.
45. Sangoi AR, McKenney JK. A tissue microarray-based comparative analysis of novel and traditional immunohistochemical markers in the distinction between adrenal cortical lesions and pheochromocytoma. Am J Surg Pathol. 2010;34:423–32.
46. Lloyd RV, Blaivas M, Wilson BS. Distribution of chromogranin and S100 protein in normal and abnormal adrenal medullary tissues. Arch Pathol Lab Med. 1985;109(7):633–5.
47. Ballav C, Naziat A, Mihai R, Karavitaki N, Ansorge O, Grossman AB. Mini-review: pheochromocytomas causing the ectopic ACTH syndrome. Endocrine. 2012;42(1):69–73.
48. Dahia PL, Ross KN, Wright ME, Hayashida CY, Santagata S, Barontini M, Kung AL, Sanso G, Powers JF, Tischler AS, Hodin R, Heitritter S, Moore F, Dluhy R, Sosa JA, Ocal IT, Benn DE, Marsh DJ, Robinson BG, Schneider K, Garber J, Arum SM, Korbonits M, Grossman A, Pigny P, Toledo SP, Nosé V, Li C, Stiles CD. A HIF1alpha regulatory loop links hypoxia and mitochondrial signals in pheochromocytomas. PLoS Geneti. 2005;1(1):72–80.
49. Gill AJ, Benn DE, Chou A, Clarkson A, Muljono A, Meyer-Rochow GY, Richardson AL, Sidhu SB, Robinson BG, Clifton-Bligh RJ. Immunohistochemistry for SDHB triages genetic

testing of SDHB, SDHC, and SDHD in paraganglioma-pheochromocytoma syndromes. Hum Pathol. 2010;41(6):805–14.
50. van Nederveen FH, Gaal J, Favier J, Korpershoek E, Oldenburg RA, de Bruyn EM, Sleddens HF, Derkx P, Rivière J, Dannenberg H, Petri BJ, Komminoth P, Pacak K, Hop WC, Pollard PJ, Mannelli M, Bayley JP, Perren A, Niemann S, Verhofstad AA, de Bruïne AP, Maher ER, Tissier F, Méatchi T, Badoual C, Bertherat J, Amar L, Alataki D, Van Marck E, Ferrau F, François J, de Herder WW, Peeters MP, van Linge A, Lenders JW, Gimenez-Roqueplo AP, de Krijger RR, Dinjens WN. An immunohistochemical procedure to detect patients with paraganglioma and pheochromocytoma with germline SDHB, SDHC, or SDHD gene mutations: a retrospective and prospective analysis. Lancet Oncol. 2009;10(8):764–71.
51. Asa SL. My approach to oncocytic tumors of the thyroid. J Clin Pathol. 2004;57:225–32.
52. Kimura N, Takayanagi R, Takizawa N, Itagaki E, Katabami T, Kakoi N, Rakugi H, Ikeda Y, Tanabe A, Nigawara T, Ito S, Kimura I, Naruse M. Pathological grading for predicting metastasis in pheochromocytoma and paraganglioma. Endocr Relat Cancer. 2014;21(3):405–14.
53. Thompson LD. Pheochromocytoma of the Adrenal gland Scaled Score (PASS) to separate benign from malignant neoplasms: a clinicopathologic and immunophenotypic study of 100 cases. Am J Surg Pathol. 2002;26(5):551–66.
54. Linnoila RI, Keiser HR, Steinberg SM, Lack EE. Histopathology of benign versus malignant sympathoadrenal paragangliomas: clinicopathologic study of 120 cases including unusual histologic features. Hum Pathol. 1990;21(11):1168–80.
55. Oudijk L, van Nederveen F, Badoual C, Tissier F, Tischler AS, Smid M, Gaal J, Lepoutre-Lussey C, Gimenez-Roqueplo AP, Dinjens WN, Korpershoek E, de Krijger R, Favier J. Vascular pattern analysis for the prediction of clinical behaviour in pheochromocytomas and paragangliomas. PLoS One. 2015;10(3):e0121361.
56. Unger P, Hoffman K, Pertsemlidis D, Thung S, Wolfe D, Kaneko M. S100 protein positive sustentacular cells in malignant and locally aggressive adrenal pheochromocytomas. Arch Pathol Lab Med. 1991;115(5):484–7.
57. Kimura N, Takekoshi K, Horii A, Morimoto R, Imai T, Oki Y, Saito T, Midorikawa S, Arao T, Sugisawa C, Yamada M, Otuka Y, Kurihara I, Sugano K, Nakane M, Fukuuchi A, Kitamoto T, Saito J, Nishikawa T, Naruse M. Clinicopathological study of SDHB mutation-related pheochromocytoma and sympathetic paraganglioma. Endocr Relat Cancer. 2014;21(3):L13–6.
58. Toledo SP, Lourenço DM, Sekiya T, Lucon AM, Baena ME, Castro CC, Bortolotto LA, Zerbini MC, Siqueira SA, Toledo RA, Dahia PL. Penetrance and clinical features of pheochromocytoma in a six-generation family carrying a germline TMEM127 mutation. J Clin Endocrinol Metab. 2015;100(2):E308–18.
59. Carney JA, Sizemore GW, Tyce GM. Bilateral adrenal medullary hyperplasia in multiple endocrine neoplasia, type 2: the precursor of bilateral pheochromocytoma. Mayo Clinic Proc. 1975;50(1):3–10.
60. Koch CA, Mauro D, Walther MM, Linehan WM, Vortmeyer AO, Jaffe R, Pacak K, Chrousos GP, Zhuang Z, Lubensky IA. Pheochromocytoma in von hippel-lindau disease: distinct histopathologic phenotype compared to pheochromocytoma in multiple endocrine neoplasia type 2. Endocr Pathol. 2002;13(1):17–27.
61. Amar L, Bertherat J, Baudin E, Ajzenberg C, Bressac-de Paillerets B, Chabre O, Chamontin B, Delemer B, Giraud S, Murat A, Niccoli-Sire P, Richard S, Rohmer V, Sadoul JL, Strompf L, Schlumberger M, Bertagna X, Plouin PF, Jeunemaitre X, Gimenez-Roqueplo AP. Genetic testing in pheochromocytoma or functional paraganglioma. J Clin Oncol Off J Am Soc Clin Oncol. 2005;23(34):8812–8.
62. Brito JP, Asi N, Bancos I, Gionfriddo MR, Zeballos-Palacios CL, Leppin AL, Undavalli C, Wang Z, Domecq JP, Prustsky G, Elraiyah TA, Prokop LJ, Montori VM, Murad MH. Testing for germline mutations in sporadic pheochromocytoma/paraganglioma: a systematic review. Clin Endocrinol. 2015;82(3):338–45.
63. Neumann HP, Bausch B, McWhinney SR, Bender BU, Gimm O, Franke G, Schipper J, Klisch J, Altehoefer C, Zerres K, Januszewicz A, Eng C, Smith WM, Munk R, Manz T, Glaesker

S, Apel TW, Treier M, Reineke M, Walz MK, Hoang-Vu C, Brauckhoff M, Klein-Franke A, Klose P, Schmidt H, MaierWoelfle M, Peçzkowska M, Szmigielski C, Eng C. Germ-line mutations in nonsyndromic pheochromocytoma. N Engl J Med. 2002;346(19):1459–66.

64. Pacak K, Wimalawansa SJ. Pheochromocytoma and paraganglioma. Endocr Pract Off J Am Coll Endocrinol Am Assoc Clin Endocrinologists. 2015;21(4):406–12.
65. Koch CA, Huang SC, Moley JF, Azumi N, Chrousos GP, Gagel RF, Zhuang Z, Pacak K, Vortmeyer AO. Allelic imbalance of the mutant and wild-type RET allele in MEN 2A-associated medullary thyroid carcinoma. Oncogene. 2001;20(53):7809–11.
66. Baysal BE, Maher ER. 15 years of paraganglioma: genetics and mechanism of pheochromocytoma-paraganglioma syndromes characterized by germline SDHB and SDHD mutations. Endocr Relat Cancer. 2015;22(4):T71–82.
67. Hoekstra AS, Devilee P, Bayley JP. Models of parent-of-origin tumorigenesis in hereditary paraganglioma. Semin Cell Dev Biol. 2015;43:117–24.
68. Luchetti A, Walsh D, Rodger F, Clark G, Martin T, Irving R, Sanna M, Yao M, Robledo M, Neumann HP, Woodward ER, Latif F, Abbs S, Martin H, Maher ER. Profiling of somatic mutations in pheochromocytoma and paraganglioma by targeted next generation sequencing analysis. Int J Endocrinol. 2015;2015:138573.
69. Burnichon N, Buffet A, Parfait B, Letouzé E, Laurendeau I, Loriot C, Pasmant E, Abermil N, ValeyrieAllanore L, Bertherat J, Amar L, Vidaud D, Favier J, Gimenez-Roqueplo AP. Somatic NF1 inactivation is a frequent event in sporadic pheochromocytoma. Hum Mol Genet. 2012;21(26):5397–405.
70. Dahia PL. Pheochromocytoma and paraganglioma pathogenesis: learning from genetic heterogeneity. Nat Rev Cancer. 2014;14(2):108–19.
71. Luchetti A, Walsh D, Rodger F, Clark G, Martin T, Irving R, Sanna M, Yao M, Robledo M, Neumann HP, Woodward ER, Latif F, Abbs S, Martin H, Maher ER. Profiling of somatic mutations in pheochromocytoma and paraganglioma by targeted next generation sequencing analysis. Int J Endocrinol. 2015;2015:138573.
72. Welander J, Söderkvist P, Gimm O. The NF1 gene: a frequent mutational target in sporadic pheochromocytomas and beyond. Endocr Relat Cancer. 2013;20(4):C13–7.
73. Geli J, Kiss N, Karimi M, Lee JJ, Bäckdahl M, Ekström TJ, Larsson C. Global and regional CpG methylation in pheochromocytomas and abdominal paragangliomas: association to malignant behavior. Clinical cancer Research: an official journal of the American Association for Cancer Research. 2008;14(9):2551–9.
74. Letouzé E, Martinelli C, Loriot C, Burnichon N, Abermil N, Ottolenghi C, Janin M, Menara M, Nguyen AT, Benit P, Buffet A, Marcaillou C, Bertherat J, Amar L, Rustin P, De Reyniès A, Gimenez-Roqueplo AP, Favier J. SDH mutations establish a hypermethylator phenotype in paraganglioma. Cancer Cell. 2013;23(6):739–52.
75. Blank A, Schmitt AM, Korpershoek E, van Nederveen F, Rudolph T, Weber N, Strebel RT, de Krijger R, Komminoth P, Perren A. SDHB loss predicts malignancy in pheochromocytomas/sympathetic paragangliomas, but not through hypoxia signalling. Endocr Relat Cancer. 2010;17(4):919–28.
76. Amar L, Baudin E, Burnichon N, Peyrard S, Silvera S, Bertherat J, Bertagna X, Schlumberger M, Jeunemaitre X, Gimenez-Roqueplo AP, Plouin PF. Succinate dehydrogenase B gene mutations predict survival in patients with malignant pheochromocytomas or paragangliomas. J Clin Endocrinol Metab. 2007;92(10):3822–8.
77. Medeiros LJ, Wolf BC, Balogh K, Federman M. Adrenal pheochromocytoma: a clinicopathologic review of 60 cases. Hum Pathol. 1985;16(6):580–9.
78. Pacak K, Eisenhofer G, Ahlman H, Bornstein SR, Gimenez-Roqueplo AP, Grossman AB, Kimura N, Mannelli M, McNicol AM, Tischler AS. Pheochromocytoma: recommendations for clinical practice from the First International Symposium. October 2005. Nat Clin Pract Endocrinol Metab. 2007;3(2):92–102.
79. Gobbi H, Barbosa AJ, Teixeira VP, Almeida HO. Immunocytochemical identification of neuroendocrine markers in human cardiac paraganglion-like structures. Histochemistry. 1991;95:337–40.

80. Paraganglia TAS. In: Mills SE, editor. Histology for pathologists. 4th ed. Philadelphia: Lippincott-Raven; 2012. p. 1277–99.
81. Zhou M, Epstein JI, Young RH. Paraganglioma of the urinary bladder: a lesion that may be misdiagnosed as urothelial carcinoma in transurethral resection specimens. Am J Surg Pathol. 2004;28(1):94–100.
82. Mannelli M, Castellano M, Schiavi F, Filetti S, Giacchè M, Mori L, Pignataro V, Bernini G, Giachè V, Bacca A, Biondi B, Corona G, Di Trapani G, Grossrubatscher E, Reimondo G, Arnaldi G, Giacchetti G, Veglio F, Loli P, Colao A, Ambrosio MR, Terzolo M, Letizia C, Ercolino T, Opocher G. Clinically guided genetic screening in a large cohort of italian patients with pheochromocytomas and/or functional or nonfunctional paragangliomas. J Clin Endocrinol Metab. 2009;94(5):1541–7.
83. Sykes JM, Ossoff RH. Paragangliomas of the head and neck. Otolaryngol Clin North Am. 1986;19(4):755–67.
84. Chapman DB, Lippert D, Geer CP, Edwards HD, Russell GB, Rees CJ, Browne JD. Clinical, histopathologic, and radiographic indicators of malignancy in head and neck paragangliomas. Otolaryngol Head Neck Surg Off J Am Acad Otolaryngol Head Neck Surg. 2010;143(4):531–7.
85. Mediouni A, Ammari S, Wassef M, Gimenez-Roqueplo AP, Laredo JD, Duet M, Tran Ba Huy P, Oker N. Malignant head/neck paragangliomas. Comparative study. Eur Ann Otorhinolaryngol Head Neck Dis. 2014;131(3):159–66.
86. Lee JH, Barich F, Karnell LH, Robinson RA, Zhen WK, Gantz BJ, Hoffman HT. National Cancer Data Base report on malignant paragangliomas of the head and neck. Cancer. 2002;94(3):730–7.
87. Rodríguez-Cuevas S, López-Garza J, Labastida-Almendaro S. Carotid body tumors in inhabitants of altitudes higher than 2000 meters above sea level. Head Neck. 1998;20(5):374–8.
88. Erickson D, Kudva YC, Ebersold MJ, Thompson GB, Grant CS, van Heerden JA, Young WF. Benign paragangliomas: clinical presentation and treatment outcomes in 236 patients. J Clin Endocrinol Metab. 2001;86(11):5210–6.
89. Zheng X, Wei S, Yu Y, Xia T, Zhao J, Gao S, Li Y, Gao M. Genetic and clinical characteristics of head and neck paragangliomas in a Chinese population. Laryngoscope. 2012;122(8):1761–6.
90. Burnichon N, Rohmer V, Amar L, Herman P, Leboulleux S, Darrouzet V, Niccoli P, Gaillard D, Chabrier G, Chabolle F, Coupier I, Thieblot P, Lecomte P, Bertherat J, Wion-Barbot N, Murat A, Venisse A, Plouin PF, Jeunemaitre X, Gimenez-Roqueplo AP. The succinate dehydrogenase genetic testing in a large prospective series of patients with paragangliomas. J Clin Endocrinol Metab. 2009;94(8):2817–27.
91. Capatina C, Ntali G, Karavitaki N, Grossman AB. The management of head-and-neck paragangliomas. Endocr Relat Cancer. 2013;20(5):291–305.
92. Moskovic DJ, Smolarz JR, Stanley D, Jimenez C, Williams MD, Hanna EY, Kupferman ME. Malignant head and neck paragangliomas: is there an optimal treatment strategy? Head Neck Oncol. 2010;2:23.
93. Opotowsky AR, Moko LE, Ginns J, Rosenbaum M, Greutmann M, Aboulhosn J, Hageman A, Kim Y, Deng LX, Grewal J, Zaidi AN, Almansoori G, Oechslin E, Earing M, Landzberg MJ, Singh MN, Wu F, Vaidya A. Pheochromocytoma and paraganglioma in cyanotic congenital heart disease. J Clin Endocrinol Metab. 2015;100(4):1325–34.
94. Lima J, Feijão T, Ferreira da Silva A, Pereira-Castro I, Fernandez-Ballester G, Máximo V, Herrero A, Serrano L, Sobrinho-Simões M, Garcia-Rostan G. High frequency of germline succinate dehydrogenase mutations in sporadic cervical paragangliomas in northern Spain: mitochondrial succinate dehydrogenase structure-function relationships and clinical-pathological correlations. J Clin Endocrinol Metab. 2007;92(12):4853–64.
95. Neumann HP, Erlic Z, Boedeker CC, Rybicki LA, Robledo M, Hermsen M, Schiavi F, Falcioni M, Kwok P, Bauters C, Lampe K, Fischer M, Edelman E, Benn DE, Robinson BG, Wiegand S, Rasp G, Stuck BA, Hoffmann MM, Sullivan M, Sevilla MA, Weiss MM, Peczkowska M, Kubaszek A, Pigny P, Ward RL, Learoyd D, Croxson M, Zabolotny D, Yaremchuk S, Draf

W, Muresan M, Lorenz RR, Knipping S, Strohm M, Dyckhoff G, Matthias C, Reisch N, Preuss SF, Esser D, Walter MA, Kaftan H, Stöver T, Fottner C, Gorgulla H, Malekpour M, Zarandy MM, Schipper J, Brase C, Glien A, Kühnemund M, Koscielny S, Schwerdtfeger P, Välimäki M, Szyfter W, Finckh U, Zerres K, Cascon A, Opocher G, Ridder GJ, Januszewicz A, Suarez C, Eng C. Clinical predictors for germline mutations in head and neck paraganglioma patients: cost reduction strategy in genetic diagnostic process as fall-out. Cancer Res. 2009;69(8):3650–6.
96. Ricketts CJ, Forman JR, Rattenberry E, Bradshaw N, Lalloo F, Izatt L, Cole TR, Armstrong R, Kumar VK, Morrison PJ, Atkinson AB, Douglas F, Ball SG, Cook J, Srirangalingam U, Killick P, Kirby G, Aylwin S, Woodward ER, Evans DG, Hodgson SV, Murday V, Chew SL, Connell JM, Blundell TL, Macdonald F, Maher ER. Tumor risks and genotype-phenotype-proteotype analysis in 358 patients with germline mutations in SDHB and SDHD. Hum Mutat. 2010;31(1):41–51.
97. Kimura N, Tateno H, Saijo S, Horii A. Familial cervical paragangliomas with lymph node metastasis expressing somatostatin receptor type 2A. Endocr Pathol. 2010;21(2):139–43.
98. Piccini V, Rapizzi E, Bacca A, Di Trapani G, Pulli R, Giachè V, Zampetti B, Lucci-Cordisco E, Canu L, Corsini E, Faggiano A, Deiana L, Carrara D, Tantardini V, Mariotti S, Ambrosio MR, Zatelli MC, Parenti G, Colao A, Pratesi C, Bernini G, Ercolino T, Mannelli M. Head and neck paragangliomas: genetic spectrum and clinical variability in 79 consecutive patients. Endocr Relat Cancer. 2012;19(2):149–55.
99. Elston MS, Meyer-Rochow GY, Conaglen HM, Clarkson A, Clifton-Bligh RJ, Conaglen JV, Gill AJ. Increased SSTR2A and SSTR3 expression in succinate dehydrogenase-deficient pheochromocytomas and paragangliomas. Hum Pathol. 2015;46(3):390–6.
100. Osinga TE, Korpershoek E, de Krijger RR, Kerstens MN, Dullaart RP, Kema IP, van der Laan BF, van der Horst-Schrivers AN, Links TP. Catecholamine-synthesizing enzymes are expressed in parasympathetic head and neck paraganglioma tissue. Neuroendocrinology. 2015;101(4):289–95.
101. Tischler AS. Pheochromocytoma and extra-adrenal paraganglioma: updates. Arch Pathol Lab Med. 2008;132(8):1272–84.
102. Korpershoek E, Favier J, Gaal J, Burnichon N, van Gessel B, Oudijk L, Badoual C, Gadessaud N, Venisse A, Bayley JP, van Dooren MF, de Herder WW, Tissier F, Plouin PF, van Nederveen FH, Dinjens WN, Gimenez-Roqueplo AP, de Krijger RR. SDHA immunohistochemistry detects germline SDHA gene mutations in apparently sporadic paragangliomas and pheochromocytomas. J Clin Endocrinol Metab. 2011;96(9):E1472–6.
103. Langerman A, Athavale SM, Rangarajan SV, Sinard RJ, Netterville JL. Natural history of cervical paragangliomas: outcomes of observation of 43 patients. Arch Otolaryngol Head Neck Surg. 2012;138(4):341–5.
104. Jansen JC, van den Berg R, Kuiper A, van der Mey AG, Zwinderman AH, Cornelisse CJ. Estimation of growth rate in patients with head and neck paragangliomas influences the treatment proposal. Cancer. 2000;88(12):2811–6.
105. Bradshaw JW, Jansen JC. Management of vagal paraganglioma: is operative resection really the best option? Surgery. 2005;137(2):225–8.
106. Ellis RJ, Patel D, Prodanov T, Nilubol N, Pacak K, Kebebew E. The presence of SDHB mutations should modify surgical indications for carotid body paragangliomas. Ann Surg. 2014;260:158–62.
107. Garnier S, Réguerre Y, Orbach D, Brugières L, Kalfa N. Pediatric pheochromocytoma and paraganglioma: an update. Bulletin du cancer. 2014;101(10):966–75.
108. Harari A, Inabnet WB. Malignant pheochromocytoma: a review. Am J Surg. 2011; 201(5):700–8.
109. Korevaar TI, Grossman AB. Pheochromocytomas and paragangliomas: assessment of malignant potential. Endocrine. 2011;40(3):354–65.
110. Goffredo P, Sosa JA, Roman SA. Malignant pheochromocytoma and paraganglioma: a population level analysis of long-term survival over two decades. J Surg Oncol. 2013;107(6):659–64.

111. JA B, Lawton A, Hajdenberg J, Rosser CJ. Pheochromocytoma of the urinary bladder: a systematic review of the contemporary literature. BMC Urol. 2013;13:22.
112. Henderson SJ, Kearns PJ, Tong CM, Reddy M, Khurgin J, Bickell M, Miick R, Ginsberg P, Metro MJ. Patients with urinary bladder paragangliomas: a compiled case series from a literature review for clinical management. Urology. 2015;85(4):e25–9.
113. Quist EE, Javadzadeh BM, Johannesen E, Johansson SL, Lele SM, Kozel JA. Malignant paraganglioma of the bladder: a case report and review of the literature. Pathol Res Pract. 2015;211(2):183–8.
114. Wang JG, Han J, Jiang T, Li YJ. Cardiac paragangliomas. J Cardiac Surg. 2015;30(1):55–60.
115. Millar AC, Mete O, Cusimano RJ, Fremes SE, Keshavjee S, Morgan CD, Asa SL, Ezzat S, Gilbert J. Functional cardiac paraganglioma associated with a rare SDHC mutation. Endocr Pathol. 2014;25(3):315–20.
116. Wen J, Li HZ, Ji ZG, Mao QZ, Shi BB, Yan WG. A decade of clinical experience with extra-adrenal paragangliomas of retroperitoneum: report of 67 cases and a literature review. Urol Ann. 2010;2(1):12–6.
117. Sclafani LM, Woodruff JM, Brennan MF. Extraadrenal retroperitoneal paragangliomas: natural history and response to treatment. Surgery. 1990;108(6):1124–9; discussion 1129-30
118. Kimura N, Watanabe T, Noshiro T, Shizawa S, Miura Y. Histological grading of adrenal and extra-adrenal pheochromocytomas and relationship to prognosis: a clinicopathological analysis of 116 adrenal pheochromocytomas and 30 extra-adrenal sympathetic paragangliomas including 38 malignant tumors. Endocr Pathol. 2005;16(1):23–32.
119. Elder EE, Xu D, Höög A, Enberg U, Hou M, Pisa P, Gruber A, Larsson C, Bäckdahl M. KI-67 AND hTERT expression can aid in the distinction between malignant and benign pheochromocytoma and paraganglioma. Mod Pathol Off J United States Can Acad Pathol Inc. 2003;16(3):246–55.
120. O'Riordain DS, Young WF, Grant CS, Carney JA, van Heerden JA. Clinical spectrum and outcome of functional extraadrenal paraganglioma. World J Surg. 1996;20(7):916–21; discussion 922
121. Eisenhofer G, Lenders JW, Siegert G, Bornstein SR, Friberg P, Milosevic D, Mannelli M, Linehan WM, Adams K, Timmers HJ, Pacak K. Plasma methoxytyramine: a novel biomarker of metastatic pheochromocytoma and paraganglioma in relation to established risk factors of tumor size, location and SDHB mutation status. Eur J Cancer (Oxford, England: 1990). 2012;48(11):1739–49.
122. Eisenhofer G, Timmers HJ, Lenders JW, Bornstein SR, Tiebel O, Mannelli M, King KS, Vocke CD, Linehan WM, Bratslavsky G, Pacak K. Age at diagnosis of pheochromocytoma differs according to catecholamine phenotype and tumor location. J Clin Endocrinol Metab. 2011;96(2):375–84.
123. Lam KY, Lo CY. Composite pheochromocytoma-ganglioneuroma of the adrenal gland: an uncommon entity with distinctive Clinicopathologic features. Endocr Pathol. 1999;10(4):343–52.
124. Linnoila RI, Keiser HR, Steinberg SM, Lack EE. Histopathology of benign versus malignant sympathoadrenal paragangliomas: clinicopathologic study of 120 cases including unusual histologic features. Hum Pathol. 1990;21(11):1168–80.
125. Khan AN, Solomon SS, Childress RD. Composite pheochromocytoma-ganglioneuroma: a rare experiment of nature. Endocr Pract Off J Am Coll Endocrinol Am Assoc Clin Endocrinologists. 2010;16(2):291–9.
126. Baisakh MR, Mohapatra N, Adhikary SD, Routray D. Malignant peripheral nerve sheath tumor of adrenal gland with heterologous osseous differentiation in a case of Von Recklinghausen's disease. Indian J Pathol Microbiol. 2014;57(1):130–2.
127. Ch'ng ES, Hoshida Y, Iizuka N, Morii E, Ikeda JI, Yamamoto A, Tomita Y, Hanasaki H, Katsuya T, Maeda K, Ohishi M, Rakugi H, Ogihara T, Aozasa K. Composite malignant pheochromocytoma with malignant peripheral nerve sheath tumor: a case with 28 years of tumor bearing history. Histopathology. 2007;51(3):420–2.

128. Tischler AS. Divergent differentiation in neuroendocrine tumors of the adrenal gland. Semin Diagn Pathol. 2000;17(2):120–6.
129. Loehry CA, Kingham JG, Whorwell PJ. Watery diarrhoea and hypokalaemia associated with a pheochromocytoma. Postgrad Med J. 1975;51(596):416–9.
130. Powers JF, Brachold JM, Tischler AS. Ret protein expression in adrenal medullary hyperplasia and pheochromocytoma. Endocr Pathol. 2003;14(4):351–61.
131. Tischler AS, Dayal Y, Balogh K, Cohen RB, Connolly JL, Tallberg K. The distribution of immunoreactive chromogranins, S-100 protein, and vasoactive intestinal peptide in compound tumors of the adrenal medulla. Hum Pathol. 1987;18(9):909–17.
132. Brady S, Lechan RM, Schwaitzberg SD, Dayal Y, Ziar J, Tischler AS. Composite pheochromocytoma/ganglioneuroma of the adrenal gland associated with multiple endocrine neoplasia 2A: case report with immunohistochemical analysis. Am J Surg Pathol. 1997;21(1):102–8.
133. Matias-Guiu X, Garrastazu MT. Composite pheochromocytomaganglioneuroblastoma in a patient with multiple endocrine neoplasia type IIA. Histopathology. 1998;32(3):281–2.
134. Bernini GP, Moretti A, Mannelli M, Ercolino T, Bardini M, Caramella D, Taurino C, Salvetti A. Unique association of non-functioning pheochromocytoma, ganglioneuroma, adrenal cortical adenoma, hepatic and vertebral hemangiomas in a patient with a new intronic variant in the VHL gene. J Endocrinol Invest. 2005;28(11):1032–7.
135. Kragel PJ, Johnston CA. Pheochromocytoma-ganglioneuroma of the adrenal. Arch Pathol Lab Med. 1985;109(5):470–2.
136. Kikuchi Y, Wada R, Sakihara S, Suda T, Yagihashi S. Pheochromocytoma with histologic transformation to composite type, complicated by watery diarrhea, hypokalemia, and achlorhydria syndrome. Endocr Pract Off J Am Coll Endocrinol Am Assoc Clin Endocrinologists. 2012;18(4):e91–6.
137. Fujiwara T, Kawamura M, Sasou S, Hiramori K. Results of surgery for a compound adrenal tumor consisting of pheochromocytoma and ganglioneuroblastoma in an adult: 5-year followup. Intern Med (Tokyo, Japan). 2000;39(1):58–62.
138. Pytel P, Krausz T, Wollmann R, Utset MF. Ganglioneuromatous paraganglioma of the cauda equina – a pathological case study. Hum Pathol. 2005;36(4):444–6.
139. Shankar GM, Chen L, Kim AH, Ross GL, Folkerth RD, Friedlander RM. Composite ganglioneuroma-paraganglioma of the filum terminale. J Neurosurg Spine. 2010;12(6):709–13.
140. Monclair T, Ruud E, Holmstrom H, Aagenaes I, Asplin M, Beiske K. Extra-adrenal composite pheochromocytoma/ganglioneuroblastoma in a 15 month old child. J Paediatr Surg Case Rep. 2015;3(8):348–50.
141. Chen CH, Boag AH, Beiko DT, Siemens DR, Froese A, Isotalo PA. Composite paraganglioma-ganglioneuroma of the urinary bladder: a rare neoplasm causing hemodynamic crisis at tumor resection. Can Urol Assoc J Journal de l'Association des urologues du Canada. 2009;3(5):E45–8.
142. Hu J, Wu J, Cai L, Jiang L, Lang Z, Qu G, Liu H, Yao W, Yu G. Retroperitoneal composite pheochromocytoma-ganglioneuroma: a case report and review of literature. Diagn Pathol. 2013;8:63.
143. de Montpréville VT, Mussot S, Gharbi N, Dartevelle P, Dulmet E. Paraganglioma with ganglioneuromatous component located in the posterior mediastinum. Ann Diagn Pathol. 2005;9(2):110–4.

Chapter 3
Clinical Features of Pheochromocytoma and Paraganglioma

Lewis Landsberg

Overview

Pheochromocytoma is a rare disease; it is estimated that only one in a thousand hypertensive patients has a pheochromocytoma. The rarity, however, should not obscure its importance. Promptly diagnosed and properly treated, it is almost always curable; delay in diagnosis or improper treatment usually results in death. Unselected autopsy series suggest that more than one-half of pheochromocytomas are not diagnosed during life, and retrospective review suggests that in most of these undiagnosed cases, the pheochromocytoma was responsible for the demise [1]. Many potential cases, it seems, are being missed.

Other indicia of importance include the facts that 1 in 20,000 general anesthesias for unrelated diseases uncovers an unsuspected pheochromocytoma (Dr John Hedley-Whyte, personal communication) and that a small but significant number of incidentally discovered adrenal masses turn out to be pheochromocytomas. Since pheochromocytoma is rare and many of the manifestations are common, the trick is to think of it; this requires knowing the unusual, as well as the common, modes of presentation.

The clinical features of pheochromocytoma are due predominantly to the release of biologically active compounds from the tumor. These are principally catecholamines, but a variety of peptide hormones are also occasionally produced, and these contribute importantly to the clinical features in individual cases [2]. Table 3.1 lists some of the other important biologically active moieties that may be secreted by pheochromocytomas.

L. Landsberg (✉)
Northwestern University, Feinberg School of Medicine, Chicago, IL, USA
e-mail: l-landsberg@northwestern.edu

L. Landsberg (ed.), *Pheochromocytomas, Paragangliomas and Disorders of the Sympathoadrenal System*, Contemporary Endocrinology,
https://doi.org/10.1007/978-3-319-77048-2_3

Table 3.1 Peptide hormones produced and secreted by pheochromocytomas

Hormone	Clinical association[a]
Adrenomedullin	Hypotension, shock
ACTH	Ectopic ACTH syndrome (Cushing's syndrome)
VIP	Watery diarrhea, hypokalemia, achlorhydria syndrome (WDHA)
PTHrP	Hypercalcemia
Erythropoietin	Polycythemia
Interleukin-6	Fever, systemic inflammatory response syndrome

[a]See text for details

Catecholamine Storage and Release from Pheochromocytomas and Paragangliomas

The normal adrenal contains about 75–80% epinephrine (E) and 20–25% norepinephrine (NE). In pheochromocytomas the concentration of NE is higher. Extra-adrenal pheochromocytomas (paragangliomas) by contrast contain and secrete only NE since, with vanishingly rare exceptions, they do not contain the E-forming enzyme (PNMT). Increased excretion of E, or its major metabolite metanephrine (MN), is diagnostic of an adrenal pheochromocytoma [2]. The predominant catecholamine secreted by the tumor cannot be predicted by the clinical symptoms. Increased excretion of dopamine (DA) or its major metabolite homovanillic acid (HVA) is suggestive but not diagnostic of malignancy [3].

As in the normal adrenal, catecholamines are stored in typical chromaffin granules. In distinction from the normal adrenal medulla, pheochromocytomas are not innervated; the mechanisms involved in the release of catecholamines and other biologically active compounds from these tumors are poorly understood. Changes in blood flow, external pressure, and hemorrhagic necrosis may be involved. A variety of drugs, as described later in this chapter, are also capable of stimulating catecholamine release from pheochromocytomas.

Clinical Manifestations and Pathophysiology

Hypertension

High blood pressure is the most common clinical feature of pheochromocytoma (Table 3.2) [4]. The traditional estimate is that 90% of pheochromocytoma patients are hypertensive; the normotensive ones are found incidentally during imaging for an unrelated problem or during the process of family screening in kindreds with syndromic pheochromocytomas. It is worth emphasizing that with increasing recognition of familial pheochromocytoma, those cases found by screening will likely increase. The hypertension is sustained in more than one-half of these patients and truly

Table 3.2 Hypertension in pheochromocytoma

Sustained 60%
With crises 27%
Without crises 33%
Paroxysmal 30%
Normotensive between attacks
No hypertension 10%
Discovered incidentally or through screening

paroxysmal in about one-third; in the latter group BP is not elevated between paroxysms. It is noteworthy that more than one-half of pheochromocytoma patients do not have discrete spells. This is the group that masquerades as essential hypertension. That said, it is not unusual for those with sustained hypertension to have increased BP variability and some of the metabolic features of pheochromocytoma such as sweating, weight loss, and carbohydrate intolerance.

The pathogenesis of the hypertension depends upon enhanced catecholamine stimulation of the heart, the vasculature, and the kidneys (see Chap. 1, Fig. 1.7). Both α and β receptors are involved, but the α effects on the vasculature are the most important, as indicated by the BP response to α blockade in pheochromocytoma patients.

The Paroxysm

Although hypertension is the most common manifestation of pheochromocytoma, the paroxysm is the defining feature [4]. Also known as "spells" or "pressor crises," the paroxysm is a presenting symptom in 55–60% of pheochromocytoma patients. The typical paroxysm (Table 3.3) is associated with very high BP, headache, palpitations, and sweating, the "classic" triad. Chest or abdominal pain is not infrequent, as is a sense of impending doom. Pallor is usual although sometimes flushing may occur. Paroxysms typically last 5 min to an hour but occasionally last even longer. Not all paroxysms are classic; many variations have been noted, but spells of any kind that are recurrent should raise the question of pheochromocytoma. Very rarely spells are not accompanied by hypertension; usually the opportunity to observe a spell and measure the BP will help establish the diagnosis.

The paroxysm is the pathological expression of unrestrained release of catecholamines and other bioactive compounds from the tumor.

Other Manifestations (Table 3.4)

Chest pain may reflect cardiac ischemia from either an increase in demand or a decrease in supply of blood and oxygen to the myocardium. Increased demand reflects the well-known effects of catecholamines on myocardial oxygen

Table 3.3 The typical paroxysm

Episodic, unregulated release of catecholamines
Symptoms and signs:
Headache, sweating, and palpitations
Very high BP (frequently with tachycardia)
Chest or abdominal pain
Pallor/flush
Apprehension (sense of impending doom)
Duration
5 min to an hour (or longer)
Frequency
Episodic; variable periodicity (more frequent and severe over time)

Table 3.4 Some other manifestations of pheochromocytoma

Carbohydrate intolerance
Suppression of insulin; glycogenolysis and gluconeogenesis
Increased metabolic rate
Stimulation of non-shivering thermogenesis (BAT)
Weight loss; sweating
Increased hematocrit
Decreased plasma volume ("stress polycythemia")
Erythrocytosis (erythropoietin production)
Rhabdomyolysis
Intense vasoconstriction → muscle necrosis
Myoglobinuric renal failure
Ischemic colitis
Cardiac ischemia
Increased oxygen demand; coronary artery spasm
Congestive heart failure
Hypertension, myocardial fibrosis
Cholelithiasis
Shock with multi-organ failure and ARDS (shock lung)
Adrenomedullin release
Fever with SIRS
IL-6 production

consumption: ↑ heart rate, ↑ contractile state, and ↑ wall tension. Decreased supply reflects the more unusual, but well-recognized, coronary artery spasm. Myocardial infarction has been noted in pheochromocytoma patients, sometimes with clean coronaries, a finding that suggests coronary spasm [4, 5].

Congestive heart failure in patients with pheochromocytoma may occur as a result of diastolic dysfunction (preserved ejection fraction) due to catecholamine-induced cardiac hypertrophy or as a result of myocardial fibrosis induced by catecholamine excess (diminished ejection fraction) [6]. Although CHF has long been recognized as an important manifestation of pheochromocytoma, recent reports have described an association with *Takotsubo cardiomyopathy*, a ballooning of the apical portion of the heart, first described in association with physical or emotional "stress" and concomitant sympathetic stimulation. In patients with a pheochromocytoma, ballooning of the basal or mid-ventricular portion of the heart appears to be common, an abnormality known as inverted Takotsubo syndrome. The importance of the association of pheochromocytoma with Takotsubo cardiomyopathy is twofold: (1) Takotsubo cardiomyopathy may be the presenting manifestation of pheochromocytoma, necessitating an evaluation for pheochromocytoma in all cases with ballooning cardiomyopathy; and (2) successful treatment of the pheochromocytoma usually results in complete resolution of this syndrome [7–10].

Abdominal pain, which may be associated with nausea and vomiting, often reflects hemorrhagic infarction within the tumor. Bowel ischemia from vasoconstriction is another possible cause. The incidence of *cholelithiasis* appears to be increased in patients with a pheochromocytoma and may contribute to the abdominal pain; the pathogenesis is not understood.

Sweating reflects the increase in heat production stimulated by catecholamines. The site of the ↑ thermogenesis is likely brown adipose tissue which has been known to be hypertrophied in pheochromocytoma patients for decades. The ↑ in thermogenesis does not result in fever since the temperature set point remains intact; sweating reflects the physiological response, heat dissipation, mediated by the sympathetic cholinergic nerves. It is not the direct result of catecholamines. The sweating is eccrine, that is, cholinergic, not adrenergic [2].

Weight loss in pheochromocytoma patients is another consequence of the ↑ in metabolic rate. The old saw "forget a fat pheochromocytoma" is not always applicable but serves as a reminder that most patients will have lost weight prior to their initial presentation.

Orthostatic hypotension is an important manifestation of pheochromocytoma. In fact, in an untreated hypertensive patient, a prominent fall in BP on standing (20/10 mmHg) should raise the suspicion of pheochromocytoma. The mechanism responsible depends upon the fact that the body cannot measure volume directly but is very good at measuring changes in pressure [2]. Catecholamine-induced vasoconstriction increases the pressure in the great veins (capacitance portion of the circulation), thereby transmitting impulses to the CNS that are read as volume expansion ("a full tank"). As a consequence a diuresis is initiated. But in fact the tank is not full; it is just smaller, rendering the pheochromocytoma patient unable to increase venous return upon assuming the upright position. This diminished volume reserve must be addressed in the preparation of patients for surgery, explaining the need for sodium repletion after α adrenergic blockade.

Another potential contributor to orthostatic hypotension in pheochromocytoma patients is the impact of high catecholamine levels on the sympathetic reflexes that defend the circulation during hydrostatic stress. Under these conditions, it is possible that these reflexes lose their training and no longer restore BP during standing.

Carbohydrate tolerance is diminished in many patients with pheochromocytoma [4, 11]. New onset diabetes mellitus is not infrequent in pheochromocytoma patients. Often erroneously attributed to increased β receptor-mediated stimulation of hepatic glucose output from glycolysis and gluconeogenesis, a moment's reflection will reveal the inadequacy of this explanation. Any increase in glucose level as a consequence of these mechanisms should result in a compensatory increase in insulin secretion with restoration of the glucose level providing that insulin is unrestrained. The real explanation, therefore, is that insulin secretion is suppressed by the high levels of catecholamines that inhibit the release of insulin by a well-recognized α receptor effect. The initiation of α blockade will frequently restore carbohydrate tolerance to normal.

An *elevated hematocrit* is a frequent finding in pheochromocytoma patients. This is usually attributable to diminished plasma volume ("stress polycythemia") with a normal red cell mass. Rarely, however, it reflects true erythrocytosis secondary to the ectopic production of erythropoietin by the tumor [12].

Hypercalcemia is occasionally noted in pheochromocytoma patients due to the production and secretion of parathyroid hormone-related protein (PTHrP).

Rhabdomyolysis and *ischemic colitis* are rare complications of pheochromocytoma secondary to intense vasoconstriction in the skeletal muscle and colon, respectively. *Myoglobinuric renal failure* may accompany rhabdomyolysis if the latter is sufficiently severe [4].

Hypotension or *shock* is infrequent but important manifestations of pheochromocytoma since they may be associated with significant morbidity or death. The pathogenesis was poorly understood until a potent hypotensive peptide, adrenomedullin, was found in these tumors [13, 14]. Secretion of this compound by the pheochromocytoma, coupled with the aforementioned diminished plasma volume, is the likely cause of the hypotensive reactions.

Acute respiratory distress syndrome (ARDS) or "*shock lung*" is a rare but serious complication of pheochromocytoma. In some cases it is the presenting manifestation; in others it develops in the wake of a particularly severe paroxysm. It is frequently associated with hypotension, presumably due to the release of adrenomedullin from the tumor. Damage to the pulmonary capillary endothelium is the likely cause of this noncardiac pulmonary edema [6]. Release of pro-inflammatory cytokines may also contribute (see below).

Acute abdominal catastrophe is another infrequent but well-recognized presentation. It is associated with abdominal pain, frequently shock, but sometimes with high and/or fluctuating blood pressure. The cause is usually hemorrhage into the tumor, sometime with the extravasation of blood into the peritoneal space; the amylase level may be elevated suggesting pancreatitis, with the pulmonary endothelium the likely source of the ↑ in amylase. ARDS may be associated. Abdominal imaging usually suggests the diagnosis with the demonstration of hemorrhage in an adrenal mass [15]. Bowel ischemia is another potential cause of an abdominal catastrophe in pheochromocytoma patients.

Systemic inflammatory *response syndrome (SIRS)* due to the release of interleukin-6 (IL-6) from the tumor has also been well described in patients with pheochromocytoma. This rare manifestation of pheochromocytoma presents with recurrent bouts of fever, chills, headache, and leukocytosis frequently with dyspnea and non-cardiogenic pulmonary edema. The fever here represents a cytokine-induced elevation of the core temperature set point, in distinction to the increased thermogenesis with normal core temperature described above [16–18].

Abnormal blood pressure responses (↑ or ↓) to drugs, anesthesia, or diagnostic manipulations such as needle biopsy (which should not be done unless pheochromocytoma has been excluded). Watery diarrhea with hypokalemia and achlorhydria has also been described [19] likely the result of the ectopic secretion of VIP.

Adverse Impact of Drugs and Diagnostic Tests

A number of drugs and diagnostic interventions are associated with unanticipated swings in BP which may be either up or down. As a consequence serious morbidity and even death has occurred as shown in the illustrative cases presented at the end of this chapter. Offending pharmaceuticals cause adverse effects in at least four different ways (Table 3.5): direct release of catecholamines from the tumor, blockade of neuronal uptake of catecholamines, inhibition of catecholamine metabolism, and release of catecholamines from the augmented stores in the sympathetic nerve endings [2, 4].

Table 3.5 Adverse drug reactions in patients with pheochromocytoma

Release of catecholamine from the tumor
OPIOIDS
Metoclopramide
Glucagon
Histamine
Glucocorticoids
ACTH
Intra-arterial radiographic contrast media
Blockade of neuronal uptake of catecholamines
Tricyclic antidepressants
Cocaine
Inhibition of metabolism of catecholamines
MAO inhibitors
Indirect-acting sympathomimetic amines
Nasal decongestants

Direct Release of Catecholamines from the Tumor

By far the most dangerous are those agents that directly release catecholamines from the tumor itself. First and foremost among this group are *opioids*. A not uncommon scenario often plays out as follows: a patient with an unsuspected pheochromocytoma presents to an emergency room or urgent care center with headache, and high BP is noted resulting in opioid administration; the BP rises, the headache worsens, and more opioid analgesic is administered resulting in further worsening and sometimes death. Since pheochromocytoma may also present with chest or abdominal pain, the same scenario may apply. Clinical features that should suggest the possibility of pheochromocytoma in these cases include a history of spells, tachycardia, wide swings in BP, and diaphoresis. Similarly, preanesthetic medication with fentanyl in a patient undergoing unrelated surgery may induce a severe paroxysm.

Other agents that stimulate release of catecholamines from the tumor include *glucagon, metoclopramide, histamine, glucocorticoids, ACTH, and radiographic contrast media when administered intra-arterially to the tumor* (intravenous contrast media is safe).

Release of Catecholamines from the Augmented Stores in Sympathetic Nerve Endings

In pheochromocytoma patients, the high circulating levels of catecholamines result in increased storage in sympathetic nerve terminals throughout the body. These increased stores are susceptible to release by a variety of *indirect-acting sympathomimetic amines*. Most commonly over-the-counter decongestants such as pseudoephedrine are responsible (see illustrative cases). In addition to stimulating release, many of these compounds block reuptake into the sympathetic nerve endings further potentiating the pressor response [2].

Interference with Inactivation of Catecholamines

Drugs that block the *neuronal uptake process*, the major inactivating process for NE released from sympathetic nerve endings, aggravate the manifestations of pheochromocytoma, particularly hypertension [2]. Antidepressants that block NE reuptake, particularly the *tricyclic antidepressants*, are the major offenders. *Cocaine* is a potent blocker of NE reuptake and also appears to increase central sympathetic outflow; as such it can cause pressor crises that resemble the paroxysms of pheochromocytoma as well as accentuating the symptoms in patients with pheochromocytomas.

Monoamine oxidase inhibitors (MAOI) increase the storage of NE in sympathetic terminals rendering the increased stores more susceptible to release by indirect-acting sympathomimetic amines.

Features that Warrant Screening for Pheochromocytoma in Hypertensive Patients

It is neither feasible nor necessary to screen all hypertensive patients for the presence of a pheochromocytoma; only a small minority of patients with high BP should be screened, but given the gravity of a missed diagnosis, it is important to note those characteristics that suggest the need to screen (Table 3.6).

Characteristics of the blood pressure are important: young age of the patient, recent onset of hypertension, severe or malignant hypertension, great blood pressure variability, orthostatic hypotension in the untreated state, and difficult to control hypertension. Presence of any of the *characteristic features of pheochromocytoma*: headache, sweating, palpitations, tachycardia, and weight loss; spells of any kind; carbohydrate intolerance and recent onset diabetes; unanticipated changes (↑ or ↓) in BP in response to drugs, diagnostic procedures, or unrelated surgeries; Takotsubo cardiomyopathy; high hematocrit; *adrenal mass* on unrelated imaging; and *positive family history* for pheochromocytoma syndromes.

The presence of any of these manifestations should raise the possibility of pheochromocytoma and the consideration of screening. The best way to screen is with a 24-h urine collection for free fractionated catecholamines and/or metanephrines or plasma metanephrines. Imaging should generally be reserved for those patients with positive biochemical evidence of catecholamine overproduction.

Table 3.6 Features in hypertensive patients that warrant screening for pheochromocytoma

Spells of any kind
Weight loss
Recent onset of hypertension
Young age
Severe or malignant hypertension
Tachycardia
Marked BP lability
Carbohydrate intolerance or overt new onset diabetes mellitus
Adrenal mass on imaging
Orthostatic hypotension in untreated state
Family history of pheochromocytoma
Unanticipated prominent changes in BP (up or down) in response to drugs or diagnostic manipulations

Adrenal Incidentalomas

Incidentally discovered adrenal masses larger than 1 cm. in diameter occur in about 3–5% of subjects, as judged from CT and autopsy studies. They are more common in the elderly. Pheochromocytoma accounts for about 5% of these lesions; pheochromocytoma needs to be ruled out in all incidentally discovered adrenal masses despite the absence of symptoms since even asymptomatic pheochromocytomas are potentially dangerous [20, 21]. Needle biopsy of these incidentally discovered lesions should be avoided until pheochromocytoma is excluded (see illustrative case). Twenty-four hour urine collection for catecholamines and metanephrines is the appropriate tests to rule out pheochromocytoma and should be performed despite imaging characteristics that are not suggestive of a chromaffin tumor.

Characteristics of Pheochromocytoma in Familial Syndromes

Although the major clinical features of pheochromocytoma are similar in sporadic and familial cases, some differences in location, E production, the likelihood of extra-adrenal tumors, and the incidence of malignancy in the genetic syndromes are worth pointing out (Table 3.7). It should also be noted that many pheochromocytomas in the familial syndromes are found during the screening of asymptomatic relatives [2].

MEN Syndromes

The most distinctive features of pheochromocytoma in the MEN 1 and 2 syndromes include very high incidence of bilateral adrenal tumors; multicentric tumors within each affected adrenal; predominance of E secretion, especially early in the course; the virtual absence of extra-adrenal pheochromocytomas; and the virtual absence of malignancy. The lesions begin as adrenal medullary hyperplasia

Table 3.7 Syndromic pheochromocytoma

Syndrome	Mutation	Pheochromocytoma	Associated diseases
MEN 2A	RET→↑TK	Bilateral adrenal	MTC; hyperpara
MEN 2B	RET→↑TK	Bilateral adrenal	MTC; mucosal neuromas
VHL	↑HIF→↑VEGF	Bilateral adrenal; extra-adrenal	Hemangioblastomas; renal cell carcinoma
NF1	↑RAS	Bilateral adrenal	Neurofibromas;café au lait spots; skeletal abnormalities
PGL1	SDHD→↑HIF→↑VEGF	Extra-adrenal; bilateral adrenal	
PGL4	SDHB→↑HIF→↑VEGF	Extra-adrenal; bilateral adrenal (↑ malignancy)	

See text for details

and progress to multicentric tumors. Early in the course, increase in urinary excretion of E is the only abnormality, a fact that has important ramifications for screening family members within an affected kindred: measurement of 24-h urinary excretion of E is required [22].

Approximately 50% of MEN patients either have a pheochromocytoma at presentation or will develop a pheochromocytoma later in the course necessitating follow-up screening in these patient at yearly intervals or sooner if signs or symptoms occur. Many MEN kindreds have been discovered by the diagnosis of a pheochromocytoma in the propositus. The pathogenesis involves the constitutive activation of a transmembrane tyrosine kinase by the RET proto-oncogene.

All patients with the MEN syndrome require a total thyroidectomy, but a pheochromocytoma should be excluded or removed before operating on the thyroid. In the case of bilateral pheochromocytomas, both adrenals should be removed in total; because of the adrenal medullary hyperplasia and multicentric tumor formation, sparing the adrenal cortex is not advisable. Doing so commits the patient to close follow-up for life and increases the likelihood of a difficult reoperation.

Von Hippel-Lindau (VHL) Retinal Cerebellar Hemangioblastomatosis

The incidence of pheochromocytomas in the VHL syndrome is highly variable and depends on the particular mutation in the VHL gene: some kindreds do not have pheochromocytomas, while others have a very high incidence of chromaffin tumors. If pheochromocytomas have appeared in any members of a kindred, the risk of developing a pheochromocytoma in an affected family member is high [23]. The pheochromocytomas in the VHL syndrome are often bilateral in the adrenals, and the presence of extra-adrenal tumors is not uncommon. The extra-adrenal lesions are most commonly located in the abdomen and, less frequently, in the thorax. Malignancy has been noted but is uncommon. The molecular pathogenesis involves increased activity of hypoxia inducible factor α (HIFα) which activates vascular endothelial growth factor (VEGF) and other mitogenic compounds.

Pheochromocytoma should be excluded or removed before operating on the other tumors characteristic of this syndrome. In patients with bilateral adrenal tumors, it may be feasible to spare the normal adrenal cortex in an effort to avoid lifelong steroid replacement. There is however a high incidence of recurrence (at least 10–25%) necessitating a more difficult reoperation.

Neurofibromatosis Type 1 (NF1)

NF1 is usually suspected on clinical grounds based on the presence of the usual NF stigmata including multiple café au lait spots, spinal abnormalities, axillary freckling, and neurofibromas. The incidence of pheochromocytoma in NF1 patients is estimated at about 1–3% but is higher if the patients are hypertensive. Bilateral pheochromocytomas are not uncommon, and extra-adrenal pheochromocytomas do occasionally occur. Malignancy occurs in about 10% of these tumors [24]. The pathogenesis involves impaired inactivation of the oncogene RAS.

Paraganglioma (PGL) Syndromes: Succinic Acid Dehydrogenase (SDH) Mutations

The SDH gene plays a role in the Krebs cycle and the mitochondrial electron transport system [2, 25]. Of the four subunits of the SDH gene, two have been principally identified with syndromic paragangliomas. The SDHD mutation gives rise to the PGL 1 syndrome; the SDHB mutation is associated with the PGL 4 syndrome. The molecular pathogenesis involves hypoxia inducible factor α (HIFα); the degradation of HIF is impaired in these syndromes producing a pseudo-hypoxic state with resultant increased production of vascular endothelial growth factor (VEGF) and other mitogens. The genetic mutation is expressed if and when the normal allele undergoes somatic inactivation. Although the inheritance is autosomal dominant, the SDHD (PGL 1) syndrome is virtually always inherited from the male parent.

PGL 1 (SDHD) is associated with bilateral adrenal and extra-adrenal pheochromocytomas (paragangliomas) located in the abdomen, thorax, and the head and neck. The head and neck tumors do not usually secrete catecholamines but may secrete VIP with associated diarrheal syndrome. PGL 4 (SDHB) is also associated with bilateral and extra-adrenal pheochromocytomas, mostly abdominal and thoracic; the incidence of malignancy is higher in the PGL 4 syndrome, particularly in the extra-adrenal lesions.

Pheochromocytoma of the Urinary Bladder

Extra-adrenal Pheochromocytomas (Paragangliomas)

Most extra-adrenal pheochromocytomas are located within the abdomen, principally around the pre-aortic plexuses; about 10% are located in the thorax generally around the sympathetic paravertebral ganglia. Head and neck paragangliomas constitute about 3% of the total extra-adrenal lesions; these rarely secrete catecholamines, are more common in children, and occasionally produce vasoactive intestinal protein (VIP) with a severe diarrheal syndrome. One percent of extra-adrenal pheochromocytomas are located in the urinary bladder. Very rarely pheochromocytomas may be located within a variety of other viscera.

Characteristics of Bladder Pheochromocytomas

Pheochromocytomas located in the urinary bladder are of special interest for two reasons: (1) the association of paroxysms with micturition and (2) the fact that they may, occasionally, be associated with normal catecholamine measurements. About 50% of patients with bladder pheochromocytomas have typical pressor crises during or shortly after urination [26, 27]. The prominent symptoms include headache, palpitations, and sweating in association with high blood pressure. Syncope has also been noted. The likely cause of the paroxysm is the contraction of the bladder detrusor muscle which stimulates catecholamine release. About one-half of these patients have hematuria. A minority of bladder pheochromocytomas will have normal catecholamine measurements at the time of diagnosis. This reflects, presumably, the fact that these tumors may become symptomatic at a time when they are quite small so that the impact on overall catecholamine production is trivial. Bladder pheochromocytomas may be well visualized by standard imaging techniques. Many will be visible at cystoscopy.

Differential Diagnosis

The diseases that may be confused with pheochromocytoma are summarized in Table 3.8. Most can be easily distinguished from pheochromocytoma, but occasionally difficulties present themselves [2].

Hyperthyroidism superficially resembles pheochromocytoma because of tachycardia, sweating, and palpitations. Although the systolic BP may be elevated, the diastolic pressure is usually low, the wide pulse pressure reflecting the increase in cardiac output occasioned by the hypermetabolic state. Some of the hyperadrenergic manifestations of the hyperthyroid state reflect enhanced sensitivity to the normal level of sympathetic tone in these patients. In any event thyroid function tests reveal the hyperthyroid state, and catecholamine levels are normal.

Table 3.8 Differential diagnosis

	NE/NMN	Diagnosis
Hyperthyroidism	Normal	↑T4, ↑T3, ↓TSH
Carcinoid syndrome	Normal	↑5-HIAA urinary
Hyperadrenergic Essential hypertension	Normal	Negative imaging
Pressor crises		
Cocaine	+/− ↑	Drug screen/history
MAOI + tyramine	↑ NMN	History
Clonidine withdrawal	+/− ↑	History
Intracranial catastrophe	↑	Imaging/coma
Factitious	+/− ↑	Psych history

The periodic flushes of the malignant *carcinoid syndrome* may raise the suspicion of pheochromocytoma, but the manifestations are really quite different. Pallor rather than flushing is the usual skin change during pheochromocytoma paroxysms, although occasionally flushing does occur during or after a pressor crisis in patients with a pheochromocytoma. The major difference is the BP which is low in the carcinoid syndrome due to the formation of vasodepressor kinins by kallikrein released from the carcinoid tumor. Diarrhea and hepatomegaly are also characteristic of carcinoid tumors. Catecholamine production is normal, while urinary 5-HIAA, the major metabolite of serotonin, is elevated in patients with the carcinoid syndrome.

Drug-related *pressor crises* may resemble the paroxysms of pheochromocytoma [2]. The responsible agents are *cocaine, clonidine withdrawal*, and *MAO inhibitors with indirect-acting sympathomimetic amines*. Cocaine overdose may cause intense vasoconstriction with hypertension, muscle necrosis, ischemic colitis, and occasionally myocardial infarction. Since cocaine blocks NE uptake into the SNS, there may be a small increase in catecholamine measurements. Drug screen and history secure the proper diagnosis. In patients on MAOI, indirect-acting sympathomimetic amines may cause release of NE from the enhanced stores in the sympathetic nerve endings. The resultant pressor crisis may be life threatening. Tyramine, formed in foodstuffs from the bacterial metabolism of tyrosine, is a common offender; any foods that undergo fermentation may cause the syndrome. Over-the-counter sympathomimetic amines in decongestants are also common causes. NMN is increased in these cases (deamination is blocked). The diagnosis is established from the history. Indirect-acting sympathomimetic amines may accentuate hypertension in pheochromocytoma patients without MAOI as well, because of the increased stores of NE in the sympathetic nerve endings. Abrupt withdrawal from the antihypertensive agent clonidine may cause a pressor crisis; slight elevations in catecholamine measurements are possible. Again the diagnosis is made from the history. In all of these cases, treatment should be with α adrenergic antagonists; β-blockers are to be avoided at least until the α-blockers lower the BP.

Panic attacks are episodic often without identifiable trigger. They are usually characterized by hyperventilation with attendant paresthesias of the fingers, toes, and lips and dizziness sometimes with fainting. The BP may be high or low with tachycardia. It is often possible to reproduce the attacks by voluntary hyperventilation. Frequent sighing is a tip off to the presence of hyperventilation. Catecholamine measurements are normal. The classic patient is a young female, but men and older adults may have panic attacks as well.

An *intracranial catastrophe* such as subarachnoid or cerebral hemorrhage may be associated with increased central SNS activity resulting in high BP and increased catecholamine production. In these patients an obvious calamitous CNS event has occurred.

Factitious pheochromocytoma has also been noticed with the surreptitious addition of NE or E to a 24 h urine collection. This is most common in hospital workers frequently with a psychiatric history.

The most important, and the most challenging, differential diagnosis is *essential hypertension with hyperadrenergic features*. Also called "pseudopheochromocytoma," these patients may have borderline elevations in catecholamine measurements. Tachycardia, flushing, and palpitations, along with excessive sweating, may be noted. Despite the fact that extensive imaging is negative, many of these patients are convinced that they have a small pheochromocytoma that defies diagnosis. These patients have hyperactive SNS activity; they never turn out to have an occult pheochromocytoma.

Neuroblastoma, Ganglioneuroblastoma, and Ganglioneuroma

These childhood tumors, like pheochromocytomas and paragangliomas, arise from neural crest (Fig. 3.1) and produce catecholamines and catecholamine metabolites. Measurement of these compounds is useful in diagnosis. Although these tumors almost always arise in childhood, they rarely present for the first time in adults [28]. The more differentiated ganglioneuroma, in particular, may occur in adults and is associated with clinical features resembling pheochromocytoma.

Neuroblastoma (NB) and ganglioneuroblastoma (GNB) have similar biologic properties and clinical manifestations. Histologically NB is composed of primitive neuroblasts, while GNB is composed, by definition, of at least 50% mature ganglion

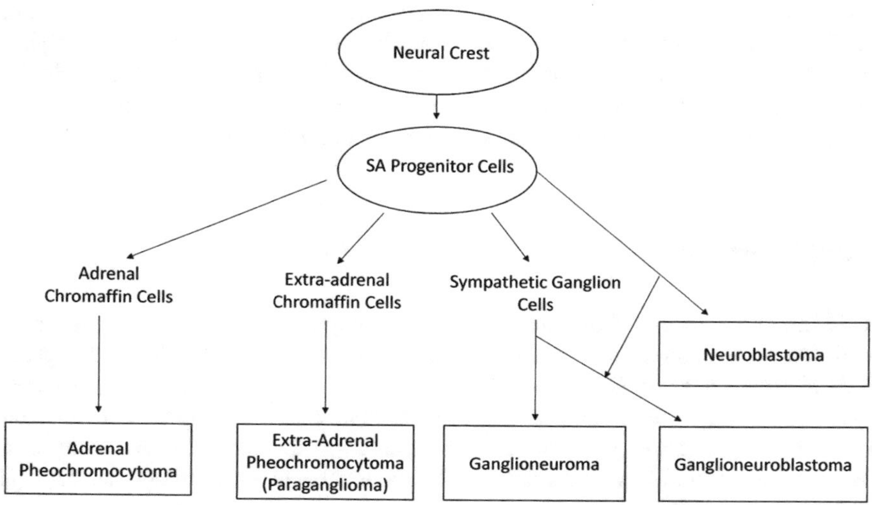

Fig. 3.1 Ontogeny of sympathoadrenal tumors (Used with permission from Landsberg [2])

cells. NB and GNB are derived from neuroblasts in the sympathetic ganglia and the adrenal medulla and usually present as mass lesions in early infancy; NB is the most common solid malignancy in children. About 50% of these lesions appear before the age of one, and these have the best prognosis. These tumors originate in the adrenal medulla in approximately 40% of cases; 25% arise from sympathetic ganglia in the abdomen and 15% in the thorax. The latter are located in the paravertebral SNS ganglia and frequently present as posterior mediastinal masses. In the cervical region, they frequently cause Horner's syndrome. The natural history of these tumors is highly variable. Spontaneous regression occasionally occurs but is poorly understood. Spontaneous maturation to mature ganglioneuromas has also been described. These tumors also have the potential for aggressive malignant spread with metastases to lymph nodes, skin, bone, and liver. A characteristic metastatic site, although not very common, is to the orbit with purplish ecchymosis and proptosis.

Catecholamine Production in NB and GNB

Like the SNS and the adrenal medulla, these tumors possess the amine uptake transport system which means they take up radiolabeled MIBG, thus permitting visualization by scintiscan. They store catecholamines in storage granules as shown in electron photomicrographs. The concentration of catecholamines is sufficient to give a bright image on T2-weighted MRI scans. Curiously, despite the catecholamine content and storage, paroxysms are rare in NB and GNB. This may reflect, at least in part, the fact that metabolism of NE and DA to VMA and HVA within these tumors is common and may take precedence over release. Over 90% of NB and GNB patients excrete increased amounts of VMA and HVA in urine thus establishing measurement of these metabolites as useful tests in confirming the diagnosis [29, 30]. The ectopic production and secretion of VIP have also been noted in association with the watery diarrhea hypokalemia achlorhydria syndrome.

Ganglioneuroma

This tumor, generally considered benign, is composed of mature ganglion cells with some Schwann cells intermixed [31]. Most common in the pediatric age group but older than NB and GNB (average age at presentation about 7 years), GN does occur in adults as well. Location is predominantly in the thoracic paravertebral sympathetic ganglia often presenting as a posterior mediastinal mass; location in or about an adrenal has also been noted. About 50% of these tumors secrete NE and concentrate MIBG; those that do resemble paragangliomas (extra-adrenal pheochromocytomas). Diagnosis and treatment are the same as for extra-adrenal pheochromocytomas. These tumors may also secrete VIP; the resulting severe diarrheal syndrome is often the clue to the diagnosis [29].

Presentation of Pheochromocytoma: Illustrative Cases

Pheochromocytoma Masquerading as Spells or Seizures

A 54-year-old woman was referred for evaluation of "spells." She was in good health until about 4 years ago when she noted peculiar sensations with lightheadedness, tremulousness, and feeling like she might faint. She said "it felt like something was taking over my whole body." These episodes occurred about once a month and lasted about 15–20 min. She was evaluated many times but defied diagnosis. Blood pressure was in the range of 140/90 mm/Hg. She was eventually diagnosed with epilepsy, although the EEG was normal and the spells were not improved with Dilantin.

Over the ensuing years, these spells increased in frequency and severity and were occurring almost weekly. She was admitted to the hospital for further evaluation. On the first hospital day, she obliged with a typical spell. Blood pressure was taken and found to be 210/140 with a pulse rate of 118. The markedly elevated BP and tachycardia suggested the proper diagnosis, and a 24-h urine for catecholamines showed markedly elevated levels. She was started on phenoxybenzamine with complete resolution of her symptoms. A left-sided pheochromocytoma was confirmed by imaging and removed uneventfully. She remains symptom free with normal catecholamine excretion.

Illustrative point *The opportunity to observe a spell and record the BP will frequently suggest the diagnosis of pheochromocytoma.*

Pheochromocytoma Presenting as Malignant Hypertension

A 38-year-old man, a carpenter in rural Maine, presented to his local hospital with headache, sweating, and palpitations. His BP was 260/170. He had lost significant weight over the preceding 6 months. On presentation he was very thin, tremulous, and diaphoretic. He had flame hemorrhages on funduscopic exam and was diagnosed with malignant hypertension. His BP failed to respond to diuretics, vasodilators, and β-blockers. One of his attending physicians considered the possibility of pheochromocytoma and managed to obtain some phenoxybenzamine which produced marked improvement in BP and sense of well-being. He was transferred to a tertiary care facility in Boston where phenoxybenzamine was continued with good BP control. He was also noted to have hard nodules in both lobes of his thyroid gland. Subsequent work-up revealed markedly elevated urinary catecholamines and very high plasma calcitonin. Imaging revealed large, bilateral, heterogeneous, adrenal masses thus securing the diagnosis of MEN 2 (Sipple's syndrome). After 2 weeks of preparation with phenoxybenzamine and, additionally, propranolol, bilateral adrenalectomies were performed; the cut surface of the adrenals showed multicentric lesions with extensive areas of hemorrhage and necrosis. After recovery from the adrenal surgery, he underwent total thyroidectomy which showed bilateral medullary carcinoma with amyloid production.

Subsequent family screening revealed a small unilateral E secreting adrenal tumor and medullary carcinoma in his 9-year-old son who was treated and apparently cured but requires long-term follow-up.

Illustrative points *(1) Malignant hypertension requires work-up for pheochromocytoma; (2) bilateral pheochromocytomas are always familial and necessitate appropriate genetic family screening.*

Pheochromocytoma Presenting as Essential Hypertension

A 47-year-old man was referred for evaluation and treatment of poorly controlled hypertension. He had been in good health except for obesity (BMI 31) and diet-controlled glucose intolerance. His blood pressure ranged between 160–170 systolic and 95–105 diastolic. There were no spells, headaches, or palpitations, but he had lost 20 pounds over the preceding 6 months. He brought with him an aortogram obtained as part of his work-up for hypertension; it revealed normal renal arteries without adrenal masses. Work-up for pheochromocytoma was undertaken because of poor response to treatment. It was a surprise when the results of a 24 h urine collection showed increased total catecholamines (550 μg, 75% NE). Subsequent imaging showed a 5 cm adrenal tumor. Further analysis revealed that the aortogram failed to show the tumor because it was shot below the superior adrenal artery (a branch of the inferior phrenic artery) which provided the blood supply to the tumor.

His BP responded to phenoxybenzamine, and his carbohydrate intolerance improved. Surgical removal was uneventful, and his blood pressure, although still elevated off treatment (150/90), was now responsive to conventional antihypertensive agents.

Illustrative points *(1) BP poorly responsive to conventional treatment warrants work-up for secondary causes including pheochromocytoma; (2) the old saw "forget a fat pheochromocytoma" may not cut much wood, but recent weight loss is characteristic.*

Adrenal Incidentaloma, Metastatic Tumor, or Pheochromocytoma?

A 45-year-old woman with history of mild hypertension underwent a mastectomy for breast cancer [32]. During the surgery her BP was note to vary between 140/80 and 160/100. After the surgery, as part of staging the malignancy, she underwent an abdominal CT which demonstrated a 4.8 by 3.7 nonhomogeneous mass above the right kidney, suggestive of a metastatic lesion. In an attempt to establish the diagnosis, a fine needle aspiration biopsy was attempted. As the needle passed into the tumor, the patient complained of pounding occipital headache and palpitations; BP rose from 120/80 to 185/90 with a significant increase in pulse rate. She then received fentanyl, and the blood pressure remained elevated for several hours. No further attempts at biopsy were undertaken. The diagnosis of pheochromocytoma was suggested by the procedure-related increase in BP and confirmed by elevated urinary catecholamines and metanephrines along with the characteristic bright appearance of the right adrenal mass on T2-weighted MRI scan.

Preoperative preparation with phenoxybenzamine and surgical resection were performed without difficulty, and she remains asymptomatic with normal follow-up of urinary catecholamines.

Illustrative points *(1) At least 5% of incidentally discovered adrenal masses turn out to be pheochromocytomas, so these should never be biopsied or manipulated before pheochromocytoma is ruled out by a 24-h collection for catecholamines and metanephrines. This is true even if the imaging characteristics are not suggestive of pheochromocytoma. (2) Fentanyl was a poor choice after symptoms began and probably explains why the BP stayed elevated for hours, emphasizing that the adverse effects of opioids in pheochromocytoma patients are insufficiently appreciated.*

Noncardiac Pulmonary Edema and Abdominal Catastrophe

A 51-year-old woman with a lifelong history of neurofibromatosis (NF1) and high blood pressure for 1 year was admitted to hospital after she presented to the emergency room with sinus congestion, nausea and vomiting, and malaise. On examination she was noted to have significant orthostatic hypotension and was admitted for further evaluation. Of note she had been admitted to hospital during the preceding month for surgical resection of neurofibromas and a schwannoma. Postoperative blood pressures were recorded at 210/92 and pulse rate of 118 [32].

She was aggressively hydrated and given sympathomimetic amines orally and intranasally in the ER and admitted. Her blood pressure remained low, although occasionally hypertensive spikes were noted. Over the next day, she became progressively dyspneic, tachypneic, and hypoxic followed by atrial fibrillation requiring cardioversion. Obtundation developed and she was intubated and placed on mechanical ventilation. Chest x-ray which had been normal in the ER now showed bilateral pulmonary consolidation with normal wedge pressure. Her deterioration continued with tachycardia to the 150 range, and occasional BP spikes as high as 210/130. Abdominal pain, spiking fever, persistent diarrhea with negative stool cultures, rising levels of transaminases, and an elevated serum amylase suggested pancreatitis or an abdominal abscess; these findings led to an abdominal CT scan which showed a 7.2 cm heterogeneous mass above the left kidney, thus clarifying the diagnosis which was confirmed with markedly elevated urinary catecholamine and catecholamine metabolite excretion. She responded well to 2 weeks of adrenergic blockade and volume expansion. Following successful surgical resection, she was discharged normotensive off all antihypertensive drugs.

Illustrative points *(1) Although only 2 or 3% of NF1 patients develop pheochromocytomas, the incidence is higher in those with hypertension; this fact, along with the elevated BPs following the preceding unrelated surgeries, were important unrecognized clues to the diagnosis. (2) The sympathomimetic amines administered as decongestants probably worsened her symptoms by releasing catecholamines from the increased NE stores in the peripheral sympathetic nerves. (3) The hypotension and pulmonary edema, although uncommon manifestations of pheochromocytoma, are well described; adrenomedullin, a hypotensive peptide released from some pheochromocytomas, is the likely explanation for the hypotension. (4) Release of interleukin-6 from the tumor is the cause of the fever and the systemic inflammatory response involving multiple organs and damaging the pulmonary endothelium. (5) The diarrhea may have reflected the ectopic production and release of vasoactive intestinal peptide (VIP) from the tumor. (6) The trick is to think of the diagnosis; confirmation is usually easy. (7) CT scan may be helpful in establishing the diagnosis. (8) The astonishing effect of appropriate treatment (although delayed in this case) is well demonstrated.*

Cushing's Syndrome and Pheochromocytoma

A 47-year-old woman with a 1 year history of resistant hypertension was admitted to hospital for evaluation. Her blood pressure was not controlled on a regimen of four agents. In addition she complained of episodic sweating, flushing, palpitations, puffiness of the face, and hirsutism. On exam BP was 220/120 and pulse 95 [33]. Noted as well were facial plethora, supraclavicular fat pads, and increased hair above the upper lip. Laboratory exam revealed a hypokalemic alkalosis and a glucose of 284 mg/dL. The diagnosis of Cushing's syndrome secondary to ectopic ACTH secretion was established by markedly increased urinary and plasma cortisol, failure to suppress on high-dose dexamethasone, and elevated ACTH levels. Interestingly, marked variation in the levels of ACTH and cortisol was noted from day to day. The diagnosis of pheochromocytoma was established by a fivefold elevation in the excretion of catecholamine metabolites. After treatment with phenoxybenzamine, the BP fell and catheterization of the adrenal veins revealed a substantial step-up of ACTH and NE on the left as well as a vascular mass in the left adrenal.

At surgery the left adrenal was removed, and pathology revealed a 3 cm pheochromocytoma with hyperplastic adrenal cortex adjacent to the medullary tumor. After surgical removal of the tumor, the ACTH levels became undetectable; catecholamine excretion returned to normal as did the BP and the plasma glucose.

Illustrative point *Pheochromocytomas may produce biologically active compounds in addition to catecholamines, and these may influence the clinical manifestations and confuse the diagnosis.*

Adverse Effects of Mistreatment and Importance of Family Screening

A 56-year-old Russian immigrant came to the ER with a severe and unrelenting headache not responsive to over-the-counter analgesics [32]. She described a 10-year history of throbbing bifrontal headaches, accompanied by pallor and visual distortions; these occurred up to three times per week and lasted about 10 min. Over the next several years, the headaches increased in severity and duration. After emigrating to the USA, the headaches worsened and were accompanied by sweating and palpitations. Two months prior to her presentation, the headaches were occurring daily, and she sought medical attention; hypertension was noted and a diuretic was prescribed. Heat intolerance worsened, and 1 week before her presentation to the ER, pseudoephedrine was prescribed for a “sinus headache.”

In the ER her BP was 210/100; hct was noted to be 45. She was given Demerol for the headache and sent home, only to return 2 h later with a much worse headache. BP was now 220/110. Demerol was repeated, and the symptoms worsened with headache, sweating, and palpitations. BP was measured at 240/140 and hct was 60! She failed to respond to morphine and nitro-vasodilators and was admitted to the ICU. In the morning light of the next day, pheochromocytoma was considered, a 24-h urine demonstrated greater than a tenfold increase in catecholamines and metanephrines, and abdominal CT scan showed bilateral adrenal masses. She responded well to adrenergic blockade and underwent surgical removal of both tumors (3.0 and 6.5 cm in diameter).

Serum calcitonin was markedly elevated, and after recovery from the adrenal surgery, on steroid replacement, total thyroidectomy was performed, and bilateral medullary carcinoma was removed. Calcium levels and PTH were normal, but after two decades nephrolithiasis developed, and hyperparathyroidism was diagnosed. She is currently awaiting surgery.

Family history revealed that her mother (deceased) and 25-year-old son suffered similar symptoms. Her son was subsequently discovered to have bilateral pheochromocytomas and MCT and underwent surgical excision of adrenals followed by total thyroidectomy.

Illustrative points *(1) Adverse effects of pseudoephedrine and particularly opiates, (2) ↑ hct secondary to hemoconcentration (“stress polycythemia”), and (3) importance of family history and necessity of lifelong screening for the syndrome components.*

High Stakes of a Missed Diagnosis: Unhappy Ending

A 42-year-old woman presented to an urgent care center with a complaint of headache. She had been without significant health problems. Her headache was occipital in location and throbbing in character. It had bothered her on and off for the last few days. On exam she appeared nervous and upset. BP was 160/105, pulse 100, with the remainder of the physical exam normal. She was given a prescription for hydrochlorothiazide and an appointment to return to clinic the next day for a complete evaluation.

She could not wait. That night she returned to the emergency ward complaining of worsening headache and chest pain. BP was 180/115. EKG was normal. She was given morphine im. Fifteen minutes later she had a seizure. BP was 210/130. She then suffered a cardiac arrest and could not be resuscitated. Postmortem exam revealed a 3.5 cm right adrenal pheochromocytoma; the cut surface revealed fresh hemorrhage and necrosis.

Illustrative points *(1) Even in retrospect it is not clear what should have been done differently; pheochromocytoma is rare and her symptoms were common. A more complete history and exam might have been revealing. (2) The adverse effects of opiates on the release of catecholamines from a pheochromocytoma were starkly demonstrated.*

References

1. Sutton MG, Sheps SG, Lie JT. Prevalence of clinically unsuspected pheochromocytoma review of a 50-year autopsy series. Mayo Clin Proc. 1981;56:354–60.
2. Landsberg L. Catecholamines. Philadelphia: Wolters-Kluwer; 2017.
3. Januszewicz W, Wocial B, Januszewicz A, et al. Dopamine and Dopa urinary excretion in patients with Pheochromocytoma – diagnostic implications. Blood Press. 2001;10:212–6.
4. Landsberg L, Young JB. Catecholamines and the adrenal medulla. In: Foster DW, Wilson JD, editors. Williams textbook of endocrinology. 7th ed. Philadelphia: W.B. Saunders; 1985. p. 891–965.
5. Landsberg L, Young JB. Pheochromocytoma. In: Harrison's principles of internal medicine. 16th ed. New York: McGraw-Hill; 2004.
6. Park M, Hyrniewicz K, Setaro JF. Pheochromocytoma presenting with myocardial infarction, cardiomyopathy, renal failure, pulmonary hemorrhage, and cyclic hypotension: case report and review of unusual presentations of pheochromocytoma. J Clin Hypertension. 2009;11:74–80.
7. Kim S, Yu A, Filippone LA, et al. Inverted-Takotsubo pattern cardiomyopathy secondary to Pheochromocytoma: a clinical case and literature review. Clin Card. 2010;33(4):200–1.
8. Zieleń P, Klisiewicz A, Januszewicz A, et al. Pheochromocytoma-related 'classic' takotsubo cardiomyopathy. J Hum Hypertens. 2010;24:363–6. https://doi.org/10.1038/jhh.2009.115; published online 4 February 2010
9. Sanchez-Recalde A, Costero O, Oliver JM, et al. Pheochromocytoma-related cardiomyopathy: inverted Takotsubo contractile pattern. Circulation. 2006;113:e738–9.
10. Chiang Y, Chen P, Lee C, Chua S. Adrenal pheochromocytoma presenting with Takotsubo-pattern cardiomyopathy and acute heart failure. A case report and literature review. Medicine. 2016;95(36):e4846.

11. Hedley JS, Law S, Phookan S, et al. Pheochromocytoma masquerading as "diabetic ketoacidosis". J Investig Med High Impact Case Rep. 2016;4(2)
12. Waldman TA, Bradley JE. Polycythemia secondary to a Pheochromocytoma with production of an erythropoiesis stimulating factor by the tumor. Proc Soc Exp Biol Med. 1961;108:425–7.
13. Kitamura K, Kangawa K, Kawamoto M, et al. Adrenomedullin: a novel hypotensive peptide isolated from human pheochromocytoma. Biochem Biophys Res Commun. 1993;192:553–60.
14. Shimosawa T, Shibagaki Y, Ishibashi K, et al. Adrenomedullin, and endogenous peptide, counteracts cardiovascular damage. Circulation. 2002;105:106–11.
15. Manger WM. The protean manifestations of Pheochromocytoma. Horm Metab Res. 2009;41:658–63.
16. Carey M, Galindo RJ, Yuan Z, et al. Interleukin-6 producing Pheochromocytoma presenting as sepsis. Endocr Rev. MON-48. 2013.
17. Ciacciarelli M, Bellini D, Laghi A, et al. IL-6-producing, noncatecholamines secreting pheochromocytoma presenting as fever of unknown origin. Case Rep Med. 2016;2016:3489046.
18. Fukumoto S, Matsumoto T, Harada SI, et al. Pheochromocytoma with pyrexia and marked inflammatory signs: a paraneoplastic syndrome with possible relation to Interleukin-6 production. J Clin Endocrinol Metab. 1991;73:877–81.
19. Ikuta S, Yasui C, Kawanaka M, et al. Watery diarrhea, hypokalemia and achlorhydria syndrome due to an adrenal pheochromocytoma. World J Gastroenterol. 2007;13:4649–52.
20. Nieman LK. Approach to the patient with an adrenal incidentaloma. J Clin Endocrinol Metab. 2010;95:4106–13.
21. Young WF Jr. The incidentally discovered adrenal mass. NEJM. 2007;356:601–10.
22. Hamilton BP, Landsberg L, Levine RJ. Measurement of urinary epinephrine in screening for pheochromocytoma in multiple endocrine neoplasia type II. Am J Med. 1978;65:1027–32.
23. Benn DE, Gimenez-Roqueplo AP, Reilly JR, et al. Clinical presentation and penetrance of pheochromocytoma/paraganglioma syndromes. J Clin Endocrinol Metab. 2006;91:827–36.
24. Gruber LM, et al. Pheochromocytoma and paraganglioma in patients with neurofibromatosis type 1. Clin Endocrinol. 2017;86:141.
25. Gill AJ, Benn DE, Chou A, et al. Immunohistochemistry for SDHB triages genetic testing of SDHB, SDHC, and SDHD in paraganglioma-pheochromocytoma syndromes. Hum Pathol. 2010;41:805–14.
26. Beilan JA, Lawton A, Hajdenberg J, Rosser CJ. Pheochromocytoma of the urinary bladder: a systematic review of the contemporary literature. UK: BioMed Central Ltd; 2013.
27. Rosenberg LM. Pheochromocytoma of the urinary bladder. Report of a Case. NEJM. 1957;257:1212–5.
28. Kaye JA, Wahol MJ, Kretschmar C, et al. Neuroblastoma in adults three case reports and a review of the literature. Cancer. 1986;58:1149–57.
29. Monsaingeon M, Perel Y, Simonnet G, Corcuff JB. Comparative values of catecholamines and metabolites for the diagnosis of neuroblastoma. Eur J Pediatr. 2003;162:397–402.
30. Laug WE, Siegel SE, Shaw KNF, et al. Initial urinary catecholamine metabolite concentrations and prognosis in neuroblastoma. Pediatrics. 1978;62:77–83.
31. Geoerger B, Hero B, Harms D, et al. Metabolic activity and clinical features of primary ganglioneuromas. Cancer. 2001;91:1905–13.
32. Gillam MP, Landsberg L. Pheochromocytoma. In: Molitch ME, editor. Contemporary endocrinology: challenging cases in endocrinology, vol. 9. Totowa: Humana Press, Inc; 2002. p. 155–83.
33. Spark RF, Connolly PB, Gluckin DS, et al. ACTH secretion form a functioning Pheochromocytoma. NEJM. 1979;301:416–8.

Chapter 4
Heritable and Syndromic Pheochromocytoma and Paraganglioma

Peter Kopp

Introduction

Pheochromocytomas (PCC) and paragangliomas (PGL) are rare neuroendocrine neoplasias that originate either in the adrenal medulla or paravertebral extra-adrenal ganglia. The majority are benign, but they can lead to significant morbidity and mortality secondary to excessive catecholamine secretion [1]. PGL are subdivided into sympathetic and parasympathetic tumors. Sympathetic chromaffin-positive PGL, which can be located in any of the ganglia in the thorax, abdomen, and pelvis, typically secrete catecholamines [2]. In contrast, most parasympathetic chromaffin-negative PGL, which are mostly found in the head and neck, are usually nonsecretory [3]. Roughly 25% of PCC/PGL have a malignant behavior and metastasize to other tissues [4]. The treatment options for metastatic PCC/PGL are scarce, and the prognosis is typically poor [5]. PCC/PGL can occur sporadically or as part of hereditary tumor syndromes [1, 6]. Remarkably, about 30% of patients with apparently sporadic PCC/PGL harbor a germline mutation in one of the predisposing susceptibility genes (Table 4.1) [7–10]. In case of a positive family history for PCC/PGL, up to 79% are positive for a germline mutation in one of these genes [8, 11].

The clinical features, diagnosis, and therapeutic management of PCC/PGL are discussed elsewhere in this book and have been outlined in detailed guidelines [12]. This chapter is focused on the discussion of the genetics of hereditary PCC/PGL and recent insights into the somatic genetic mechanisms underlying the development of these tumors.

P. Kopp (✉)
Division of Endocrinology, Metabolism and Molecular Medicine and Center for Genetic Medicine, Feinberg School of Medicine, Northwestern University, Chicago, IL, USA
e-mail: p-kopp@northwestern.edu

L. Landsberg (ed.), *Pheochromocytomas, Paragangliomas and Disorders of the Sympathoadrenal System*, Contemporary Endocrinology,
https://doi.org/10.1007/978-3-319-77048-2_4

Table 4.1 Syndromes and genes associated with hereditary PCC/PGL

Gene	Syndrome	Protein	OMIM#	Inheritance	Malignancy rate	Catecholamine secretion	Comment
VHL	Von Hippel- Lindau syndrome	VHL protein two isoforms	608537	AD	~5%	NE	Classic example of Knudson two-hit concept. multiple manifestations
RET	Multiple endocrine neoplasia type 2	RET tyrosine kinase receptor	171400	AD Gain-of-function	<5%	E	MTC, PCC, HPTH
NF1	Neurofibromatosis type 1	GTPase	162200	AD De novo mutations	~12	E	Classic example of Knudson two-hit concept
SDHD	Paraganglioma syndrome 1	SDH subunit D	602690	AD Usually paternal inheritance	<5%	NE	Gist, RCC
SDHAF2	Paraganglioma syndrome 2	SDH complex assembly factor 2	601650	AD Paternal inheritance	Low	NE (?)	
SDHC	Paraganglioma syndrome 3	SDH subunit C	602413	AD	Low	NE/NE + D/NS	GIST
SDHB	Paraganglioma syndrome 4	SDH subunit B	185470	AD	31–71%	NE/NE + D/NS	Gist, RCC
SDHA	Paraganglioma syndrome 5	SDH subunit A	600857	AD Monoallelic	Low	NE/NE + D/NS	Gist, RCC, pa Biallelic mutations > Leigh syndrome: AR juvenile encephalopathy
TMEM127		Transmembrane protein	613403	AD	Low	E	

MAX		Basic helix loop helix leucine zipper protein	154950	AD Preferential paternal transmission	?	Intermediate: NE + E	Rare
FH		Fumarate hydratase		AD		NE	Rare RCC, leiomyomatosis
MDH2		Malate dehydrogenase type 2		AD		NE	Rare
EPAS1/HIF2A		Endothelial PAS domain protein 1	603349	AD Gain-of-function		NE	Rare Somatic mosaicism possible
EGLN1(PHD2)		*C. Elegans* homolog 1/prolyl hydroxylase					Rare
MERTK		MER tyrosine kinase proto-oncogene					Rare
MET		MET proto-oncogene					Rare
H3F3A		H3 histone, family 3a					Rare Somatic mosaicism possible

SDH succinate dehydrogenase, *AD* autosomal dominant, *AR* autosomal recessive, *E* adrenergic, *NE* noradrenergic, *D* dopamine, *NS* nonsecreting, *MTC* medullary thyroid cancer, *HPTH* hyperparathyroidism, *RCC* renal cell carcinoma, *GIST* gastrointestinal tumor, *PA* pituitary adenoma

Inheritance

Von Hippel-Lindau disease (VHL) and neurofibromatosis type 1 (NF1) are classic examples of the Knudson two-hit model inactivating both alleles of a tumor suppressor gene [13]. In this instance, a germline mutation is inherited in an autosomal dominant fashion inactivating one allele of the involved tumor suppressor gene. If the second allele acquires a somatic mutation (or undergoes silencing through an epigenetic mechanism) in an affected cell, this "second hit" or "loss of heterozygosity" results in inactivation of the other allele and subsequent neoplastic growth. Thus, although the predisposing germline defect is transmitted in a dominant mode, tumorigenesis results from a biallelic loss of the tumor suppressor gene in the affected tissue. The later occurrence of the second somatic hit in one or several cells or tissues explains the variability in the time of manifestation and the spectrum of disease manifestations in the syndromic forms.

In contrast to mutations in VHL and NF1, the autosomal dominant inheritance of multiple endocrine neoplasia type 2 (MEN2) is explained by the constitutive activation of one allele of the RET tyrosine kinase receptor. Mutations in the *SDHD*, *SDHAF2*, *SDHC*, and *SDHB* genes are also associated with an autosomal dominant inheritance pattern following the two-hit concept, but in the case of *SDHD* and *SDHAF2* mutations, it is usually limited to paternal inheritance due to silencing of the maternal allele (Table 4.1). For SDHA, monoallelic mutations have been associated with PGL, whereas biallelic mutations lead to Leigh syndrome (autosomal recessive juvenile encephalopathy).

In addition to classic germline transmission, PCC/PGL can also occur in patients in whom a postzygotic mutation leads to somatic mosaicism as, for example, in the case of EPAS1/HIF2A mutations [14]. Similarly, mosaic mutations leading to a syndrome involving PCC/PGL and giant-cell bone tumors of the bone were reported in association with the *H3F3A* gene [15]. Whether mosaicism occurs in PCC/PGL in other susceptibility genes has not been systematically examined. Of note, however, *VHL* and *NF1* mutations have been detected as mosaic mutations in patients affected by VHL and NF1 [16–19]. Taken together, mosaicism and somatic transmission might occur more frequently in PCC/PGL [14].

Von Hippel-Lindau Disease

Von Hippel-Lindau (VHL) disease is an autosomal dominant syndrome characterized by the presence of a broad spectrum of tumors [20]. Characteristic manifestations include hemangioblastomas, renal cysts and clear cell renal carcinoma (RCC), pancreatic cysts, neuroendocrine tumors of the pancreas, endolymphatic sac tumors, meningiomas, and epididymal cystadenomas [21]. The incidence of VHL has been estimated at about 1:36,000 [22]. PCC occur in 10–20% of VHL patients; they are usually located in the adrenal glands and frequently bilateral [23–25].

Extra-adrenal and neck PGL are uncommon [24, 25]. The malignancy rate is approximately 5% [21].

The *VHL* tumor suppressor gene is located on chromosome 3p25–26 and consists of three exons [26]. It encodes two VHL proteins consisting of 213 or 160 amino acids. These proteins are involved in regulating the transcription of hypoxia-inducible genes [27, 28]. The predominant function of the VHL protein consists in its E3 ubiquitin ligase activity that marks protein for degradation. Hypoxia-inducible factor 1α (HIF1α), a transcription factor that regulates the expression of several factors involved in angiogenesis [29], is its best characterized target. Under conditions with normal oxygen levels, VHL binds to HIF1α through two hydroxylated prolines and then ubiquinates its target, which leads to HIF1α degradation in the proteasome. Under conditions of hypoxia, the proline residues on HIF1α are no longer hydroxylated, which disrupts the binding of VHL. Alternatively, the interaction between VHL and HIF1α can be disrupted by mutations in the *VHL* gene, which subsequently alters the expression of genes regulated by HIF1α through its binding to hypoxia response elements (HRE) [27]. More than 1000 mutations have been described in the *VHL* gene [30]. Among mutations in the *VHL* gene, there is a clear genotype-phenotype correlation in terms of the risk for developing a PCC [30, 31]. Type 1 mutations consist of truncations, which are associated with a high risk for RCC but a low risk of PCC; type 2 mutations consist of missense mutations, which can be associated with either an increased risk for RCC or PCC depending on their location [30]. Mutations that disrupt the VHL-HIF1α interaction are associated with an increased risk for RCC, whereas mutations in other regions of the VHL protein increase the risk for PCC [26, 32, 33]. This suggests that the development of PCC occurs independently of primary HIF1α regulation.

Clinical Vignette

Figure 4.1 shows a characteristic pedigree of family affected by von Hippel-Lindau disease (VHL). The transmission is autosomal dominant. The index patient was diagnosed with bilateral pheochromocytomas at the age of 12 years. At age 35, she presented with cardiac decompensation due to Takotsubo cardiomyopathy. The biochemical work-up showed a 24-h norepinephrine level of 4142 mcg/24 h (<80), an epinephrine level of 104 mcg/24 h (<20), and a dopamine level of 1016 mcg/24 h (<500). Imaging studies revealed a 6.4 cm retrocaval heterogeneous mass of 6.5 cm. She was treated with doxazosin. Against medical advice, she conceived her fifth child. Pregnancy and Cesarean section was completed successfully under close blood pressure control. The patient was then lost to follow-up. The patient illustrates the risk for bilateral PCC, an increased risk for aggressive behavior, and a predominant noradrenergic secretory phenotype associated with VHL mutations.

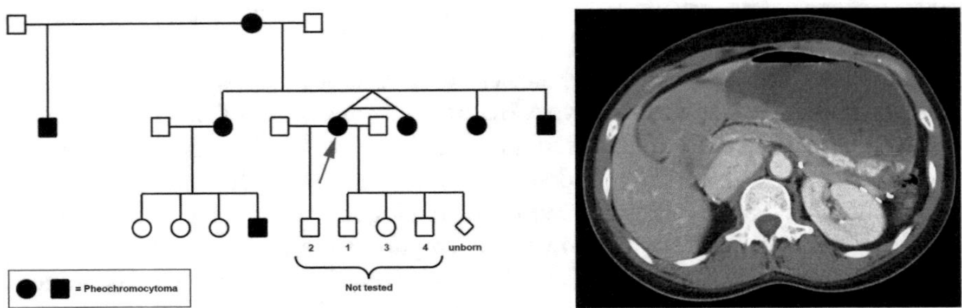

Fig. 4.1 Pedigree of a family with von Hippel-Lindau disease with exclusive pheochromocytomas. (**Left panel**) The pedigree is consistent with autosomal dominant transmission. The patient (arrow) underwent bilateral adrenalectomy for PCC at the age of 12 years. (**Right panel**) At the age of 35, the index patient presented with cardiac decompensation to Takotsubo cardiomyopathy. The biochemical work-up showed a predominant noradrenergic phenotype, CT imaging demonstrates an enhancing mass measuring cm consistent with recurrent pheochromocytoma, the left adrenal gland is surgically absent. The patient illustrates the risk for bilateral PCC, an increased risk for aggressive behavior, and a predominant noradrenergic secretory phenotype associated with VHL mutations.

Neurofibromatosis Type 1

Neurofibromatosis type 1 (NF1) or Recklinghausen's disease is characterized by a wide and variable spectrum of manifestations that includes, among others, neurofibromas, café-au-lait spots with a regular border, freckling, hamartomas of the iris (Lisch nodules), optic nerve gliomas, macrocephaly and bone malformations, and peripheral nerve sheath tumors [34]. NF1 is caused by mutations in the *NF1* tumor suppressor gene located on chromosome 17q12. It includes 60 exons and encodes neurofibromin, a large 2818 amino acid protein that functions as a GTPase-inactivating RAS and thus the MAPK signaling pathway [35].

Mutations in NF1 lead to a loss of function and subsequent constitutive activation of RAS and the MAPK, PI3K, and mTOR pathways [36]. While NF1 can be inherited in an autosomal dominant way, about 50% of patients have de novo germline mutations. Penetrance (manifestation of the phenotype in individuals with a mutant genotype) and expressivity (severity of the phenotype in individuals expressing the phenotype) vary even among patients with the same mutation [34, 35]. Because of the incomplete penetrance, individuals who carry the mutation but have no evidence of the disease can still transmit the disorder to subsequent generations [13].

The diagnosis of NF1 is based on clinical manifestations [34]. Screening for PCC is only recommended for patients with hypertension [37]. PCC occur in about 5–7% of patients with NF1 and are usually unilateral; the malignancy rate is roughly 12% [38]. Genetic testing and mutational analysis are performed only rarely because the diagnosis can be made on clinical grounds and the fact that the analysis of the NF1 gene is labor-intensive, at least with traditional sequencing methods.

Multiple Endocrine Neoplasia Type 2

Multiple endocrine neoplasia type 2 (MEN2) is an autosomal tumor syndrome caused by missense mutations in the *RET* proto-oncogene located on chromosome 10q11.2 [39]. It encodes the RET tyrosine kinase receptor, which is involved in regulating cell proliferation and apoptosis through the PI3 kinase pathway. The missense mutations result in a gain-of-function, and therefore a mutation in a single allele is sufficient to cause aberrant signaling and autosomal dominant transmission of the disease.

MEN2 is divided into several subtypes based on the phenotypic manifestations [39, 40]. MEN2A consists of medullary thyroid cancer (MTC), PCC, and hyperparathyroidism (HPTH). If the phenotype is limited to MTC, it is also designated as familial medullary thyroid cancer (FMTC). In MEN2B, patients present with MTC, PCC, ganglioneuromas, and a marfanoid habitus. Of note, while the penetrance of MTC is complete, this is not the case for the other manifestations such as PCC and hyperparathyroidism.

There is a strong genotype-phenotype correlation, and *RET* gene mutations are classified into three risk categories (moderate, high, highest) for the development of MTC (Table 4.2) [40]. In addition, the incidence of PCC and HPTH, as well as less common manifestations such as cutaneous lichen amyloidosis and Hirschsprung disease, is variable depending on the specific mutation (Table 4.2) [40, 41].

Table 4.2 Common RET mutations and risk of MTC, PCC, and HPTH

RET mutation	MTC risk	Incidence of PCC	Incidence of HPTH	CLA	HD
G533C	Moderate	+	–	No	No
C609F/G/R/S/Y	Moderate	+/++	+	No	Yes
C611F/G/S/W	Moderate	+/++	+	No	Yes
C618F/R/S	Moderate	+/++	+	No	Yes
C620F/R/S	Moderate	+/++	+	No	Yes
C630Y	Moderate	+/++	+	No	Yes
D631Y	Moderate	+++	–	No	No
C634F/G/R/S/W/Y	High	+++	++	Yes	No
K666E	Moderate	+	–	No	No
E768D	Moderate	–	–	No	No
L790F	Moderate	+	–	No	No
V804L	Moderate	+	+	No	No
V804M	Moderate	+	+	Yes	No
A883F	High	+++	–	No	No
S891A	Moderate	+	+	No	No
R912P	Moderate	–	–	No	No
M918T	Highest	+++	–	No	No

Modified from 2015 Revised American Thyroid Association guidelines for the management of medullary thyroid carcinoma [40] with permission.

MTC medullary thyroid cancer, *PCC* pheochromocytoma, *HPTH* hyperparathyroidism, *CLA* lichen amyloidosis, *HD* Hirschsprung disease, + corresponds to risk of ~10%, ++ ~20–30%, +++ ~50%

Certain mutations are associated with a PCC risk of ~50%; others have a lower or no risk for the development of PCC (Table 4.2). PCC are frequently bilateral [42] but rarely malignant (<5%) [43]. The implementation of genetic testing had a significant impact for the management of families affected by MEN2 and allows early identification of carriers and subsequent testing for MTC, PCC, and HPTH according to the risk levels of individual mutations [40].

Clinical Vignette

Figure 4.2 illustrates a FMTC/MEN2A pedigree. The transmission is autosomal dominant, but in contrast to VHL or NF1, this is due to a gain-of-function mutation. In this family, all affected individuals developed MTC. The affected individuals are positive for the V804 L mutation in the RET tyrosine kinase receptor. This mutation is associated with a moderate risk for MTC according to the 2015 Revised American Thyroid Association guidelines for the management of medullary thyroid carcinoma and a low risk of PCC and HPTH [40]. Carriers of the mutation need to be screened for (paroxysmal) hypertension and abnormal hypersecretion of plasma metanephrines and normetanephrines or 24-h urinary metanephrines and normetanephrines.

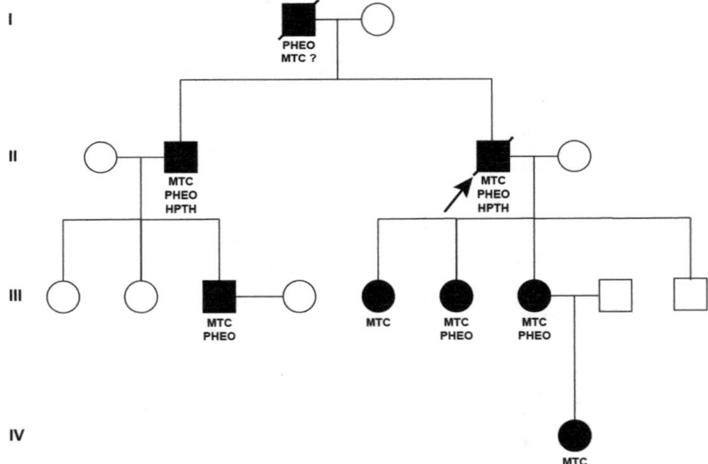

Fig. 4.2 Pedigree of a family with Familial Medullary Thyroid Cancer/Multiple Endocrine Neoplasia Type 2A. The individuals shown with black filled symbols all carry a C643R mutation in the RET tyrosine kinase receptor first detected in the index patient (III-3; arrow). The transmission is autosomal dominant, but in contrast to VHL or NF1, this is due to a gain-of-function mutation. In this family, all affected individuals developed MTC. The C643R mutation is associated with a high risk for PCC (Table 2). The index patient has been diagnosed with bilateral PCC at age 20 and died secondary to metastatic disease. He and several other individuals also developed HPTH. Two of his daughters (individuals III-6 and III-7) also developed bilateral PCC. Carriers of the mutation need to be screened for (paroxysmal) hypertension and abnormal hypersecretion of plasma metanephrines and normetanephrines or 24-hour urinary metanephrines and normetanephrines

Paraganglioma (PGL) Syndromes

The paraganglioma syndromes types 1–5 (PGL 1–5) are autosomal dominant disorders with a predisposition for developing PGL, less commonly PCC, RCC, gastrointestinal tumors (GIST), more rarely pituitary adenomas, and other neoplasias [44]. The PGL syndromes are caused by mutations in genes encoding the four subunits of succinate dehydrogenase (SDH) or the assembly factor SDHAF2 (Fig. 4.3) [44, 45]. SDH, also referred to as mitochondrial complex II, is a heterotetrameric protein that transfers electrons directly to the ubiquinone pool as a member of the respiratory chain at the inner membrane of mitochondria, and it is involved in the Krebs cycle [46]. The penetrance of disease is highly variable, and there are divergent phenotypes among the PGL syndromes [44].

PGL1: SDHD Mutations

PGL1 is caused by mutations in SDHD [44, 47–49]. The *SDHD* gene is located on chromosome 11q23, spans 4 exons, and encodes a 103 amino acid protein which forms the anchoring subunit of SDH [50]. It contains a ubiquinone binding site which accepts electrons from the SDHB subunit.

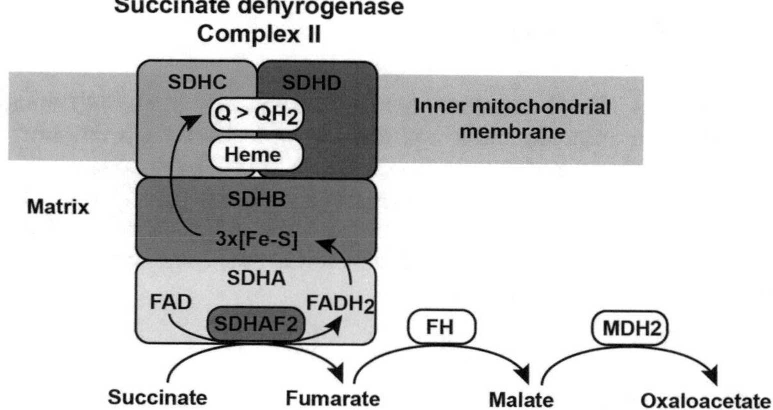

Fig. 4.3 Succinate dehydrogenase. Succinate dehydrogenase (SDH), also referred to as complex II, consists of four subunits (A–D); the succinate dehydrogenase assembly factor 2 exerts flavination of SDHA. SDH is a component of the tricarboxylic acid (TCA) cycle and the mitochondrial electron transport chain. The PGL syndromes 1–5 are caused by mutations in genes encoding the four subunits of succinate dehydrogenase (SDH) or the assembly factor SDHAF2. Fumarate hydratase (or fumarase) (FH) catalyzes the reversible hydration/dehydration of fumarate to malate; malate dehydrogenase 2 catalyzes the reversible oxidation of malate to oxaloacetate. Germline mutations in FH confer predisposition to malignant PCC/PGL; mutation of MDH2 has been found in malignant PGL

The inheritance of PGL1 is autosomal dominant, and predisposition to tumor development occurs usually only if the mutated allele is inherited from the father [51]. One possible explanation is that the maternal copy of the gene is imprinted and inactive, but the data supporting this model remain controversial [52–54]. Some studies have documented monoallelic paternal SDHD expression in tumor tissue [52], whereas other studies documented biallelic expression [47, 53, 54]. Moreover, possible maternal transmission has been reported in isolated cases [55, 56]. The penetrance increases with age, and by age 70, it is 90% or higher [51, 57]. The main manifestation includes multiple head and neck PGL, but adrenal PCC can also occur, and the malignancy rate is below 5% [51, 58].

PGL2: SDHAF2 Mutations

The *SDHAF2* gene is located on chromosome 11q12.2 and encodes a 167 amino acid mitochondrial protein that exerts flavination of SDHA. SDHAF2 mutations are uncommon but should be considered in PGL patients negative for mutations in the *SDHB*, *SDHC*, or *SDHD* subunit genes [44, 59]. The inheritance of PGL2 susceptibility is also autosomal dominant, and similar to SDHD mutations, it is associated with paternal inheritance [59–61]. The clinical manifestation includes predominantly multiple head and neck PGL, penetrance is high and up to 100%, and the malignancy rate is low [61].

PGL3: SDHC Mutations

The *SDHC* gene is located on chromosome 1q23.3 and encodes the 140 amino acid subunit carrying the cytochrome b, and together with SDHD it is one of the two hydrophobic membrane anchor subunits (Fig. 4.3) [50]. Compared to mutations in *SDHD* and *SDHB*, mutations in *SDHC* are less common [11, 62–64]. They are inherited in an autosomal dominant fashion without parent-of-origin effect. The characteristic tumor manifestation consists of solitary head and neck PGL, and the malignancy risk is very low [11, 65].

PGL4: SDHB Mutations

The *SDHB* gene, located on chromosome 1p36.1–35, encodes the hydrophilic iron sulfur subunit of the SDH complex. Tumor predisposition is inherited in an autosomal dominant way, and the tumorigenic mechanism involves inactivation of the second allele in a somatic way according to the Knudson two-hit model [66]. The loss of both alleles results in overexpression of HIF1α [67, 68]. Patients develop often unifocal PGL located anywhere between the neck and the bladder [11, 51, 69].

Penetrance is age dependent but as high as 80–100% by age 70 [11, 51, 69]. The malignancy risk is substantial and has been estimated to be as high as 71% [1, 51, 57, 70]. More than 200 *SDHB* mutations occurring in all eight coding exons have been described, and there is no evidence for a genotype-phenotype correlation [44]. Carriers of *SDHB* mutations have an increased risk for RCC and GIST [69, 71, 72].

Clinical Vignette

A 35-year-old male patient with uncontrolled non-paroxymal hypertension and diabetes mellitus type 1 since the age of 18 years developed proteinuria [73]. Computerized tomography (CT) of the abdomen and pelvis revealed a bladder mass. A PGL was not suspected. During a cystoscopy, the patient developed a hypertensive crisis. Biochemical evaluation demonstrated increased norepinephrine and normetanephrine levels. A ^{123}iodine-meta-iodobenzylguanidine (MIBG) scan showed intense uptake in the mass (Fig. 4.4). The family history was negative for PCC/PGL. Surgical resection was performed after appropriate alpha- and beta-blockade. The surgical pathology showed a bladder PGL with aggressive features, and mutational analysis revealed a novel SDHB mutation (W200R) [73].

PGL5: SDHA Mutations

The *SDHA* gene is located on chromosome 5p15 and encodes the 621 amino acid catalytic flavoprotein subunit of SDH (Fig. 4.3). Individuals with biallelic mutations in SDHA develop autosomal recessive juvenile encephalopathy (Leigh syndrome) [74]. A monoallelic mutation has first been identified in a patient with an abdominal

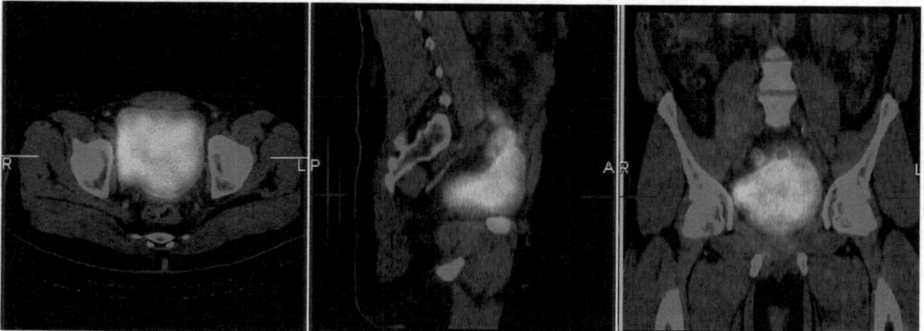

Fig. 4.4 Paraganglioma in the bladder in a patient with PGL syndrome 4 with a SDHB mutation. A ^{123}iodine-meta-iodobenzylguanidine (MIBG) scan fused with CT shows intense uptake in the mass. The tumor was detected incidentally in a patient with non-paroxysmal hypertension, diabetes mellitus, and proteinuria. Cystoscopy led to a hypertensive crisis. Surgical pathology showed aggressive histology and mutational analysis revealed a novel SDHB mutation (W200R) [73]. (MIBG image courtesy of Dr. Grazia Aleppo, Northewestern University, Chicago)

PGL, and subsequently a few additional patients were found to harbor SDHA mutations [75]. *SDHA* mutations are thought to be a rare cause of PGL accounting for roughly 3% of all cases, and the penetrance may be low, which suggests that alterations in modifier genes or other contributing factors need to be present for the development of the phenotype [76]. GIST and pituitary adenomas have also been described in patients with PGL5 [77–79]. Mutational analysis of the *SDHA* gene is complicated by the presence of three pseudogenes (*SDHAP1*, *SDHAP2*, *SDHAP3*) – similar but nonfunctional sequences – but immunohistochemistry can be useful for the identification of tumors harboring SDHA mutations [75].

TMEM127

TMEM127 is a more recently identified PCC/PGL susceptibility gene located on chromosome 2q11.2 encoding a 238 amino acid transmembrane protein [80]. The exact pathophysiological role of TMEM127 is still poorly defined. It is a tumor suppressor gene, and tumor susceptibility is inherited in an autosomal dominant way, and tumor development requires a second somatic hit. Mutations in *TMEM127* have been found in patients with bilateral, extra-adrenal PCC and head and neck PGL [81–83]. The penetrance is incompletely defined, and the malignancy rate is very low [81, 82].

MAX

Exome sequencing of three unrelated individuals with hereditary PCC has led to the identification of mutations in the *MAX (MYC associated factor X)* gene as PCC/PGL susceptibility gene [84]. Subsequent analysis identified additional mutations as well as gene rearrangements involving *MAX* [84, 85, 86]. The inheritance is autosomal dominant with preferential paternal transmission [84]. MAX-mutated PCC/PGL are rare, typically bilateral, and associated with a distinct biochemical phenotype with larger increases in normetanephrine and an intermediate metanephrine level, not typical of the adrenergic or noradrenergic phenotype [2, 85].

Mutations in Other Elements of the Tricarboxylic Acid (TCA) Krebs Cycle: Fumarate Hydratase (FH) and Malate Dehydrogenase Type 2 (MDH2)

Several novel PCC/PGL susceptibility genes have been recently discovered through whole-exome sequencing [87, 88]. In addition to the mutations in the *SDHx* and *SDHAF2* genes, loss-of-function mutations in other elements of the tricarboxylic acid (TCA) Krebs cycle, FH (fumarate hydratase) and MDH2 (malate dehydrogenase type 2), predispose to PCC/PGL [87, 88]. FH catalyzes the hydroxylation of fumarate to malate, and MDH2 catalyzes the oxidation of malate to oxaloacetate. Accumulation of fumarate through FH mutations inhibits the action of prolyl hydroxylase domain proteins that hydroxylate HIF1α and thus leads to activation of the HIF signaling pathway [88]. Remarkably, PCC/PGL that are deficient in FH show an identical pattern of epigenetic deregulation as SDHB-mutated tumors [87].

Mutations in Endothelial PAS Domain Protein 1/Hypoxia-Inducible Factor Type 2A

(EPAS1/HIF2A)

Somatic gain-of-function EPAS1/HIF2A (endothelial PAS domain protein 1/ hypoxia-inducible factor type 2A) mutations have first been described in patients with multiple PGL, somatostatinoma, and polycythemia [89]. Although initially considered to be nonheritable, recent studies have shown that these mutations may be present in numerous locations through somatic mosaicism acquired through postzygotic mutations occurring in early developmental stages and, occasionally, also as germline mutations [90, 91]. Patients with EPAS1/HIF2A mutations present with significantly elevated plasma norepinephrine and normetanephrine levels due to involvement of HIF-2α in catecholamine synthesis [89, 92].

Other Susceptibility Genes

A growing list of other genes has been implicated in conferring a risk for developing PCC/PGL along with other neoplasias. They include, among others, *PDH1, PDH2, KIF1B, MERTK, MET* and *H3F3A* (Table 4.1) [14, 15]. Their rare occurrence makes it in part difficult to establish a causative link in all instances. The detection of these less common variants can, however, be of great value for a better understanding of the pathways involved in the development of these tumors.

Correlation Between Genetic Mutation and Biochemical Phenotype

The details surrounding the biochemical work-up of patients with PCC/PGL are discussed elsewhere in this book (Chapter 5). Measurements of catecholamine metabolites, plasma-free metanephrines, or urinary fractionated metanephrines are the recommended initial tests [2, 93–95]; the measurement of plasma 3-methoxytyramine

(3-MT) can be used to further characterize the secretory phenotype of the tumor [96–98]. About 50% of PCC/PGL almost exclusively secrete norepinephrine, while the other 50% secrete both epinephrine and norepinephrine [2, 99]. Based on the biochemical profile, PCC/PGL can be divided into three biochemical subtypes: (1) a noradrenergic phenotype with predominant secretion of norepinephrine, (2) an adrenergic phenotype with predominant secretion of epinephrine, and (3) a rare subtype secreting predominantly dopamine.

The noradrenergic phenotype is associated with tumors that are primarily located in extra-adrenal areas, but they can occasionally also occur in the adrenal gland [99]. Clinically, these patients present more commonly with non-episodic hypertension [100]. The noradrenergic phenotype is usually associated with the so-called cluster 1 mutations, i.e., mutations resulting in stabilization of hypoxia-inducible factors and activating the hypoxia signaling pathways (Table 4.3) [9]. The expression of the *phenylethanolamine N-methyltransferase (PNMT)* gene and protein is reduced, resulting in a decreased or absent conversion of norepinephrine to epinephrine. Mechanistically, this has been explained by epigenetic silencing of the *PNMT* gene through hypermethylation of the promoter region [101]. Patients with the adrenergic phenotype present more frequently with paroxysmal events (Chap. 3). These tumors tend to be located in the adrenal glands and are more differentiated [102]. The expression of PNMT is high [100, 103]. They are associated with mutations resulting in the activation of kinase signaling pathways and are referred to as cluster 2 mutations (Table 4.3). Cluster 2 includes MEN2 and NF1, as well as mutations in the *TMEM127* and *MAX* genes [2], although PCC/PGL with MAX mutations can have an intermediate phenotype (normetaepinephrine > metanephrines; metanephrines intermediate) [85, 86].

The dopaminergic phenotype, with very low increases in norepinephrine and epinephrine, is extremely rare and can be characterized by measuring dopamine and 3-MT [96, 97]. The tumors are most commonly extra-adrenal, and they can be malignant [98]. They have reduced levels of dopamine β-hydroxylase, which results in decreased production of norepinephrine and accumulation of dopamine [2]. Lastly, silent PGL without secretion of catecholamines or metanephrines can occur very rarely [104]. They can become clinical apparent because of mass effects.

Table 4.3 Gene clusters and associated phenotypes

	Genes	Mechanisms	Biochemical phenotype	Tumor location
Cluster 1 mutations	*VHL, SDHA, SDHB, SDHC, SDHD, FH, MDH2, EPAS1/HIF2A, (SDHAF2)*	Induction of pseudohypoxic condition	Predominantly noradrenergic	Predominantly extra-adrenal. Can occur within the adrenal gland, particularly in VHL
Cluster 2 mutations	*MEN2, NF1, TMEM127, MAX*	Alterations in kinase signaling pathways: activation of proliferation, inhibition of apoptosis	Predominantly adrenergic	Predominantly adrenal

Characteristics of Pediatric Compared to Adult PCC/PGL

PCC/PGL in children have a higher prevalence of hereditary disease associated with germline mutations in susceptibility genes than adults [7, 105–107]. Secondly, children with PCC/PGL have more frequently bilateral, multiple, and extra-adrenal tumors [108]. In a recent study including 748 patients with PCC/PGL, including 95 patients with a first presentation during childhood, the prevalence of hereditary causes was 80.4% in children versus 52.6% in adults, extra-adrenal manifestations occurred in 66.3 versus 35.1%, multifocal tumors in 32.6 versus 13.5%, metastatic disease was found in 49.5 versus 29.1%, and recurrences in 29.5 versus 14.2% (Fig. 4.5) [6]. Biochemically, there was a higher prevalence of noradrenergic tumors with a relative lack of plasma metanephrine secretion, which confirms the observation by Hume published in 1960 demonstrating that most pediatric PCC/PGL predominantly secrete norepinephrine [105]. Six hundred eleven patients included in this study underwent genetic testing; 74/92 children (80.4%) and 273/519 (52.6%) adults were found to have a germline mutation in one of the tumor susceptibility genes. Mutations in cluster 1 genes were more common in children compared to adults with 76.1 versus 39.3% [6]. These findings strongly support that that all children with PCC/PGL should undergo genetic testing and be managed at specialized centers with appropriate expertise [6, 12]. Because of the higher risk for extra-adrenal tumors, Pamporaki et al. recommend that children should be evaluated with high-signal intensity on T2-weighted magnetic resonance imaging (MRI), rather than with CT as suggested by the Endocrine Society guidelines [12]. In pediatric mutation carriers, biochemical surveillance is indicated in all mutation carriers beginning at an early age of 5 years, and clinical surveillance needs to be tailored to the specific mutation and associated syndrome [6].

Mutational Analysis

PCC/PGL have a very high degree of heritability of close to 50%, and genetic testing has been recommended for all patients independent of a positive family history [12]. The genetic heterogeneity, i.e., a similar phenotype caused by mutations in more than 15 susceptibility genes, is, however, a challenge for genetic testing [109]. Several algorithms for genetic testing based on the clinical and biochemical presentation have been proposed in the recent past [8, 9, 12, 110]. In patients with a syndromic or familial presentation, targeted sequencing of the most plausible candidate gene is often the first step, as, e.g., in VHL and MEN2.

However, in the absence of other clinical clues, targeted sequencing of single genes may not be readily informative, and it is cost- and labor-intensive. Advances in next-generation sequencing (NGS) techniques now permit sequencing of comprehensive validated gene panels, and this is ideally suited for the mutational analysis of patients with PCC/PGL [111]. A recent consensus statement on next-generation

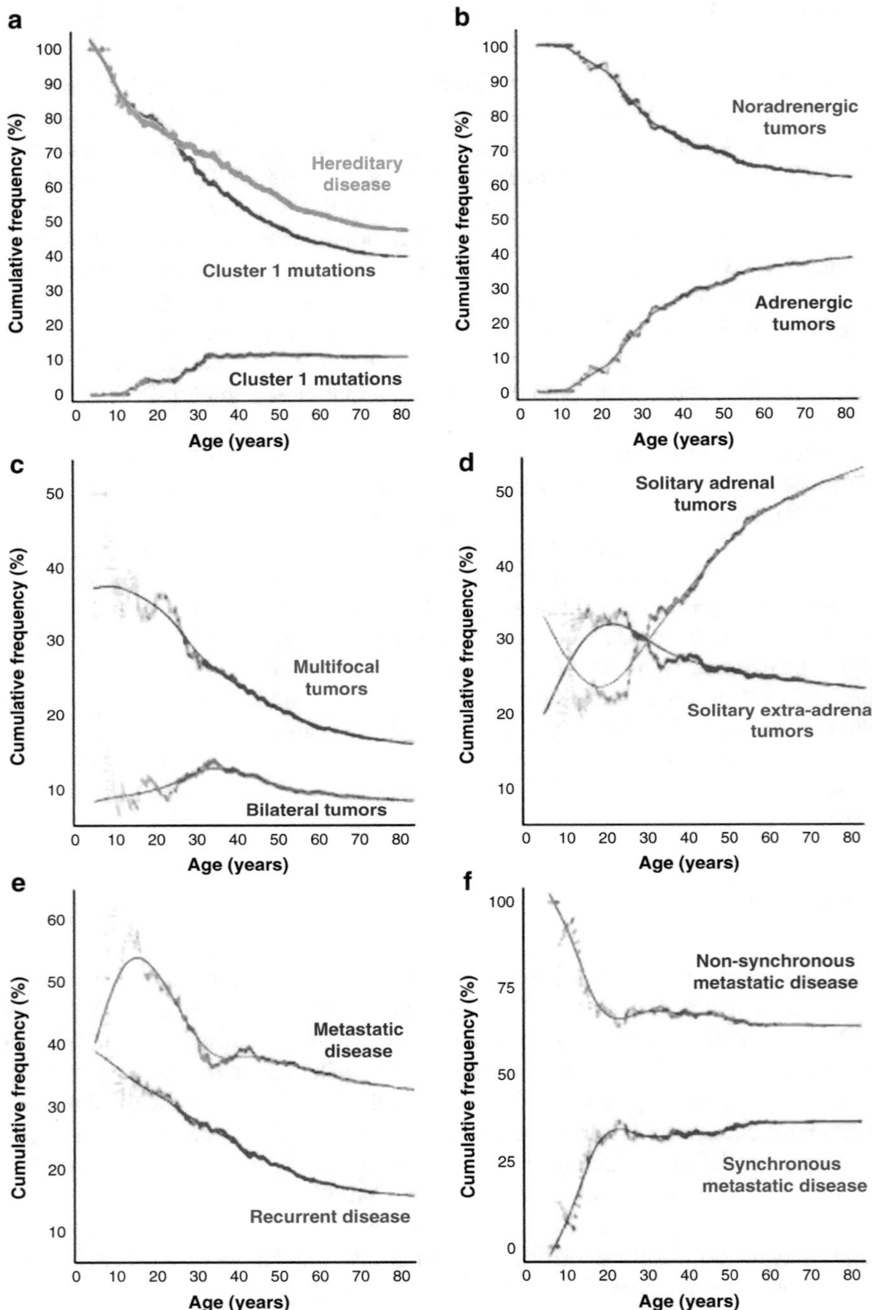

Fig. 4.5 Cumulative frequencies as a function of age in hereditary disease. (**a**) Tumors due to cluster 1 versus cluster 2 mutations, (**b**) noradrenergic versus adrenergic tumors, (**c**) multifocal versus bilateral adrenal tumors, (**d**) solitary adrenal versus extra-adrenal tumors, (**e**) metastatic disease versus recurrent nonmetastatic disease, and (**f**) nonsynchronous versus synchronous metastatic disease. (From Pamporaki et al. [6] with permission)

sequencing-based diagnostic testing of hereditary pheochromocytomas and paragangliomas provides a detailed overview on this rapidly evolving approach and associated challenges [14]. While NGS is greatly facilitating genetic testing in this setting, it must be recognized that access to these platforms and insurance coverage vary widely. Hence, careful and thorough clinical and biochemical evaluations, in combination with traditional Sanger sequencing of candidate genes, continue to be essential first steps and of high value in the characterization of patients affected by PCC/PGL.

PCC/PGL

Somatic Mutations in the Pathogenesis of PCC/PGL

The understanding of the somatic alterations in the genomic landscape of PCC/PGL have fundamentally changed with the recent publication of the Comprehensive Molecular Characterization of Pheochromocytoma and Paraganglioma study as a part of The Cancer Genome Atlas (TCGA) initiative of the National Cancer Institute [10]. This had been preceded by a number of studies that identified mutations in several genes (e.g., *EPAS1 (HIF2α), RET, VHL, RAS, NF1,* and *ATRX*) and recurrent copy number variations [10, 112, 113].

In the PCC/PGL TCGA, 173 PCC/PGL were submitted to a comprehensive integrated analysis using a multiplatform approach including whole-exome DNA sequencing, DNA copy number analysis, mRNA sequencing, miRNA sequencing, DNA methylation, and protein array analysis. The age range of the included patients was 19–83 years (median 47 years), 16 had aggressive tumors, and 11 had distant metastatic events. The integrated analysis identified a genetic alteration in 95% of the tumors. The analysis revealed that PCC/PGL exhibit a low somatic mutation rate but a remarkably diverse spectrum of driver mutations disrupting distinct biological pathways through germline and somatic mutations (Fig. 4.6), as well as somatic gene rearrangements and copy number variations. The integration of the mutational profile and gene expression patterns allowed to classify PCC/PGL into four distinct molecular subtypes based on the mutational profile and gene expression patterns: (1) kinase signaling (cluster 2), (2) pseudohypoxia (cluster 1), (3) WNT-altered, and (4) cortical admixture subtype. In addition to the confirmation of known driver genes (*HRAS, RET, EPAS1, NF1*), the TCGA has identified loss-of-function mutations in the *CSDE1 (cold shock domain containing E1)* gene as a new important driving mechanism and discovered several somatic gene fusions involving genes such as *MAML3, BRAF, NGFR*, and *NF1*. Somatic mutations were also found in *RET, NF1,* and *VHL*. Usually, the mutations were limited to one of the affected pathways indicating mutual exclusivity among these mutations. Markers associated with a poor outcome included, among others, the presence of *MAML3* gene fusions, *SDHB* germline mutations, somatic mutations in *SETD2* or *ATRX*, a high mutation rate within the tumor, hypermethylation, extra-adrenal tumor manifestation, and a nonsecretory phenotype.

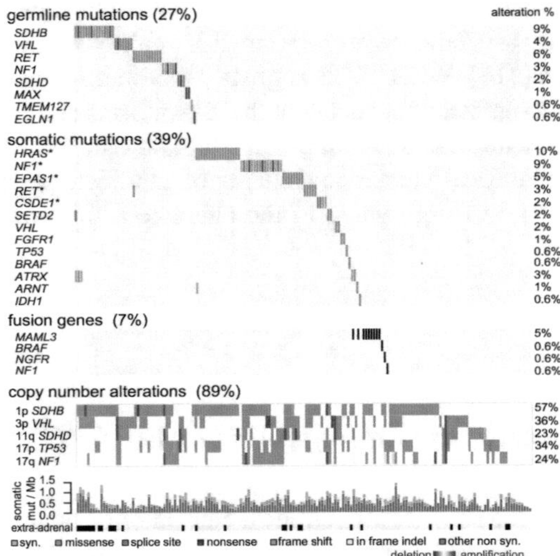

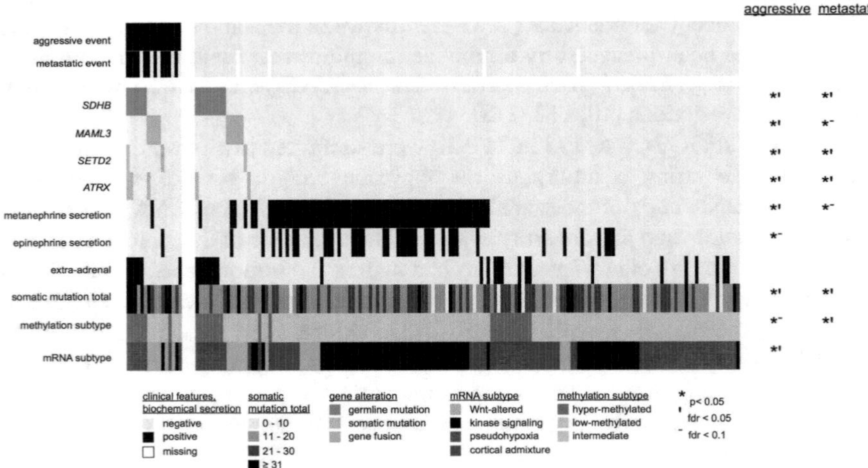

Fig. 4.6 Germline and somatic genome mutations in the TCGA of PCC/PGL. (**a**) Genomic features in rows and primary tumors ($n = 173$) in columns; shading indicates the effect of a mutation on protein sequence. Significant somatically mutated genes are indicated by an asterisk (*). (**b**) Molecular discriminants of clinical outcomes. Primary tumors appear in columns ($n = 173$). Molecular and clinical features appear in rows. Somatic mutation total is the number of somatic mutations in a tumor. Marker and outcome associations were determined by log rank tests (p). (Modified with permission from Fishbein et al. [10])

Mutations in the Kinase Subtype

Cluster 2 mutations in Table 4.3 were associated with better outcomes.

Conclusion

In patients presenting with PCC/PGL, the elucidation of the underlying genetic predisposition can have important clinical ramifications. It assists in identifying patients at risk for developing multifocal or malignant lesions, or associated neoplasias, and it has impact for the identification of carriers within the family and genetic counseling. For these reasons and the fact that about 30–40% with supposedly sporadic PCC/PGL and more than 50% with PGL carry germline mutations in one of the susceptibility genes, recent recommendations emphasize that the threshold for genetic testing should be low [1, 8, 110]. In particular, all patients with multiple lesions or presenting at a young age should undergo formal genetic testing [1, 6]. The advent of NGS permitting to analyze gene panels now allows more efficient analysis of all potential candidate genes [14]. Moreover, the elucidation of the genomic landscape of the germline and somatic mutations present in PCC/PGL may also permit identifying patients at risk for developing metastatic disease, and these insights are crucial for the development of novel targeted therapeutic modalities for metastatic tumors [10].

References

1. Fishbein L, Nathanson KL. Pheochromocytoma and paraganglioma: understanding the complexities of the genetic background. Cancer Genet. 2012;205(1–2):1–11.
2. Gupta G, Pacak K, AACE Adrenal Scientific Committee. Precision medicine: an update on genotype- biochemical phenotype relationships in Pheochromocytoma/Paraganglioma patients. Endoc Pract Off J Am Coll Endocrinol Am Assoc Clin Endocrinologists. 2017;23:690–704.
3. Lenders JW, Eisenhofer G, Mannelli M, Pacak K. Phaeochromocytoma. Lancet. 2005; 366(9486):665–75.
4. Ayala-Ramirez M, Feng L, Johnson MM, Ejaz S, Habra MA, Rich T, et al. Clinical risk factors for malignancy and overall survival in patients with pheochromocytomas and sympathetic paragangliomas: primary tumor size and primary tumor location as prognostic indicators. J Clin Endocrinol Metab. 2011;96(3):717–25.
5. Hescot S, Leboulleux S, Amar L, Vezzosi D, Borget I, Bournaud-Salinas C, et al. One- year progression-free survival of therapy-naive patients with malignant pheochromocytoma and paraganglioma. J Clin Endocrinol Metab. 2013;98(10):4006–12.
6. Pamporaki C, Hamplova B, Peitzsch M, Prejbisz A, Beuschlein F, Timmers H, et al. Characteristics of pediatric vs adult pheochromocytomas and paragangliomas. J Clin Endocrinol Metab. 2017;102(4):1122–32.
7. Neumann HP, Bausch B, McWhinney SR, Bender BU, Gimm O, Franke G, et al. Germ- line mutations in nonsyndromic pheochromocytoma. N Engl J Med. 2002;346(19):1459–66.
8. Neumann HP, Erlic Z, Boedeker CC, Rybicki LA, Robledo M, Hermsen M, et al. Clinical predictors for germline mutations in head and neck paraganglioma patients: cost reduction strategy in genetic diagnostic process as fall-out. Cancer Res. 2009;69(8):3650–6.
9. Favier J, Amar L, Gimenez-Roqueplo AP. Paraganglioma and phaeochromocytoma: from genetics to personalized medicine. Nat Rev Endocrinol. 2015;11(2):101–11.
10. Fishbein L, Leshchiner I, Walter V, Danilova L, Robertson AG, Johnson AR, et al. Comprehensive molecular characterization of Pheochromocytoma and Paraganglioma. Cancer Cell. 2017;31(2):181–93.

11. Burnichon N, Rohmer V, Amar L, Herman P, Leboulleux S, Darrouzet V, et al. The succinate dehydrogenase genetic testing in a large prospective series of patients with paragangliomas. J Clin Endocrinol Metab. 2009;94(8):2817–27.
12. Lenders JW, Duh QY, Eisenhofer G, Gimenez-Roqueplo AP, Grebe SK, Murad MH, et al. Pheochromocytoma and paraganglioma: an Endocrine Society clinical practice guideline. J Clin Endocrinol Metab. 2014;99(6):1915–42.
13. Jameson J, Kopp P. Principles of human genetics. In: Braunwald E, Fauci A, Kasper D, Hauser S, Longo D, Jameson J, editors. Harrison's principles of internal medicine. 19th ed. New York: McGraw-Hill; 2015. p. 425–45.
14. NGS in PPGL (NGSnPPGL) Study Group, Toledo RA, Burnichon N, Cascon A, Benn DE, Bayley JP, et al. Consensus statement on next-generation-sequencing-based diagnostic testing of hereditary phaeochromocytomas and paragangliomas. Nat Rev Endocrinol. 2017;13(4):233–47.
15. Toledo RA, Qin Y, Cheng ZM, Gao Q, Iwata S, Silva GM, et al. Recurrent mutations of chromatin-remodeling genes and kinase receptors in pheochromocytomas and paragangliomas. Clin Cancer Res Off J Am Assoc Cancer Res. 2016;22(9):2301–10.
16. Murgia A, Martella M, Vinanzi C, Polli R, Perilongo G, Opocher G. Somatic mosaicism in von Hippel-Lindau disease. Hum Mutat. 2000;15(1):114.
17. Santarpia L, Sarlis NJ, Santarpia M, Sherman SI, Trimarchi F, Benvenga S. Mosaicism in von Hippel-Lindau disease: an event important to recognize. J Cell Mol Med. 2007;11(6):1408–15.
18. Kaplan L, Foster R, Shen Y, Parry DM, McMaster ML, O'Leary MC, et al. Monozygotic twins discordant for neurofibromatosis 1. Am J Med Genet A. 2010;152A(3):601–6.
19. Vogt J, Kohlhase J, Morlot S, Kluwe L, Mautner VF, Cooper DN, et al. Monozygotic twins discordant for neurofibromatosis type 1 due to a postzygotic NF1 gene mutation. Hum Mutat. 2011;32(6):E2134–47.
20. Nielsen SM, Rhodes L, Blanco I, Chung WK, Eng C, Maher ER, et al. Von Hippel-Lindau disease: genetics and role of genetic Counseling in a multiple Neoplasia syndrome. J Clin Oncol Off J Am Soc Clin Oncol. 2016;34(18):2172–81.
21. Maher ER, Neumann HP, von Richard S. Hippel-Lindau disease: a clinical and scientific review. Eur J Hum Genet EJHG. 2011;19(6):617–23.
22. Maher ER, Iselius L, Yates JR, Littler M, Benjamin C, Harris R, et al. Von Hippel- Lindau disease: a genetic study. J Med Genet. 1991;28(7):443–7.
23. Delman KA, Shapiro SE, Jonasch EW, Lee JE, Curley SA, Evans DB, et al. Abdominal visceral lesions in von Hippel-Lindau disease: incidence and clinical behavior of pancreatic and adrenal lesions at a single center. World J Surg. 2006;30(5):665–9.
24. Boedeker CC, Erlic Z, Richard S, Kontny U, Gimenez-Roqueplo AP, Cascon A, et al. Head and neck paragangliomas in von Hippel-Lindau disease and multiple endocrine neoplasia type 2. J Clin Endocrinol Metab. 2009;94(6):1938–44.
25. Gaal J, van Nederveen FH, Erlic Z, Korpershoek E, Oldenburg R, Boedeker CC, et al. Parasympathetic paragangliomas are part of the Von Hippel-Lindau syndrome. J Clin Endocrinol Metab. 2009;94(11):4367–71.
26. Gossage L, Eisen T, Maher ER. VHL, the story of a tumour suppressor gene. Nat Rev Cancer. 2015;15(1):55–64.
27. Kaelin WG Jr. Molecular basis of the VHL hereditary cancer syndrome. Nat Rev Cancer. 2002;2(9):673–82.
28. Min JH, Yang H, Ivan M, Gertler F, Kaelin WG Jr, Pavletich NP. Structure of an HIF-1alpha-pVHL complex: hydroxyproline recognition in signaling. Science. 2002;296(5574):1886–9.
29. Czyzyk-Krzeska MF, Meller J. von Hippel-Lindau tumor suppressor: not only HIF's executioner. Trends Mol Med. 2004;10(4):146–9.
30. Nordstrom-O'Brien M, van der Luijt RB, van Rooijen E, van den Ouweland AM, Majoor-Krakauer DF, Lolkema MP, et al. Genetic analysis of von Hippel-Lindau disease. Hum Mutat. 2010;31(5):521–37.
31. Chen F, Slife L, Kishida T, Mulvihill J, Tisherman SE, Zbar B. Genotype-phenotype correlation in von Hippel-Lindau disease: identification of a mutation associated with VHL type 2A. J Med Genet. 1996;33(8):716–7.

32. Rechsteiner MP, von Teichman A, Nowicka A, Sulser T, Schraml P, Moch H. VHL gene mutations and their effects on hypoxia inducible factor HIFalpha: identification of potential driver and passenger mutations. Cancer Res. 2011;71(16):5500–11.
33. Forman JR, Worth CL, Bickerton GR, Eisen TG, Blundell TL. Structural bioinformatics mutation analysis reveals genotype-phenotype correlations in von Hippel-Lindau disease and suggests molecular mechanisms of tumorigenesis. Proteins. 2009;77(1):84–96.
34. Ferner RE, Huson SM, Thomas N, Moss C, Willshaw H, Evans DG, et al. Guidelines for the diagnosis and management of individuals with neurofibromatosis 1. J Med Genet. 2007;44(2):81–8.
35. Gutmann DH, Ferner RE, Listernick RH, Korf BR, Wolters PL, Johnson KJ. Neurofibromatosis type 1. Nat Rev Dis Primers. 2017;3:17004.
36. Johannessen CM, Johnson BW, Williams SM, Chan AW, Reczek EE, Lynch RC, et al. TORC1 is essential for NF1-associated malignancies. Curr Biol. 2008;18(1):56–62.
37. Williams VC, Lucas J, Babcock MA, Gutmann DH, Korf B, Maria BL. Neurofibromatosis type 1 revisited. Pediatrics. 2009;123(1):124–33.
38. Bausch B, Borozdin W, Neumann HP. European-American Pheochromocytoma study G. Clinical and genetic characteristics of patients with neurofibromatosis type 1 and pheochromocytoma. N Engl J Med. 2006;354(25):2729–31.
39. Hyde SM, Cote GJ, Grubbs EG. Genetics of multiple endocrine Neoplasia type 1/multiple endocrine Neoplasia type 2 syndromes. Endocrinol Metab Clin N Am. 2017;46(2):491–502.
40. Wells SA Jr, Asa SL, Dralle H, Elisei R, Evans DB, Gagel RF, et al. Revised American Thyroid Association guidelines for the management of medullary thyroid carcinoma. Thyroid Off J Am Thyroid Assoc. 2015;25(6):567–610.
41. Brandi ML, Gagel RF, Angeli A, Bilezikian JP, Beck-Peccoz P, Bordi C, et al. Guidelines for diagnosis and therapy of MEN type 1 and type 2. J Clin Endocrinol Metab. 2001;86(12):5658–71.
42. Pacak K, Ilias I, Adams KT, Eisenhofer G. Biochemical diagnosis, localization and management of pheochromocytoma: focus on multiple endocrine neoplasia type 2 in relation to other hereditary syndromes and sporadic forms of the tumour. J Intern Med. 2005;257(1):60–8.
43. Wohllk N, Schweizer H, Erlic Z, Schmid KW, Walz MK, Raue F, et al. Multiple endocrine neoplasia type 2. Best Pract Res Clin Endocrinol Metab. 2010;24(3):371–87.
44. Benn DE, Robinson BG, Clifton-Bligh RJ. 15 YEARS OF PARAGANGLIOMA: clinical manifestations of paraganglioma syndromes types 1-5. Endocr Relat Cancer. 2015;22(4):T91–103.
45. Boedeker CC, Hensen EF, Neumann HP, Maier W, van Nederveen FH, Suarez C, et al. Genetics of hereditary head and neck paragangliomas. Head Neck. 2014;36(6):907–16.
46. Bezawork-Geleta A, Rohlena J, Dong L, Pacak K, Neuzil J. Mitochondrial complex II: at the crossroads. Trends Biochem Sci. 2017;42(4):312–25.
47. Baysal BE, Ferrell RE, Willett-Brozick JE, Lawrence EC, Myssiorek D, Bosch A, et al. Mutations in SDHD, a mitochondrial complex II gene, in hereditary paraganglioma. Science. 2000;287(5454):848–51.
48. Gimm O, Armanios M, Dziema H, Neumann HP, Somatic EC. Occult germ-line mutations in SDHD, a mitochondrial complex II gene, in nonfamilial pheochromocytoma. Cancer Res. 2000;60(24):6822–5.
49. Astuti D, Douglas F, Lennard TW, Aligianis IA, Woodward ER, Evans DG, et al. Germline SDHD mutation in familial phaeochromocytoma. Lancet. 2001;357(9263):1181–2.
50. Hirawake H, Taniwaki M, Tamura A, Amino H, Tomitsuka E, Kita K. Characterization of the human SDHD gene encoding the small subunit of cytochrome b (cybS) in mitochondrial succinate-ubiquinone oxidoreductase. Biochim Biophys Acta. 1999;1412(3):295–300.
51. Ricketts CJ, Forman JR, Rattenberry E, Bradshaw N, Lalloo F, Izatt L, et al. Tumor risks and genotype-phenotype-proteotype analysis in 358 patients with germline mutations in SDHB and SDHD. Hum Mutat. 2010;31(1):41–51.
52. Badenhop RF, Cherian S, Lord RS, Baysal BE, Taschner PE, Schofield PR. Novel mutations in the SDHD gene in pedigrees with familial carotid body paraganglioma and sensorineural hearing loss. Genes Chromosomes Cancer. 2001;31(3):255–63.

53. Cascon A, Ruiz-Llorente S, Fraga MF, Leton R, Telleria D, Sastre J, et al. Genetic and epigenetic profile of sporadic pheochromocytomas. J Med Genet. 2004;41:3):e30.
54. Yamashita R, Usui T, Hashimoto S, Suzuki H, Takahashi M, Honkura K, et al. Predominant expression of mutated allele of the succunate dehydrogenase D (SDHD) gene in the SDHD-related paragangliomas. Endocr J. 2009;56(9):1129–35.
55. Pigny P, Vincent A, Cardot Bauters C, Bertrand M, de Montpreville VT, Crepin M, et al. Paraganglioma after maternal transmission of a succinate dehydrogenase gene mutation. J Clin Endocrinol Metab. 2008;93(5):1609–15.
56. Yeap PM, Tobias ES, Mavraki E, Fletcher A, Bradshaw N, Freel EM, et al. Molecular analysis of pheochromocytoma after maternal transmission of SDHD mutation elucidates mechanism of parent-of-origin effect. J Clin Endocrinol Metab. 2011;96(12):E2009–13.
57. Neumann HP, Pawlu C, Peczkowska M, Bausch B, McWhinney SR, Muresan M, et al. Distinct clinical features of paraganglioma syndromes associated with SDHB and SDHD gene mutations. JAMA. 2004;292(8):943–51.
58. Dannenberg H, van Nederveen FH, Abbou M, Verhofstad AA, Komminoth P, de Krijger RR, et al. Clinical characteristics of pheochromocytoma patients with germline mutations in SDHD. J Clin Oncol Off J Am Soc Clin Oncol. 2005;23(9):1894–901.
59. Bayley JP, Kunst HP, Cascon A, Sampietro ML, Gaal J, Korpershoek E, et al. SDHAF2 mutations in familial and sporadic paraganglioma and phaeochromocytoma. Lancet Oncol. 2010;11(4):366–72.
60. Hao HX, Khalimonchuk O, Schraders M, Dephoure N, Bayley JP, Kunst H, et al. SDH5, a gene required for flavination of succinate dehydrogenase, is mutated in paraganglioma. Science. 2009;325(5944):1139–42.
61. Kunst HP, Rutten MH, de Monnink JP, Hoefsloot LH, Timmers HJ, Marres HA, et al. SDHAF2 (PGL2-SDH5) and hereditary head and neck paraganglioma. Clin Cancer Res Off J Am Assoc Cancer Res. 2011;17(2):247–54.
62. Badenhop RF, Jansen JC, Fagan PA, Lord RS, Wang ZG, Foster WJ, et al. The prevalence of SDHB, SDHC, and SDHD mutations in patients with head and neck paraganglioma and association of mutations with clinical features. J Med Genet. 2004;41(7):e99.
63. Baysal BE, Willett-Brozick JE, Lawrence EC, Drovdlic CM, Savul SA, McLeod DR, et al. Prevalence of SDHB, SDHC, and SDHD germline mutations in clinic patients with head and neck paragangliomas. J Med Genet. 2002;39(3):178–83.
64. Schiavi F, Boedeker CC, Bausch B, Peczkowska M, Gomez CF, Strassburg T, et al. Predictors and prevalence of paraganglioma syndrome associated with mutations of the SDHC gene. JAMA. 2005;294(16):2057–63.
65. Peczkowska M, Cascon A, Prejbisz A, Kubaszek A, Cwikla BJ, Furmanek M, et al. Extra-adrenal and adrenal pheochromocytomas associated with a germline SDHC mutation. Nat Clin Pract Endocrinol Metab. 2008;4(2):111–5.
66. Astuti D, Latif F, Dallol A, Dahia PL, Douglas F, George E, et al. Gene mutations in the succinate dehydrogenase subunit SDHB cause susceptibility to familial pheochromocytoma and to familial paraganglioma. Am J Hum Genet. 2001;69(1):49–54.
67. Gimenez-Roqueplo AP, Favier J, Rustin P, Rieubland C, Kerlan V, Plouin PF, et al. Functional consequences of a SDHB gene mutation in an apparently sporadic pheochromocytoma. J Clin Endocrinol Metab. 2002;87(10):4771–4.
68. Pollard PJ, El-Bahrawy M, Poulsom R, Elia G, Killick P, Kelly G, et al. Expression of HIF-1alpha, HIF-2alpha (EPAS1), and their target genes in paraganglioma and pheochromocytoma with VHL and SDH mutations. J Clin Endocrinol Metab. 2006;91(11):4593–8.
69. Benn DE, Gimenez-Roqueplo AP, Reilly JR, Bertherat J, Burgess J, Byth K, et al. Clinical presentation and penetrance of pheochromocytoma/paraganglioma syndromes. J Clin Endocrinol Metab. 2006;91(3):827–36.
70. Brouwers FM, Eisenhofer G, Tao JJ, Kant JA, Adams KT, Linehan WM, et al. High frequency of SDHB germline mutations in patients with malignant catecholamine-producing paragangliomas: implications for genetic testing. J Clin Endocrinol Metab. 2006;91(11):4505–9.

71. Ricketts C, Woodward ER, Killick P, Morris MR, Astuti D, Latif F, et al. Germline SDHB mutations and familial renal cell carcinoma. J Natl Cancer Inst. 2008;100(17):1260–2.
72. Gill AJ, Chou A, Vilain R, Clarkson A, Lui M, Jin R, et al. Immunohistochemistry for SDHB divides gastrointestinal stromal tumors (GISTs) into 2 distinct types. Am J Surg Pathol. 2010;34(5):636–44.
73. Heller M, Elaraj D, Aleppo G, Sturgeon C. Novel Germline SDHB mutation in a 35-year-old male with malignant bladder Paraganglioma. World J Endocr Surg. 2010;2(3):135–8.
74. Bourgeron T, Rustin P, Chretien D, Birch-Machin M, Bourgeois M, Viegas-Pequignot E, et al. Mutation of a nuclear succinate dehydrogenase gene results in mitochondrial respiratory chain deficiency. Nat Genet. 1995;11(2):144–9.
75. Burnichon N, Briere JJ, Libe R, Vescovo L, Riviere J, Tissier F, et al. SDHA is a tumor suppressor gene causing paraganglioma. Hum Mol Genet. 2010;19(15):3011–20.
76. Korpershoek E, Favier J, Gaal J, Burnichon N, van Gessel B, Oudijk L, et al. SDHA immunohistochemistry detects germline SDHA gene mutations in apparently sporadic paragangliomas and pheochromocytomas. J Clin Endocrinol Metab. 2011;96(9):E1472–6.
77. Dwight T, Benn DE, Clarkson A, Vilain R, Lipton L, Robinson BG, et al. Loss of SDHA expression identifies SDHA mutations in succinate dehydrogenase-deficient gastrointestinal stromal tumors. Am J Surg Pathol. 2013;37(2):226–33.
78. Dwight T, Mann K, Benn DE, Robinson BG, McKelvie P, Gill AJ, et al. Familial SDHA mutation associated with pituitary adenoma and pheochromocytoma/paraganglioma. J Clin Endocrinol Metab. 2013;98(6):E1103–8.
79. Dénes J, Swords F, Rattenberry E, Stals K, Owens M, Cranston T, et al. Heterogeneous genetic background of the association of pheochromocytoma/paraganglioma and pituitary adenoma: results from a large patient cohort. J Clin Endocrinol Metab. 2015;100(3):E531–41.
80. Qin Y, Yao L, King EE, Buddavarapu K, Lenci RE, Chocron ES, et al. Germline mutations in TMEM127 confer susceptibility to pheochromocytoma. Nat Genet. 2010;42(3):229–33.
81. Yao L, Schiavi F, Cascon A, Qin Y, Inglada-Perez L, King EE, et al. Spectrum and prevalence of FP/TMEM127 gene mutations in pheochromocytomas and paragangliomas. JAMA. 2010;304(23):2611–9.
82. Burnichon N, Lepoutre-Lussey C, Laffaire J, Gadessaud N, Molinie V, Hernigou A, et al. A novel TMEM127 mutation in a patient with familial bilateral pheochromocytoma. Eur J Endocrinol. 2011;164(1):141–5.
83. Neumann HP, Sullivan M, Winter A, Malinoc A, Hoffmann MM, Boedeker CC, et al. Germline mutations of the TMEM127 gene in patients with paraganglioma of head and neck and extraadrenal abdominal sites. J Clin Endocrinol Metab. 2011;96(8):E1279–82.
84. Comino-Mendez I, Gracia-Aznarez FJ, Schiavi F, Landa I, Leandro-Garcia LJ, Leton R, et al. Exome sequencing identifies MAX mutations as a cause of hereditary pheochromocytoma. Nat Genet. 2011;43(7):663–7.
85. Burnichon N, Cascon A, Schiavi F, Morales NP, Comino-Mendez I, Abermil N, et al. MAX mutations cause hereditary and sporadic pheochromocytoma and paraganglioma. Clin Cancer Res. 2012;18(10):2828–37.
86. Korpershoek E, Koffy D, Eussen BH, Oudijk L, Papathomas TG, van Nederveen FH, et al. Complex MAX rearrangement in a family with malignant pheochromocytoma, renal oncocytoma, and erythrocytosis. J Clin Endocrinol Metab. 2016;101(2):453–60.
87. Castro-Vega LJ, Buffet A, De Cubas AA, Cascon A, Menara M, Khalifa E, et al. Germline mutations in FH confer predisposition to malignant pheochromocytomas and paragangliomas. Hum Mol Genet. 2014;23(9):2440–6.
88. Cascon A, Comino-Mendez I, Curras-Freixes M, de Cubas AA, Contreras L, Richter S, et al. Whole-exome sequencing identifies MDH2 as a new familial paraganglioma gene. J Natl Cancer Inst. 2015;107(5)
89. Pacak K, Jochmanova I, Prodanov T, Yang C, Merino MJ, Fojo T, et al. New syndrome of paraganglioma and somatostatinoma associated with polycythemia. J Clin Oncol Off J Am Soc Clin Oncol. 2013;31(13):1690–8.

90. Buffet A, Smati S, Mansuy L, Menara M, Lebras M, Heymann MF, et al. Mosaicism in HIF2A-related polycythemia-paraganglioma syndrome. J Clin Endocrinol Metab. 2014;99(2):E369–73.
91. Lorenzo FR, Yang C, Ng Tang Fui M, Vankayalapati H, Zhuang Z, Huynh T, et al. A novel EPAS1/HIF2A germline mutation in a congenital polycythemia with paraganglioma. J Mol Med. 2013;91(4):507–12.
92. Zhuang Z, Yang C, Lorenzo F, Merino M, Fojo T, Kebebew E, et al. Somatic HIF2A gain-of-function mutations in paraganglioma with polycythemia. N Engl J Med. 2012;367(10):922–30.
93. Pacak K, Eisenhofer G, Ahlman H, Bornstein SR, Gimenez-Roqueplo AP, Grossman AB, et al. Pheochromocytoma: recommendations for clinical practice from the First International Symposium. October 2005. Nat Clin Pract Endocrinol Metab. 2007;3(2):92–102.
94. Lenders JW, Pacak K, Walther MM, Linehan WM, Mannelli M, Friberg P, et al. Biochemical diagnosis of pheochromocytoma: which test is best? JAMA. 2002;287(11):1427–34.
95. Lenders JW, Pacak K, Eisenhofer G. New advances in the biochemical diagnosis of 895 pheochromocytoma: moving beyond catecholamines. Ann N Y Acad Sci. 2002;970:29–40.
96. Eisenhofer G, Lenders JW, Siegert G, Bornstein SR, Friberg P, Milosevic D, et al. Plasma methoxytyramine: a novel biomarker of metastatic pheochromocytoma and paraganglioma in relation to established risk factors of tumour size, location and SDHB mutation status. Eur J Cancer. 2012;48(11):1739–49.
97. van Duinen N, Corssmit EP, de Jong WH, Brookman D, Kema IP, Romijn JA. Plasma levels of free metanephrines and 3-methoxytyramine indicate a higher number of biochemically active HNPGL than 24-h urinary excretion rates of catecholamines and metabolites. Eur J Endocrinol. 2013;169(3):377–82.
98. Van Der Horst-Schrivers AN, Osinga TE, Kema IP, Van Der Laan BF, Dullaart RP. Dopamine excess in patients with head and neck paragangliomas. Anticancer Res. 2010;30(12):5153–8.
99. Eisenhofer G, Lenders JW, Goldstein DS, Mannelli M, Csako G, Walther MM, et al. Pheochromocytoma catecholamine phenotypes and prediction of tumor size and location by use of plasma free metanephrines. Clin Chem. 2005;51(4):735–44.
100. Eisenhofer G, Walther MM, Huynh TT, Li ST, Bornstein SR, Vortmeyer A, et al. Pheochromocytomas in von Hippel-Lindau syndrome and multiple endocrine neoplasia type 2 display distinct biochemical and clinical phenotypes. J Clin Endocrinol Metab. 2001;86(5):1999–2008.
101. Castro-Vega LJ, Letouze E, Burnichon N, Buffet A, Disderot PH, Khalifa E, et al. Multi-omics analysis defines core genomic alterations in pheochromocytomas and paragangliomas. Nat Commun. 2015;6:6044.
102. van der Harst E, de Herder WW, de Krijger RR, Bruining HA, Bonjer HJ, Lamberts SW, et al. The value of plasma markers for the clinical behaviour of phaeochromocytomas. Eur J Endocrinol. 2002;147(1):85–94.
103. Eisenhofer G, Lenders JW, Timmers H, Mannelli M, Grebe SK, Hofbauer LC, et al. Measurements of plasma methoxytyramine, normetanephrine, and metanephrine as discriminators of different hereditary forms of pheochromocytoma. Clin Chem. 2011;57(3):411–20.
104. Timmers HJ, Pacak K, Huynh TT, Abu-Asab M, Tsokos M, Merino MJ, et al. Biochemically silent abdominal paragangliomas in patients with mutations in the succinate dehydrogenase subunit B gene. J Clin Endocrinol Metab. 2008;93(12):4826–32.
105. Hume DM. Pheochromocytoma in the adult and in the child. Am J Surg. 1960;99:458–96.
106. Cascon A, Inglada-Perez L, Comino-Mendez I, de Cubas AA, Leton R, Mora J, et al. Genetics of pheochromocytoma and paraganglioma in Spanish pediatric patients. Endocr Relat Cancer. 2013;20(3):L1–6.
107. Bausch B, Wellner U, Bausch D, Schiavi F, Barontini M, Sanso G, et al. Long-term prognosis of patients with pediatric pheochromocytoma. Endocr Relat Cancer. 2014;21(1):17–25.
108. Caty MG, Coran AG, Geagen M, Thompson NW. Current diagnosis and treatment of pheochromocytoma in children. Experience with 22 consecutive tumors in 14 patients. Arch Surg. 1990;125(8):978–81.

109. Dahia PL. Pheochromocytoma and paraganglioma pathogenesis: learning from genetic heterogeneity. Nat Rev Cancer. 2014;14(2):108–19.
110. Amar L, Bertherat J, Baudin E, Ajzenberg C, Bressac-de Paillerets B, Chabre O, et al. Genetic testing in pheochromocytoma or functional paraganglioma. J Clin Oncol Off J Am Soc Clin Oncol. 2005;23(34):8812–8.
111. Curras-Freixes M, Pineiro-Yanez E, Montero-Conde C, Apellaniz-Ruiz M, Calsina B, Mancikova V, et al. PheoSeq: a targeted next-generation sequencing assay for pheochromocytoma and paraganglioma diagnostics. J Mol Diagn JMD. 2017;19(4):575–88.
112. Fishbein L, Khare S, Wubbenhorst B, DeSloover D, D'Andrea K, Merrill S, et al. Whole-exome sequencing identifies somatic ATRX mutations in pheochromocytomas and paragangliomas. Nat Commun. 2015;6:6140.
113. Flynn A, Benn D, Clifton-Bligh R, Robinson B, Trainer AH, James P, et al. The genomic landscape of phaeochromocytoma. J Pathol. 2015;236(1):78–89.

Chapter 5
Pheochromocytoma and Paraganglioma in the Pediatric Population

Rachel Kadakia, Monica Bianco, Elizabeth Dabrowski, and Donald Zimmerman

Introduction

Pheochromocytomas (PHEO) and paragangliomas (PGL) are neural crest-derived tumors that can arise from both the sympathetic and parasympathetic paraganglia from the base of the skull to the pelvis. PHEO refers specifically to a catecholamine-secreting tumor originating in the adrenal medulla, while PGL are extra-adrenal in location and can be catecholamine secreting (functional PGL) or dormant (non-functional PGL).

PHEO and PGL are rare lesions in pediatrics. The overall incidence of PHEO and PGL is <0.3 cases per million per year with 10–20% of these cases diagnosed during childhood. These tumors are slightly more common in boys and are diagnosed at an average age of 11 years [1–3].

In contrast to PHEO and PGL in adults, in pediatric patients these tumors are far more likely to be due to a genetic condition than a sporadic occurrence. 50–80% of individuals presenting with PHEO or PGL in childhood had germline mutations [4–6]. Genetic mutations giving rise to PHEO or PGL are most likely to occur in the following genes: *VHL*, *RET*, *NF1*, *SDHA*, *SDHB*, *SDHC*, *SDHD*, *SDHAF2*, *MAX*, and *TMEM127*. Furthermore, hereditary PHEO or PGL are more likely than sporadic tumors to be multifocal, to present at an earlier age, to be extra-adrenal in location, and to be malignant [4]. Genetic testing is essential for any child presenting with a PHEO or PGL, even in the absence of a family history, given the impact it may have on the development of malignancy risk or additional related disease.

R. Kadakia (✉) · M. Bianco · E. Dabrowski · D. Zimmerman
Department of Pediatrics, Northwestern University Feinberg School of Medicine, Chicago, IL, USA

Division of Endocrinology, Ann and Robert H. Lurie Children's Hospital of Chicago, Chicago, IL, USA
e-mail: rkadakia@luriechildrens.org

L. Landsberg (ed.), *Pheochromocytomas, Paragangliomas and Disorders of the Sympathoadrenal System*, Contemporary Endocrinology,
https://doi.org/10.1007/978-3-319-77048-2_5

Clinical Presentation

The presentation of PHEO and PGL is variable and depends on whether the lesion is catecholamine producing. Typical symptoms in pediatrics include hypertension, headaches, palpitations, diaphoresis, syncope, orthostatic hypotension, anxiety, and tremor. Hypertension in pediatric patients is more often sustained as compared to paroxysmal in adults [2]. In addition, 1–2% of pediatric patients who are diagnosed with hypertension have a PHEO or functional PGL [7, 8]. Children can also present with nonspecific symptoms such as abdominal pain, fatigue, worsening school performance, behavioral problems, difficulty concentrating, blurry vision, diarrhea, weight changes, or low-grade fever. Hematuria can signify a bladder lesion. Both functional and nonfunctional lesions can present with signs and symptoms of mass effect such as hearing loss, tinnitus, voice hoarseness, dysphagia, and cough for head and neck lesions.

In a pediatric case review of 30 patients with PHEO or PGL over a 30-year period, 30% presented with signs and symptoms related to mass effect, and 57% presented with one or more typical symptoms such as sweating, nausea, vomiting, or diarrhea. Sixty-four percent of patients had hypertension. Forty-seven percent of cases were malignant, with PGL more commonly malignant than PHEO [9]. Another case review of seven patients demonstrated that only two patients presented with hypertension, while the remainder had nonspecific symptoms such as sweating, nausea, visual disturbances, or mental status changes [10]. These cases highlight that a high index of suspicion is necessary to make the diagnosis of a PHEO or PGL in the pediatric population.

The European-American Pheochromocytoma-Paraganglioma Registry includes 2001 patients with PHEO or PGL of whom 177 or 9% were diagnosed before age 18. 81% of these patients had one of the following hereditary syndromes: von Hippel-Lindau (53%), PGL1 (10%), PGL4 (14%), neurofibromatosis type 1 (3%), multiple endocrine neoplasia type 2 (1%), PGL3 (1%), and familial pheochromocytoma syndrome (1%) [11]. Follow-up of all pediatric patients showed that 38% of patients with a PGL developed a second PGL with a mean interval of 25 years from initial diagnosis and that a significantly higher percentage of patients with hereditary syndromes developed second tumors compared with patients with sporadic disease. A retrospective study of 748 patients with PHEO or PGL of whom 95 presented in childhood demonstrated that lesions in children were more likely to be extra-adrenal, noradrenergic, were twice as likely to have recurrent primary tumors, and 1.7 times as likely to have metastatic disease [6].

Syndromes Associated with PHEO and PGL

We will briefly review the hereditary conditions associated with PHEO and PGL in the pediatric population.

Von Hippel-Lindau

Case *An 11-year-old boy with a 2-week history of nausea and vomiting was seen by his PCP for evaluation. He was noted to have tachycardia and a heart murmur, so an echocardiogram was obtained revealing moderate concentric hypertrophy and mildly decreased left ventricular systolic and diastolic dysfunction. He was referred to cardiology where his HR was 120 beats per minute. Due to weakness and elevation of brain natriuretic peptide (BNP) to 402.65 pg/ml (<100 pg/ml), he was admitted for observation. Upon admission, his blood pressure increased to 200/100 mmHg, and he was started on doxazosin and intravenous nicardipine, with the later addition of propranolol. Prior to this admission, he denied any episodes of headaches, chest pain, or palpitations, though he did endorse episodes of sweating when playing video games. The patient's father and paternal aunt both had a history of pheochromocytoma.*

An MRI of the abdomen revealed a 4.6 × 4.1 × 5.7 cm well-circumscribed mass in the right adrenal gland and a 3.3 × 2.9 × 3.2 cm rounded lesion in the left adrenal gland. Plasma metanephrines were 35 pg/ml (<57), plasma normetanephrines were 19,693 pg/ml (<148), and 24 h urine normetanephrines were 532 mcg/24 h (67–503). MIBG scan showed MIBG localization in bilateral retroperitoneal masses, compatible with bilateral pheochromocytoma.

The patient underwent a bilateral adrenalectomy and was subsequently placed on glucocorticoid and mineralocorticoid replacement. He was weaned off of his antihypertensive medications over time. Genetic testing was pursued and revealed a c.250G > A (Val84Met) missense mutation in VHL. Interestingly, this patient's mutation had not previously been characterized but was consistent with a diagnosis of von Hippel-Lindau syndrome in the patient's clinical context. An ophthalmology examination was notable only for hypertensive retinopathy. Routine surveillance for additional VHL manifestations was performed. Two years later, his plasma metanephrines became elevated, and imaging revealed a right paraspinal paraganglioma which was subsequently resected. The patient is now 17 years old and has not yet developed any other clinical manifestations of VHL.

Von Hippel-Lindau (VHL) is caused by a mutation in the *VHL* gene which is transmitted in an autosomal dominant pattern of inheritance with variable penetrance. VHL is responsible for 50% of all PHEO in pediatric patients and is associated with noradrenergic PHEO/PGL, CNS and retinal hemangioblastomas, renal cysts and clear cell renal cell carcinoma, pancreatic cysts and cystadenomas, endolymphatic sac tumors, papillary cystadenomas of the epididymis in males and of the round ligament in females, and nonfunctioning pancreatic endocrine tumors. While PHEO typically presents in the third decade in patients with VHL, it can be the first manifestation of VHL in the pediatric population [12]. In a study of 273 patients with VHL, 25% initially presented with a PHEO in childhood, with the youngest age at diagnosis being 5.5 years [13]. In pediatric patients with known VHL, screening for PHEO should begin at age 5. Patients with VHL are at a 38% risk for developing a recurrence or a second PGL [11].

VHL can be characterized into four subtypes. VHL type 1 is typically due to mutations related to disrupted folding of the VHL protein. Clinical manifestations include retinal angioma, CNS hemangioblastoma, renal cell carcinoma, pancreatic cysts, and neuroendocrine tumors. The risk of PHEO in VHL type 1 is quite low. In contrast, VHL type 2 is characterized by a high risk for PHEO and is often due to a missense mutation. VHL type 2 can be divided into three subtypes: type 2A has a low risk for renal carcinoma; type 2B has a high risk for renal carcinoma; and type 2C is typically associated only with pheochromocytoma and an absence of other VHL manifestations [14].

Familial PGL Syndromes

Case *A 13-year-old male was referred to a pediatric endocrinologist for management of an SDHD gene mutation identified on genetic screening. His father had recently died secondary to complications from bilateral carotid paraganglioma resection. Postmortem genetic diagnosis in the father revealed the presence of an SDHD mutation. At the patient's initial visit, he denied headaches, diaphoresis, palpitations, anxiety, flushing, hematuria, hoarse voice, tinnitus, or diarrhea. His heart rate was noted to be 128 beats per minute, and his blood pressure was 115/75 mmHg. Screening labs revealed elevated plasma normetanephrines of 957 pg/mL (<146 pg/mL), elevated total plasma metanephrines of 999 ng/mL (<205 pg/mL), elevated 24 h urine normetanephrine of 1916 mcg/24 h (67–503 mcg/24 h), and elevated chromogranin A of 36 ng/mL (<15 ng/mL).*

The patient underwent a whole-body MRI which uncovered a T2 hyperintense and T1 isointense 2.4 cm right periaortic mass with mild mass effect and anterolateral displacement of the inferior vena cava with narrowing of the right renal artery. The presence of the periaortic mass was atypical in this patient; 40–50% of PGL in SDHD mutations are located in the head and neck, and 15% are located in the chest, abdomen, and pelvis. Compared to patients with SDHB mutations, patients with an SDHD mutation have an odds ratio of 24 for a head and neck PGL. Additionally, in SDHD mutations, tumors are less likely to produce catecholamines than with other genetic mutations. Given the unusual location of the mass that would require an open laparotomy for resection, a PET scan was obtained to further characterize the lesion which revealed an avid focus of increased radiotracer uptake corresponding to the mass identified on MRI. Preoperatively, the patient was started on doxazosin, and the mass was resected uneventfully. At follow-up, urine and plasma catecholamine levels were within or lower than the normal ranges, and blood pressure and heart rate remained normal off medication.

Familial PGL syndromes (PGL1-4) are due to mutations in one of the subunits of the mitochondrial complex II succinate dehydrogenase (SDH) enzyme gene. All of these syndromes are associated with PGL, and some include a risk of PHEO as well. PGL1 and PGL3 are due to mutations in *SDHD* and *SDHC*, respectively. Both conditions are associated primarily with parasympathetic head and neck paragangliomas. PGL2 is caused by mutations in *SDH5* (also known as *SDHAF2*) and is associated with parasympathetic head and neck PGL. PGL4 is due to an *SDHB* mutation and most commonly causes sympathetic PGLs in the thorax, abdomen, or pelvis. PGLs associated with the *SDHB* mutation have the highest likelihood of malignant potential [15].

Neurofibromatosis Type 1

Neurofibromatosis type 1 (NF1) is an autosomal dominant disease characterized by at least two of the following: six or more café au lait macules, two or more neurofibromas of one plexiform neurofibroma, axillary or inguinal freckling, optic glioma, two or more Lisch nodules, bony lesions such as thickening of the long-bone cortex or pseudoarthrosis, and a first-degree relative with NF1. Approximately 3% of individuals with NF1 have PHEO or PGL, and these lesions are more likely to be malignant than are sporadic PHEO or PGL [16, 17]. Prevalence estimates may be higher in those undergoing active surveillance for PHEO/PGL.

Multiple Endocrine Neoplasia Types 2A and 2B

Multiple endocrine neoplasia types 2A and 2B (MEN2A and MEN2B) are caused by a mutation in one of several codons of the *RET* proto-oncogene. MEN2A is comprised of medullary thyroid carcinoma, hyperparathyroidism secondary to parathyroid gland hyperplasia, PHEO, and Hirschsprung's disease. The phenotype of MEN2B includes medullary thyroid carcinoma in virtually all patients, PHEO, gastrointestinal ganglioneuromatosis, and a marfanoid body habitus. Up to 50% of individuals with *MEN2* will manifest a PHEO [18]. PHEO can be the first clinical manifestation of MEN2A [19]. The risk of development of PHEO in patients with MEN2A and MEN2B is mutation dependent. Those with mutations in codon 634, exon 11 have a particularly high risk of PHEO [20].

Diagnosis

Diagnosis of PHEO and PGL in pediatrics can be challenging as symptoms are often vague and the lesions are relatively rare. Evaluation begins with the measurement of plasma metanephrines or 24 h urine metanephrines [3, 21]. Liquid chromatography-tandem mass spectrometric (LC-MS/MS) methodology is preferred for these assays as it is more sensitive than the enzyme-linked immunoassay method and it is less prone to interference by other drugs compared to the high-performance liquid chromatography method [22]. Furthermore, age-specific reference ranges should be used, as there are age and body size related increases in normal catecholamine levels [23]. The upper limit of the pediatric reference range is lower than that of the adult range and could lead to a missed diagnosis if only adult ranges are used [24]. Levels that are four times higher than the upper limit of the reference range are considered highly suspicious of a PHEO or functional PGL with nearly 100% probability. Several drugs, including acetaminophen, tricyclic antidepressants, phenoxybenzamine, and decongestants, are known to interfere with plasma and urine metanephrine testing, and these medications should be avoided prior to sample collection. Blood samples should be collected after lying in a supine position for 30 min to avoid and false positive results from stress or exercise. Careful instructions must be given in order to ensure that urine samples are collected for a full 24 h.

Chromogranin A is a protein present in the chromaffin cells of the adrenal medulla and co-secreted from storage granules with catecholamines. It serves as a tumor marker for PHEO and may correlate with malignant potential [3, 25, 26]. In addition, it may be a useful marker of SDH-related paragangliomas which are often clinically silent [3].

Children who have positive biochemical results should undergo imaging studies to determine the location of the lesion. While PHEO and PGL can be imaged via CT or MRI, MRI is preferable in children due to the substantial radiation exposure associated with CT scans. MRI of the abdomen and pelvis is recommended first, followed by imaging of the head and neck if the initial MRI does not yield a diagnosis. MIBG scanning can be considered if no lesion is identified on MRI; however, care should be taken to ensure the patient is not on medications that can impair MIBG uptake.

Malignancy

Though rare, PHEO and PGL can be malignant, with malignancy more common in pediatric versus adult patients. Malignancy is defined as distant metastatic lesions in locations where PGL no not typically occur. Twelve percent of PHEO and PGL in pediatrics are malignant [2]. Features more commonly associated with malignancy are extra-adrenal location, tumor necrosis, coarse nodularity of the primary tumor, absence of hyaline nodules, high proliferative index, and size larger than 5 cm [27].

Treatment

Treatment of pediatric PHEO and PGL requires a careful and thoughtful medical and surgical management plan in order to reduce risk of complications. There is a lack of pediatric-specific evidence-based recommendations on which to guide treatment.

Functional lesions require initiation of medical therapy prior to surgery, and a comprehensive preoperative plan should be created in collaboration with an experienced pediatric surgeon and pediatric anesthesiologist. The major preoperative goals are to normalize blood pressure and heart rate, restore volume depletion, and prevent intra- and postoperative hemodynamic instability and cardiac dysrhythmias that can result from surgical manipulation of the lesion.

Typically, medical therapy should be initiated 1–2 weeks prior to the planned surgery and start with an α-adrenergic blocker. α blockade will lower blood pressure and decrease vascular tone; however, postoperatively there is risk for hypotension. The use of a noncompetitive α blocker, such as phenoxybenzamine, is associated with a higher postoperative risk of hypotension than the use of a selective α_1 blocker. However, selective α_1 blockers can cause postural hypotension after just one dose but are associated with less reflex tachycardia than a noncompetitive α blocker. If α blockade fails to achieve normotension, addition of a calcium channel blocker can be considered [3, 28, 29].

After adequate α blockade is achieved, therapy with a β-blocker should be initiated if reflex tachycardia is present. β-blockers should never be used in isolation due to unopposed catecholamine effects at α receptors that could lead to worsening hypertension [21]. Fluids or volume expansion is important in the immediate preoperative period in an attempt to reduce severe postoperative hypotension [29].

There is also risk of hyperglycemia preoperatively as pancreatic α stimulation inhibits insulin release. All patient should have glucose levels monitored and insulin therapy initiated if necessary [28].

Surgical resection can proceed once preoperative hemodynamic stability is achieved. Intraoperatively, careful management of the patient's hemodynamic and fluid status by an experienced anesthesiologist is necessary. Postoperatively, patients should be monitored closely for hypotension, hypoglycemia, and in the case of bilateral PHEO resection – glucocorticoid and mineralocorticoid deficiency [21, 28]. Cortical-sparing procedures are favored in the clinical scenario of bilateral PHEO to minimize the chance that the patient will require lifelong glucocorticoid and mineralocorticoid replacement [30].

For patients with malignant disease or distant metastasis, additional techniques such as radiation therapy, radiofrequency ablation, MIBG, and chemotherapy can be considered but are not well studied in children [3].

For nonfunctional lesions, surgical resection remains the mainstay, but careful attention remains necessary as the location of PGLs can be near important structures such as the carotid sheath.

Genetic Testing Considerations

As there are many hereditary disorders associated with PHEO and PGL, genetic testing should proceed in a systematic manner. In patients presenting with PHEO, mutations in VHL are most common. In patients presenting with PGL or malignant disease, *SDHB* should be considered. Testing for RET mutation is recommended in patients with PHEO and an adrenergic predominance. Screening for genetic mutations in the context of a family history should occur in all first-degree relatives by age 10 years or at least 10 years prior to the earliest age at diagnosis in the family [15]. If the mutation is known, directed testing can be pursued in family members. Those who are found to have a pathogenic variant can proceed with screening per recommended surveillance protocols. Testing should always be ordered in consultation with an experienced geneticist or genetic counselor.

Conclusions

PHEO and PGL are very rare in the pediatric population, and a high index of suspicion is necessary to make the diagnosis. Knowledge of the strong association with genetic mutations is imperative as this can have direct impact on a patient's management and risk of associated conditions. A multidisciplinary team inclusive of endocrinologists, surgeons, anesthesiologists, and genetic counselors specifically trained in the management of pediatric PHEO and PGL is necessary for optimal patient care.

References

1. Beltsevich DG, Kuznetsov NS, Kazaryan AM, Lysenko MA. Pheochromocytoma surgery: epidemiologic peculiarities in children. World J Surg. 2004;28(6):592–6.
2. Barontini M, Levin G, Sanso G. Characteristics of pheochromocytoma in a 4- to 20-year-old population. Ann N Y Acad Sci. 2006;1073:30–7.
3. Waguespack SG, Rich T, Grubbs E, et al. A current review of the etiology, diagnosis, and treatment of pediatric pheochromocytoma and paraganglioma. J Clin Endocrinol Metab. 2010;95(5):2023–37.
4. Neumann HP, Bausch B, McWhinney SR, et al. Germ-line mutations in nonsyndromic pheochromocytoma. N Engl J Med. 2002;346(19):1459–66.
5. Babic B, Patel D, Aufforth R, et al. Pediatric patients with pheochromocytoma and paraganglioma should have routine preoperative genetic testing for common susceptibility genes in addition to imaging to detect extra-adrenal and metastatic tumors. Surgery. 2017;161(1):220–7.
6. Pamporaki C, Hamplova B, Peitzsch M, et al. Characteristics of Pediatric vs adult Pheochromocytomas and Paragangliomas. J Clin Endocrinol Metab. 2017;102(4):1122–32.
7. Wyszynska T, Cichocka E, Wieteska-Klimczak A, Jobs K, Januszewicz PA. Single pediatric center experience with 1025 children with hypertension. Acta Paediatr (Oslo, Norway : 1992). 1992;81(3):244–6.
8. Grinsell MM, Norwood VF. At the bottom of the differential diagnosis list: unusual causes of pediatric hypertension. Pediatr Nephrol (Berlin, Germany). 2009;24(11):2137–46.
9. Pham TH, Moir C, Thompson GB, et al. Pheochromocytoma and paraganglioma in children: a review of medical and surgical management at a tertiary care center. Pediatrics. 2006;118(3):1109–17.
10. Sullivan J, Groshong T, Tobias JD. Presenting signs and symptoms of pheochromocytoma in pediatric-aged patients. Clin Pediatr. 2005;44(8):715–9.

11. Bausch B, Wellner U, Bausch D, et al. Long-term prognosis of patients with pediatric pheochromocytoma. Endocr Relat Cancer. 2014;21(1):17–25.
12. Barontini M, Dahia PL. VHL disease. Best Pract Res Clin Endocr Metab. 2010;24(3):401–13.
13. Aufforth RD, Ramakant P, Sadowski SM, et al. Pheochromocytoma screening initiation and frequency in von Hippel-Lindau syndrome. J Clin Endocrinol Metab. 2015;100(12):4498–504.
14. Glasker S, Neumann HPH, Koch CA, Vortmeyer AO. Von Hippel-Lindau disease. In: De Groot LJ, Chrousos G, Dungan K, et al., editors. Endotext. South Dartmouth: MDText.com, Inc.; 2000.
15. Kirmani S, Young WF. Hereditary paraganglioma-pheochromocytoma syndromes. In: Pagon RA, Adam MP, Ardinger HH, et al., editors. GeneReviews(R). Seattle: University of Washington, Seattle University of Washington, Seattle. GeneReviews is a registered trademark of the University of Washington, Seattle. All rights reserved; 1993.
16. Gruber LM, Erickson D, Babovic-Vuksanovic D, Thompson GB, Young WF Jr, Bancos I. Pheochromocytoma and paraganglioma in patients with neurofibromatosis type 1. Clin Endocrinol. 2017;86(1):141–9.
17. Bausch B, Borozdin W, Clinical NHP. Genetic characteristics of patients with neurofibromatosis type 1 and pheochromocytoma. N Engl J Med. 2006;354(25):2729–31.
18. Marquard J, Eng C. Multiple endocrine neoplasia type 2. In: Pagon RA, Adam MP, Ardinger HH, et al., editors. GeneReviews(R). Seattle: University of Washington, Seattle University of Washington, Seattle. All rights reserved; 1993.
19. Pacak K, Ilias I, Adams KT, Eisenhofer G. Biochemical diagnosis, localization and management of pheochromocytoma: focus on multiple endocrine neoplasia type 2 in relation to other hereditary syndromes and sporadic forms of the tumour. J Intern Med. 2005;257(1):60–8.
20. Eng C, Clayton D, Schuffenecker I, et al. The relationship between specific RET proto- oncogene mutations and disease phenotype in multiple endocrine neoplasia type 2. International RET mutation consortium analysis. JAMA. 1996;276(19):1575–9.
21. Lenders JW, Duh QY, Eisenhofer G, et al. Pheochromocytoma and paraganglioma: an endocrine society clinical practice guideline. J Clin Endocrinol Metab. 2014;99(6):1915–42.
22. Weismann D, Peitzsch M, Raida A, et al. Measurements of plasma metanephrines by immunoassay vs liquid chromatography with tandem mass spectrometry for diagnosis of pheochromocytoma. Eur J Endocrinol. 2015;172(3):251–60.
23. Parra A, Ramirez del Angel A, Cervantes C, Sanchez M. Urinary excretion of catecholamines in healthy subjects in relation to body growth. Acta Endocrinol. 1980;94(4):546–51.
24. Weise M, Merke DP, Pacak K, Walther MM, Eisenhofer G. Utility of plasma free metanephrines for detecting childhood pheochromocytoma. J Clin Endocrinol Metab. 2002;87(5):1955–60.
25. Grossrubatscher E, Dalino P, Vignati F, et al. The role of chromogranin a in the management of patients with phaeochromocytoma. Clin Endocrinol. 2006;65(3):287–93.
26. Bilek R, Safarik L, Ciprova V, Vlcek P, Lisa L, Chromogranin A. A member of neuroendocrine secretory proteins as a selective marker for laboratory diagnosis of pheochromocytoma. Physiol Res. 2008;57(Suppl 1):S171–9.
27. Chrisoulidou A, Kaltsas G, Ilias I, Grossman AB. The diagnosis and management of malignant phaeochromocytoma and paraganglioma. Endocr Relat Cancer. 2007;14(3):569–85.
28. Hack HA. The perioperative management of children with phaeochromocytoma. Paediatr Anaesth. 2000;10(5):463–76.
29. Pacak K. Preoperative management of the pheochromocytoma patient. J Clin Endocrinol Metab. 2007;92(11):4069–79.
30. Ludwig AD, Feig DI, Brandt ML, Hicks MJ, Fitch ME, Cass DL. Recent advances in the diagnosis and treatment of pheochromocytoma in children. Am J Surg. 2007;194(6):792–6. discussion 796–7

Chapter 6
Diagnosis of Pheochromocytoma and Paraganglioma

William F. Young

Evolution in the Clinical Presentation of Pheochromocytoma and Paraganglioma

There has been a dramatic evolution in both the clinical presentation and the methods used to diagnose pheochromocytoma and paraganglioma (PPGL) over the past nine decades. From 1926 to 1945, the diagnosis of PPGL was suspected based on signs and symptoms of catecholamine hypersecretion and confirmed with exploratory laparotomy [1, 2]. In an effort to preoperatively diagnose PPGL in symptomatic patients, provocative stimulation tests (e.g., with histamine) were developed in the 1940s and suppression tests (e.g., with phentolamine) in the 1950s [2–6]. The first reliable biochemical tests to detect PPGL were developed in the 1960s—measurement of 24-h urinary excretion of the catecholamine metabolites vanillylmandelic acid and total metanephrines [7–9]. Additional biochemical testing advances followed and included high-performance liquid chromatography (HPLC) with electrochemical detection (EC) for measurement of catecholamines in blood and urine in the 1970s [10], measurement of plasma fractionated metanephrines by HPLC-EC in the 1990s [11, 12], and the stable isotope dilution liquid chromatography/tandem mass spectrometry method preceded by solid phase extraction of metanephrines in 2002 [13, 14].

Advances in imaging studies to localize PPGL paralleled the development of biochemical testing and included aortography and selective angiography before 1960 [15, 16], intravenous pyelography and adrenal vein sampling from 1960 to 1980 [17–20], cross-sectional imaging with computed tomography starting in the mid-1970s [21, 22], ^{131}I-metaiodobenzylguanidine scintigraphy in 1981 [23],

W. F. Young (✉)
Division of Endocrinology, Diabetes, Metabolism, and Nutrition, Mayo Clinic, Rochester, MN, USA
e-mail: young.william@mayo.edu

L. Landsberg (ed.), *Pheochromocytomas, Paragangliomas and Disorders of the Sympathoadrenal System*, Contemporary Endocrinology,
https://doi.org/10.1007/978-3-319-77048-2_6

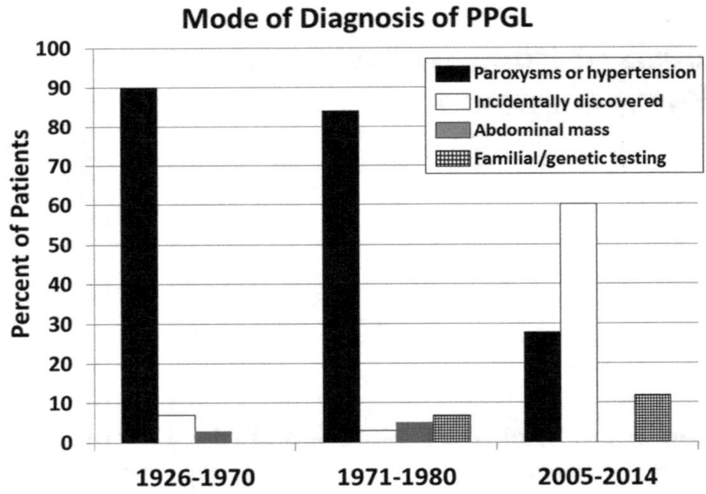

Fig. 6.1 The mode of diagnosis of pheochromocytoma and paraganglioma at Mayo Clinic has evolved over the nine decades since the first patient was operated in 1926 [1]. Before 1980, incidental discovery was very infrequent (3–7%) and occurred at surgery [29, 30]. In the most recent patient series (2005–2014), incidental discovery occurred prior to surgery on cross-sectional imaging in 60% of patients [31]

abdominal magnetic resonance imaging in the 1980s [24, 25], positron emission tomography (PET) with 18F-flurodexoyglucose in the 1990s, and gallium 68 (68-Ga) 1,4,7,10-tetraazacyclododecane-1,4,7,10-tetraacetic acid (DOTA)-octreotate PET-CT in 2015 [26–28].

The advances in biochemical testing and imaging have dramatically impacted how PPGLs are detected and diagnosed in 2018. For example, in the Mayo Clinic series of 138 patients with PPGL who were treated surgically between 1926 and 1970, 90% were detected because of symptoms (paroxysms or hypertension) (Fig. 6.1) [29]. That experience is contrasted with the 106 patients with PPGL who were treated surgically at Mayo Clinic between 1971 and 1980, where 84% were detected because of either paroxysms or hypertension and 7% were diagnosed because of family testing for familial forms of PPGL [30]. Whereas, in the most recent report from Mayo Clinic on 222 patients with PPGL who were treated surgically between 2005 and 2014, the most common (60%) reason for detecting PPGL was incidental discovery on cross-sectional imaging done for other reasons (Fig. 6.1) [31]. A symptom-based (paroxysms or hypertension) diagnosis of PPGL was made in only 28% of patients, followed by genetic case detection testing in 12% [31]. PPGLs discovered due to symptoms were larger than those discovered incidentally or by genetic case detection testing (5.3 vs. 4.7 vs. 3.6 cm, respectively; $P = 0.04$) [31]. In addition, some of the patients with PPGL who were diagnosed based on an incidental finding on cross-sectional imaging actually had normal biochemical testing but went to surgery based on the adrenal mass imaging phenotype (Fig. 6.2).

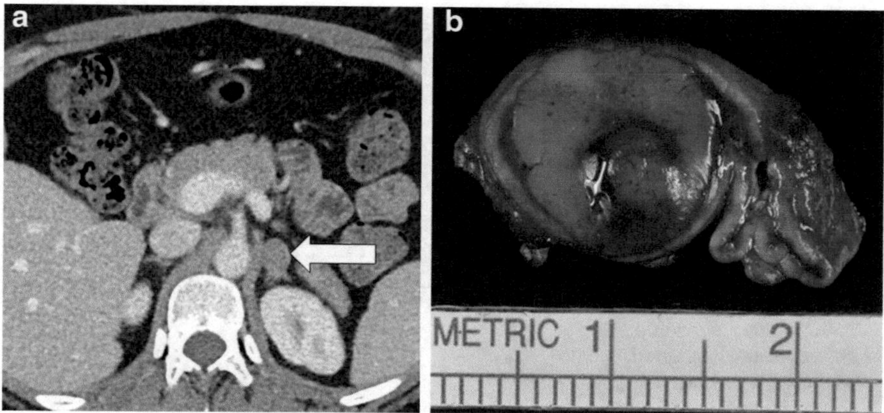

Fig. 6.2 An incidentally discovered "prebiochemical" adrenal pheochromocytoma. This 39-year-old woman had a computed tomographic (CT) scan of the abdomen performed for the evaluation of small bowel ileus following an ectopic pregnancy. She was normotensive and asymptomatic. *Panel A*, CT scan axial image shows a 1.9 × 1.3 cm left adrenal mass with a precontrast CT attenuation of 39 Hounsfield units and a 40% contrast washout at 10 min. The biochemical testing for pheochromocytoma was normal and included plasma metanephrine, 0.44 nmol/L (normal, <0.5); plasma normetanephrine, 0.82 nmol/L (normal, <0.9); and 24-h urine norepinephrine, 29 μg (normal, <170); epinephrine, 8.6 μg (normal, <35); dopamine, 22 μg (normal, <700); metanephrine, 325 μg (normal, <400); and normetanephrine, 557 μg (normal, <900). However, because the CT imaging phenotype was consistent with pheochromocytoma and because the plasma and urine metanephrine levels were high-normal, she was advised to have laparoscopic left adrenalectomy. *Panel B*, cut section of a 2.0 × 1.4 × 1.2 cm left adrenal pheochromocytoma. The postoperative plasma fractionated metanephrines dropped further into the reference ranges: metanephrine, <0.3 nmol/L (normal, <0.5) and normetanephrine, 0.53 nmol/L (normal, <0.9)

Differential Diagnosis for Patients with Symptomatic Presentations

Numerous disorders can cause signs and symptoms that may prompt the clinician to test for PPGL. The disorders span much of medicine and include endocrine disorders (e.g., primary hypogonadism), cardiovascular disorders (e.g., idiopathic orthostatic hypotension), psychologic disorders (e.g., panic disorder), pharmacologic causes (e.g., withdrawal from an adrenergic inhibitor), neurologic disorders (e.g., postural orthostatic tachycardia syndrome), and a wide variety of other disorders (e.g., mast cell disease) (Table 6.1) [32]. Indeed, most patients tested for a catecholamine-secreting tumor do not have it. In addition, levels of fractionated catecholamines and metanephrines may be elevated in several clinical scenarios, including withdrawal from medications or drugs (e.g., clonidine, alcohol), acute illness (e.g., subarachnoid hemorrhage, migraine headache, preeclampsia), and administration of many medications (e.g., tricyclic antidepressants, buspirone, and antipsychotic agents) (Table 6.2) [33].

Table 6.1 Differential diagnosis of pheochromocytoma-type spells

Endocrine causes
Carbohydrate intolerance
Hyperadrenergic spells
Hypoglycemia
Pancreatic tumors (e.g., insulinoma)
Pheochromocytoma
Primary hypogonadism (menopausal syndrome)
Thyrotoxicosis
Cardiovascular causes
Angina
Cardiovascular deconditioning
Labile essential hypertension
Orthostatic hypotension
Paroxysmal cardiac arrhythmia
Pulmonary edema
Renovascular disease
Syncope (e.g., vasovagal reaction)
Psychological causes
Factitious (e.g., drugs, Valsalva)
Hyperventilation
Severe anxiety and panic disorders
Somatization disorder
Pharmacologic causes
Chlorpropamide alcohol flush
Combination of a monoamine oxidase inhibitor and a decongestant
Illegal drug ingestion (cocaine, phencyclidine, lysergic acid diethylamide)
Sympathomimetic drug ingestion
Vancomycin ("red man syndrome")
Withdrawal of adrenergic inhibitor
Neurologic causes
Autonomic neuropathy
Cerebrovascular insufficiency
Diencephalic epilepsy (autonomic seizures)
Migraine headache
Postural orthostatic tachycardia syndrome
Stroke
Other causes
Carcinoid syndrome
Mast cell disease
Recurrent idiopathic anaphylaxis
Unexplained flushing spells

Table 6.2 Medications that may increase measured levels of fractionated catecholamines and metanephrines

Tricyclic antidepressants (including cyclobenzaprine)
Levodopa
Buspirone and antipsychotic agents
Serotonin and noradrenaline reuptake inhibitors
Monoamine oxidase inhibitors
Drugs containing adrenergic receptor agonists (e.g., decongestants)
Amphetamines
Prochlorperazine
Reserpine
Withdrawal from clonidine and other drugs (e.g., illicit drugs, ethanol)
Illicit drugs (e.g., cocaine, heroin)

Case Detection Testing

Pheochromocytoma should be suspected in patients who have one or more of the following:

- Hyperadrenergic spells (e.g., self-limited episodes of nonexertional forceful palpitations, diaphoresis, headache, tremor, or pallor)
- Resistant hypertension
- A familial syndrome that predisposes to catecholamine-secreting tumors (e.g., multiple endocrine neoplasia type 2, neurofibromatosis type 1, and von Hippel-Lindau disease)
- A family history of pheochromocytoma
- An incidentally discovered adrenal mass with imaging characteristics consistent with pheochromocytoma [34, 35]
- Pressor response during anesthesia, surgery, or angiography
- Onset of hypertension at a young age (e.g., <20 years)
- Idiopathic dilated cardiomyopathy [36]

Measurement of Fractionated Metanephrines and Catecholamines in Blood and Urine

The diagnosis of PPGL should be confirmed biochemically by the presence of increased concentrations of fractionated metanephrines and catecholamines in urine or plasma [33, 37, 38]. The metabolism of catecholamines is primarily intratumoral, with formation of metanephrine from epinephrine and normetanephrine from norepinephrine [39]. Most laboratories now measure fractionated catecholamines (dopamine, norepinephrine, and epinephrine) and fractionated metanephrines (metanephrine and normetanephrine) by high-performance liquid chromatography with electrochemical detection or by tandem mass spectrometry [13]. These techniques have overcome the problems with fluorometric analysis, which include false-positive results caused by α-methyldopa, labetalol, sotalol, and imaging contrast agents.

At Mayo Clinic, the most reliable case-detection strategy is measurement of fractionated metanephrines and catecholamines in a 24-h urine collection (sensitivity, 98%; specificity, 98%) [37, 38, 40]. Some groups have advocated that plasma fractionated metanephrines should be a first-line test for PPGL [41, 42] because the predictive value of a negative test is extremely high, and a normal result excludes PPGL except in patients with early preclinical disease (Fig. 6.2) and those with strictly dopamine-secreting neoplasms [40]. A plasma test is also attractive because of simplicity. Although measurement of plasma fractionated metanephrines has a diagnostic sensitivity of 96% to 100%, the diagnostic specificity at some centers is suboptimal at 85–89%; the diagnostic specificity falls to 77% in patients older than 60 years [40, 43, 44]. Because of the suboptimal specificity, it has been estimated that 97% of patients with hypertension seen in a tertiary care clinic who have plasma normetanephrine measurements above the reference range will not have a PPGL, resulting in excessive healthcare expenditures because of subsequent imaging and potentially inappropriate surgery [43, 45]. The suboptimal specificity of plasma fractionated metanephrines may be due in part to the setting used for blood sampling—most centers use seated venipuncture in non-fasting patients. Whereas, obtaining blood from an indwelling cannula after 30 min of supine rest in a fasted patient improves specificity [33, 46–48]. However, the supine rested indwelling cannula approach to testing plasma fractionated metanephrines is associated with increased cost and simply not available at most clinics and hospitals. Thus, the most reliable initial case detection test for PPGL is a 24-h urine for fractionated metanephrines and catecholamines (Fig. 6.3) [38, 42].

The 24-h urine collection for fractionated metanephrines and catecholamines should include measurement of urinary creatinine to verify an adequate collection. The diagnostic cutoffs for most 24-h urinary fractionated metanephrines assays are based on normal ranges derived from normotensive volunteer reference groups, and this can result in excessive false-positive test results. For example, in normotensive laboratory volunteers, the 95th percentiles are 428 μg for normetanephrine and 200 μg for metanephrine, whereas the corresponding values in individuals who are being tested for pheochromocytoma as part of routine clinical practice but who do not have the neoplasm are, respectively, 71% and 51% higher than those of the normal volunteers (<900 μg for normetanephrine and <400 μg for metanephrines) [38]. These higher cutoffs for normality are what is used at Mayo Clinic, and levels above these cutoffs are considered abnormal, and those patients merit further investigation for PPGL.

Although it is preferred that patients not receive any medication during the diagnostic evaluation, treatment with most medications may be continued. Tricyclic antidepressants are the drugs that interfere most frequently with the interpretation of

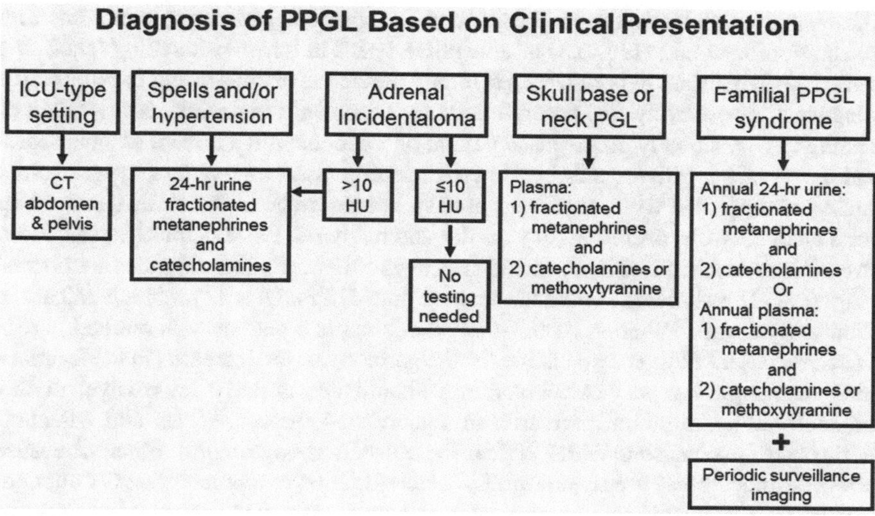

Fig. 6.3 Diagnostic pathways for detection of pheochromocytoma and paraganglioma based on clinical presentation and setting. Abbreviations used: *HU* Hounsfield units, *ICU* intensive care unit, *PGL* paraganglioma, and *PPGL* pheochromocytoma and paraganglioma

24-h urinary catecholamines and metabolites. To effectively screen for catecholamine-secreting tumors, treatment with tricyclic antidepressants and other psychoactive agents listed in Table 6.2 should be tapered and discontinued at least 2 weeks before any hormonal assessments. There are clinical situations for which it is contraindicated to discontinue certain medications (e.g., antipsychotics), and if case-detection testing is positive, then CT or MRI of the abdomen and pelvis would be needed to exclude a catecholamine-secreting tumor. Furthermore, catecholamine secretion may be appropriately increased in situations of physical stress or illness (e.g., stroke, myocardial infarction, congestive heart failure) [49, 50]. There are no reliable reference ranges for fractionated metanephrines or catecholamines in patients requiring intensive care unit hospitalization. Thus, the best case detection test for PPGL in the patient in the intensive care unit is CT with contrast of the abdomen and pelvis (Fig. 6.3) [50].

Test Selection and Clinical Context

The clinician should assess the relative likelihood of pheochromocytoma in each patient. Decisions for the type of test performed may be subject to clinical availability, cost, clinical experience of the ordering physician, and the local laboratory. If measurement of plasma fractionated metanephrines is performed, a positive test result in a high-risk setting (such as a genetically predisposed individual or an individual with a known adrenal mass with imaging characteristics consistent with pheochromocytoma) (Fig. 6.3) or a negative result in a low-risk setting (such as a patient with resistant hypertension) is highly predictive of confirming or refuting the diagnosis, respectively. However, a negative result in a high-risk setting (such as testing of a genetically predisposed patient or a patient with a known vascular adrenal mass) or a positive result in a low-risk setting (such as resistant hypertension) must be interpreted with some caution [51]. For example, in the clinical context of an incidentally discovered 2-cm vascular adrenal mass, PPGL should be suspected even if measurements of fractionated metanephrines and catecholamines are normal (Fig. 6.2). The clinician should understand that all PPGLs are "prebiochemical" in their early stages. Whereas, if the clinical context is a patient with marked paroxysms, then if a PPGL is responsible for the paroxysms, the increases in the fractionated metanephrines and catecholamines should be similarly impressive; in this clinical setting, minimal increases in fractionated metanephrines and catecholamines are not consistent with PPGL as the cause for the symptoms. Finally, because pheochromocytomas are lipid poor, lipid-rich (defined as a precontrast CT attenuation of $\leq$10 Hounsfield units) adrenal incidentalomas cannot be pheochromocytomas, and biochemical testing is not needed (Fig. 6.3).

Most of the false-positive test results are due to mild elevations in plasma normetanephrine or 24-hr urinary normetanephrine (the later when the reference range is based on normotensive laboratory volunteers rather than patients proven to not have PPGL). When appropriate cutoffs are used, all patients with abnormal test results should be evaluated further for possible PPGL. If a patient is taking a medication (Table 6.2) that could result in the abnormal laboratory value, it should be tapered and discontinued. Testing can be repeated 3–4 weeks later.

Measurement of 24-h urinary dopamine or plasma dopamine and methoxytyramine can be very useful in detecting the rare tumor with selective dopamine hypersecretion, because plasma and urine metanephrine fractions are not direct metabolites of dopamine and may be normal in the setting of a dopamine-secreting tumor [40, 52–54]. Two additional clinical pearls regarding dopamine-secreting tumors include the following: they tend to be located in the skull base and neck (Fig. 6.3), and because of the renal sulfation of dopamine, the 24-h urinary dopamine may be falsely normal, and measurement of plasma catecholamines or methoxytyramine is indicated (Fig. 6.3).

Other Tests That Have Been Used to Assess for Pheochromocytoma and Paraganglioma

Because of poor overall accuracy in testing for pheochromocytoma, measurement of plasma catecholamines no longer has a role except to detect dopamine-secreting paragangliomas [12]. Chromogranin A is stored and released from dense-core secretory granules of neuroendocrine cells and is increased in 80% of patients with pheochromocytoma [55]. Chromogranin A is not specific for pheochromocytoma, and elevations may be seen with other neuroendocrine tumors [56–58]. The 24-h urinary vanillylmandelic acid excretion has poor diagnostic sensitivity and specificity compared with fractionated 24-h urinary metanephrines.

The high false-positive rate for plasma fractionated catecholamines and fractionated metanephrines triggered the development of a confirmatory test, the clonidine suppression test [59]. This test is intended to distinguish between PPGL and false-positive increases in plasma fractionated catecholamines and metanephrines. Clonidine is a centrally acting α2-adrenergic receptor agonist that normally suppresses the release of catecholamines from neurons but does not affect the catecholamine secretion from a pheochromocytoma. Clonidine (0.3 mg) is administered orally, and plasma fractionated catecholamines or metanephrines are measured before and 3 h after the dose [60, 61]. In patients with essential hypertension, plasma catecholamine concentrations decrease (norepinephrine + epinephrine <500 pg/mL or >50% decrease in norepinephrine), as do plasma normetanephrine concentrations (into the normal range or >40% decrease) [62]. However, these concentrations remain increased in patients with pheochromocytoma.

Special Situations

Renal Failure Measurements of urinary catecholamines and metabolites may be invalid if the patient has advanced kidney disease [63]. Serum chromogranin A levels have poor diagnostic specificity in these patients [64]. In patients without PPGL who are receiving hemodialysis, plasma norepinephrine and dopamine concentrations are increased threefold and twofold above the upper limit of normal, respectively [65]. However, standard reference ranges can be used for interpreting plasma epinephrine concentrations [66]. Therefore, when patients with renal failure have plasma norepinephrine concentrations more than threefold above the upper normal limit or epinephrine concentrations greater than the upper normal limit, PPGL should be suspected. The findings of one study suggested that plasma concentrations of fractionated metanephrines are increased approximately twofold in patients with renal failure and may be useful in the biochemical evaluation of patients with marked chronic kidney disease or renal failure [67]. However, the results of an earlier study suggested that concentrations of plasma fractionated metanephrines could not distinguish between 10 patients with pheochromocytoma and 11 patients with end-stage renal disease who required long-term hemodialysis [68].

Factitious Pheochromocytoma As with other similar disorders, factitious pheochromocytoma can be very difficult to confirm [69, 70]. The patient usually has a medical background. The patient may "spike" the 24-h urine container, or the catecholamines may be administered systemically [71, 72].

References

1. Mayo CH. Paroxysmal hypertension with tumor of retroperitoneal nerve. JAMA. 1927;89:1047–50.
2. Young WF Jr. Endocrine hypertension: then and now. Endocr Pract. 2010;16(5):888–902.
3. Kvale WF. Headache and paroxysmal hypertension: observations before and after the surgical removal of a pheochromocytoma. Sug Clin North Am. 1944;24:922–33.
4. Gifford RW Jr, Roth GM, Kvale WF. Evaluation of new adrenolytic drug (regitine) as test for pheochromocytoma. J Am Med Assoc. 1952;149(18):1628–34.
5. Grimson KS, Longino FH, et al. Treatment of a patient with a pheochromocytoma; use of an adrenolytic drug before and during operation. J Am Med Assoc. 1949;140(16):1273.
6. Roth GM, Flock EV, Kvale WF, Waugh JM, Ogg J. Pharmacologic and chemical tests as an aid in the diagnosis of pheochromocytoma. Circulation. 1960;21:769–78.
7. Pisano JJ. A simple analysis for normetanephrine and metanephrine in urine. Clin Chim Acta. 1960;5:406–14.
8. Sheps SG, Tyce GM, Flock EV, Maher FT. Current experience in the diagnosis of pheochromocytoma. Circulation. 1966;34(3):473–83.
9. Armstrong MD, Mc MA, Shaw KN. 3-Methoxy-4-hydroxy-D-mandelic acid, a urinary metabolite of norepinephrine. Biochim Biophys Acta. 1957;25(2):422–3.
10. Moyer TP, Jiang NS, Tyce GM, Sheps SG. Analysis for urinary catecholamines by liquid chromatography with amperometric detection: methodology and clinical interpretation of results. Clin Chem. 1979;25(2):256–63.
11. Lenders JW, Eisenhofer G, Armando I, Keiser HR, Goldstein DS, Kopin IJ. Determination of metanephrines in plasma by liquid chromatography with electrochemical detection. Clin Chem. 1993;39(1):97–103.
12. Lenders JW, Keiser HR, Goldstein DS, Willemsen JJ, Friberg P, Jacobs MC, et al. Plasma metanephrines in the diagnosis of pheochromocytoma. Ann Intern Med. 1995;123(2):101–9.
13. Taylor RL, Singh RJ. Validation of liquid chromatography-tandem mass spectrometry method for analysis of urinary conjugated metanephrine and normetanephrine for screening of pheochromocytoma. Clin Chem. 2002;48(3):533–9.
14. Singh RJ. Advances in metanephrine testing for the diagnosis of pheochromocytoma. Clin Lab Med. 2004;24(1):85–103.
15. Snyder CH, Rutledge LJ. Pheochromocytoma: localization by aortography. Pediatrics. 1955;15(3):312–6.
16. Pendergrass HP, Tristan TA, Blakemore WS, Sellers AM, Jannetta PJ, Murphy JJ. Roentgen technics in the diagnosis and localization of pheochromocytoma. Radiology. 1962;78:725–37.
17. Pickering RS, Hartman GW, Weeks RE, Sheps SG, Hattery RR. Excretory urographic localization of adrenal cortical tumors and pheochromocytomas. Radiology. 1975;114(2):345–9.
18. Hardy JD, Carter T, Turner MD. Catechol amine metabolism: peripheral plasma levels of epinephrine (E) and norepinephrine (NE) during laparotomy under different types of anesthesia in dogs, during operation in man (including adrenal vein sampling), and before and following resection of a pheochromocytoma associated with von Recklinghausen's neurofibromatosis. Ann Surg. 1959;150:666–83.
19. Mahoney EM, Friend DG, Dexter L, Harrison JH. Localization of (adrenal and extra-adrenal) Pheochromocytomas by vena Caval blood sampling. Surg Forum. 1963;14:495–6.
20. Harrison TS, Freier DT. Pitfalls in the technique and interpretation of regional venous sampling for localizing pheochromocytoma. Surg Clin North Am. 1974;54(2):339–47.
21. Stewart BH, Bravo EL, Haaga J, Meaney TF, Tarazi R. Localization of pheochromocytoma by computed tomography. N Engl J Med. 1978;299(9):460–1.
22. Laursen K, Damgaard-Pedersen K. CT for pheochromocytoma diagnosis. AJR Am J Roentgenol. 1980;134(2):277–80.
23. Sisson JC, Frager MS, Valk TW, Gross MD, Swanson DP, Wieland DM, et al. Scintigraphic localization of pheochromocytoma. N Engl J Med. 1981;305(1):12–7.

24. Moon KL Jr, Hricak H, Crooks LE, Gooding CA, Moss AA, Engelstad BL, et al. Nuclear magnetic resonance imaging of the adrenal gland: a preliminary report. Radiology. 1983;147(1):155–60.
25. Fink IJ, Reinig JW, Dwyer AJ, Doppman JL, Linehan WM, Keiser HR. MR imaging of pheochromocytomas. J Comput Assist Tomogr. 1985;9(3):454–8.
26. Janssen I, Blanchet EM, Adams K, Chen CC, Millo CM, Herscovitch P, et al. Superiority of [68Ga]-DOTATATE PET/CT to other functional imaging modalities in the localization of SDHB-associated metastatic Pheochromocytoma and Paraganglioma. Clin Cancer Res. 2015;21(17):3888–95.
27. Janssen I, Chen CC, Millo CM, Ling A, Taieb D, Lin FI, et al. PET/CT comparing (68) Ga-DOTATATE and other radiopharmaceuticals and in comparison with CT/MRI for the localization of sporadic metastatic pheochromocytoma and paraganglioma. Eur J Nucl Med Mol Imaging. 2016;43(10):1784–91.
28. Janssen I, Chen CC, Taieb D, Patronas NJ, Millo CM, Adams KT, et al. 68Ga-DOTATATE PET/CT in the localization of head and neck Paragangliomas compared with other functional imaging modalities and CT/MRI. J Nucl Med. 2016;57(2):186–91.
29. Remine WH, Chong GC, Van Heerden JA, Sheps SG, Harrison EG Jr. Current management of pheochromocytoma. Ann Surg. 1974;179(5):740–8.
30. van Heerden JA, Sheps SG, Hamberger B, Sheedy PF 2nd, Poston JG, ReMine WH. Pheochromocytoma: current status and changing trends. Surgery. 1982;91(4):367–73.
31. Gruber L, Young WF. Bancos I. Pheochromocytoma characteristics and behavior differ depending on method of discovery 2017 Endocrine Society Annual Meeting. 2017.
32. Young WF Jr, Maddox DE. Spells: in search of a cause. Mayo Clin Proc. 1995;70(8):757–65.
33. Lenders JW, Duh QY, Eisenhofer G, Gimenez-Roqueplo AP, Grebe SK, Murad MH, et al. Pheochromocytoma and paraganglioma: an endocrine society clinical practice guideline. J Clin Endocrinol Metab. 2014;99(6):1915–42.
34. Young WF Jr. Clinical practice. The incidentally discovered adrenal mass. N Engl J Med. 2007;356(6):601–10.
35. Wachtel H, Cerullo I, Bartlett EK, Roses RE, Cohen DL, Kelz RR, et al. Clinicopathologic characteristics of incidentally identified pheochromocytoma. Ann Surg Oncol. 2015;22(1):132–8.
36. Brilakis ES, Young WF Jr, Wilson JW, Thompson GB, Munger TM. Reversible catecholamine-induced cardiomyopathy in a heart transplant candidate without persistent or paroxysmal hypertension. J Heart Lung Transplant. 1999;18(4):376–80.
37. Kudva YC, Sawka AM, Young WF Jr. Clinical review 164: the laboratory diagnosis of adrenal pheochromocytoma: the Mayo Clinic experience. J Clin Endocrinol Metab. 2003;88(10):4533–9.
38. Perry CG, Sawka AM, Singh R, Thabane L, Bajnarek J, Young WF Jr. The diagnostic efficacy of urinary fractionated metanephrines measured by tandem mass spectrometry in detection of pheochromocytoma. Clin Endocrinol. 2007;66(5):703–8.
39. Eisenhofer G, Kopin IJ, Goldstein DS. Catecholamine metabolism: a contemporary view with implications for physiology and medicine. Pharmacol Rev. 2004;56(3):331–49.
40. Sawka AM, Jaeschke R, Singh RJ, Young WF Jr. A comparison of biochemical tests for pheochromocytoma: measurement of fractionated plasma metanephrines compared with the combination of 24-hour urinary metanephrines and catecholamines. J Clin Endocrinol Metab. 2003;88(2):553–8.
41. Lenders JW, Pacak K, Walther MM, Linehan WM, Mannelli M, Friberg P, et al. Biochemical diagnosis of pheochromocytoma: which test is best? JAMA. 2002;287(11):1427–34.
42. Eisenhofer G, Pacak K, Maher ER, Young WF, de Krijger RR. Pheochromocytoma. Clin Chem. 2013;59(3):466–72.
43. Sawka AM, Thabane L, Gafni A, Levine M, Young WF Jr. Measurement of fractionated plasma metanephrines for exclusion of pheochromocytoma: can specificity be improved by adjustment for age? BMC Endocr Disord. 2005;5(1):1.

44. Chen Y, Xiao H, Zhou X, Huang X, Li Y, Xiao H, et al. Accuracy of plasma free Metanephrines in the diagnosis of Pheochromocytoma and Paraganglioma: a systematic review and meta-analysis. Endocr Pract. 2017;23(10):1169–77.
45. Sawka AM, Gafni A, Thabane L, Young WF Jr. The economic implications of three biochemical screening algorithms for pheochromocytoma. J Clin Endocrinol Metab. 2004;89(6):2859–66.
46. Darr R, Pamporaki C, Peitzsch M, Miehle K, Prejbisz A, Peczkowska M, et al. Biochemical diagnosis of phaeochromocytoma using plasma-free normetanephrine, metanephrine and methoxytyramine: importance of supine sampling under fasting conditions. Clin Endocrinol. 2014;80(4):478–86.
47. Darr R, Kuhn M, Bode C, Bornstein SR, Pacak K, Lenders JWM, et al. Accuracy of recommended sampling and assay methods for the determination of plasma-free and urinary fractionated metanephrines in the diagnosis of pheochromocytoma and paraganglioma: a systematic review. Endocrine. 2017;56(3):495–503.
48. de Jong WH, Eisenhofer G, Post WJ, Muskiet FA, de Vries EG, Kema IP. Dietary influences on plasma and urinary metanephrines: implications for diagnosis of catecholamine-producing tumors. J Clin Endocrinol Metab. 2009;94(8):2841–9.
49. Wortsman J, Frank S, Cryer PE. Adrenomedullary response to maximal stress in humans. Am J Med. 1984;77(5):779–84.
50. Amar L, Eisenhofer G. Diagnosing phaeochromocytoma/paraganglioma in a patient presenting with critical illness: biochemistry versus imaging. Clin Endocrinol. 2015;83(3):298–302.
51. Sawka AM, Prebtani AP, Thabane L, Gafni A, Levine M, Young WF Jr. A systematic review of the literature examining the diagnostic efficacy of measurement of fractionated plasma free metanephrines in the biochemical diagnosis of pheochromocytoma. BMC Endocr Disord. 2004;4(1):2.
52. Eisenhofer G, Goldstein DS, Sullivan P, Csako G, Brouwers FM, Lai EW, et al. Biochemical and clinical manifestations of dopamine-producing paragangliomas: utility of plasma methoxytyramine. J Clin Endocrinol Metab. 2005;90(4):2068–75.
53. Peitzsch M, Prejbisz A, Kroiss M, Beuschlein F, Arlt W, Januszewicz A, et al. Analysis of plasma 3-methoxytyramine, normetanephrine and metanephrine by ultraperformance liquid chromatography-tandem mass spectrometry: utility for diagnosis of dopamine-producing metastatic phaeochromocytoma. Ann Clin Biochem. 2013;50(Pt 2):147–55.
54. Rao D, Peitzsch M, Prejbisz A, Hanus K, Fassnacht M, Beuschlein F, et al. Plasma methoxytyramine: clinical utility with metanephrines for diagnosis of pheochromocytoma and paraganglioma. Eur J Endocrinol. 2017;177(2):103–13.
55. Algeciras-Schimnich A, Preissner CM, Young WF Jr, Singh RJ, Grebe SK. Plasma chromogranin a or urine fractionated metanephrines follow-up testing improves the diagnostic accuracy of plasma fractionated metanephrines for pheochromocytoma. J Clin Endocrinol Metab. 2008;93(1):91–5.
56. Wang YH, Yang QC, Lin Y, Xue L, Chen MH, Chen J. Chromogranin a as a marker for diagnosis, treatment, and survival in patients with gastroenteropancreatic neuroendocrine neoplasm. Medicine (Baltimore). 2014;93(27):e247.
57. Young WF Jr. Phaeochromocytoma: how to catch a moonbeam in your hand. Eur J Endocrinol. 1997;136(1):28–9.
58. Stridsberg M, Husebye ES. Chromogranin a and chromogranin B are sensitive circulating markers for phaeochromocytoma. Eur J Endocrinol. 1997;136(1):67–73.
59. Bravo EL, Tarazi RC, Fouad FM, Vidt DG, Gifford RW Jr. Clonidine-suppression test: a useful aid in the diagnosis of pheochromocytoma. N Engl J Med. 1981;305(11):623–6.
60. Sjoberg RJ, Simcic KJ, Kidd GS. The clonidine suppression test for pheochromocytoma. A review of its utility and pitfalls. Arch Intern Med. 1992;152(6):1193–7.
61. McHenry CM, Hunter SJ, McCormick MT, Russell CF, Smye MG, Atkinson AB. Evaluation of the clonidine suppression test in the diagnosis of phaeochromocytoma. J Hum Hypertens. 2011;25(7):451–6.

62. Eisenhofer G, Goldstein DS, Walther MM, Friberg P, Lenders JW, Keiser HR, et al. Biochemical diagnosis of pheochromocytoma: how to distinguish true- from false-positive test results. J Clin Endocrinol Metab. 2003;88(6):2656–66.
63. Godfrey JA, Rickman OB, Williams AW, Thompson GB, Young WF Jr. Pheochromocytoma in a patient with end-stage renal disease. Mayo Clin Proc. 2001;76(9):953–7.
64. Bech PR, Ramachandran R, Dhillo WS, Martin NM, Bloom SR. Quantifying the effects of renal impairment on plasma concentrations of the neuroendocrine neoplasia biomarkers chromogranin a, chromogranin B, and cocaine- and amphetamine-regulated transcript. Clin Chem. 2012;58(5):941–3.
65. Stumvoll M, Radjaipour M, Seif F. Diagnostic considerations in pheochromocytoma and chronic hemodialysis: case report and review of the literature. Am J Nephrol. 1995;15(2):147–51.
66. Morioka M, Yuihama S, Nakajima T, Kobayashi T, Sone A, Furukawa Y, et al. Incidentally discovered pheochromocytoma in long-term hemodialysis patients. Int J Urol. 2002;9(12):700–3.
67. Eisenhofer G, Huysmans F, Pacak K, Walther MM, Sweep FC, Lenders JW. Plasma metanephrines in renal failure. Kidney Int. 2005;67(2):668–77.
68. Marini M, Fathi M, Vallotton M. Determination of serum metanephrines in the diagnosis of pheochromocytoma. Ann Endocrinol (Paris). 1994;54(5):337–42.
69. Stern TA, Cremens CM. Factitious pheochromocytoma. One patient history and literature review. Psychosomatics. 1998;39(3):283–7.
70. Pessina AC, Bisogni V, Fassina A, Rossi GP. Munchausen syndrome: a novel cause of drug-resistant hypertension. J Hypertens. 2013;31(7):1473–6.
71. Sawka AM, Singh RJ, Young WF Jr. False positive biochemical testing for pheochromocytoma caused by surreptitious catecholamine addition to urine. Endocrinologist. 2001;11:421–3.
72. Chidakel AR, Pacak K, Eisenhofer G, Lawrence JE, Ayala AR. Utility of plasma free metanephrines in diagnosis of factitious pheochromocytoma. Endocr Pract. 2006;12(5):568–71.

Chapter 7
Localization of Pheochromocytoma and Paraganglioma

Carla B. Harmath and Hatice Savas

Introduction

Located above the kidneys, the adrenal glands are usually inverted Y, V, or T shaped, routinely identified on computed tomography (CT) and magnetic resonance (MR). If a pheochromocytoma is clinically suspected or diagnosed, the goal of imaging is lesion localization, and there are anatomical and functional imaging modalities used for it. CT is the anatomical modality of choice to identify an adrenal lesion or the less common extra-adrenal paragangliomas, and MIBG is the most widely used functional modality. Paragangliomas are frequently intra-abdominal [1], located in the retroperitoneum near the level of the SMA origin or aortic bifurcation (organ of Zuckerkandl) [2]. However, they may be encountered anywhere from the base of the skull to the urinary bladder, as they develop in the chromaffin tissue of the sympathetic nervous system [1], and other common extra-adrenal locations include the bladder wall, other parts of the retroperitoneum, heart, mediastinum, carotid body, and glomus jugulare body. MR is an alternate anatomical imaging localization modality; however, due to the greater availability, better spatial resolution and lower cost, CT remains the preferred initial anatomical imaging modality. The functional imaging modalities include nuclear medicine exams with a variety of radiotracers, including more specific tracers being developed as the biochemical characteristics of the tumors are better understood.

C. B. Harmath (✉)
Department of Radiology, Section of Abdominal Imaging, The University of Chicago Medicine, Chicago, IL, USA
e-mail: CHarmath@radiology.bsd.uchicago.edu

H. Savas
University of Chicago Medicine, Chicago, IL, USA

L. Landsberg (ed.), *Pheochromocytomas, Paragangliomas and Disorders of the Sympathoadrenal System*, Contemporary Endocrinology,
https://doi.org/10.1007/978-3-319-77048-2_7

Adrenal pheochromocytomas are rarely found as incidental lesions on imaging exams, and usually if so, they are larger than 4 cm and most with subclinical hyperfunction [3, 4]. Functional tumors can be very small, found to be as small as 5 mm [5]. Both CT and MR can be used as initial modalities to investigate for a pheochromocytoma or a paraganglioma given their optimal spatial resolution which facilitates surgical planning and can be helpful in evaluating metastasis and multifocal abdominal lesions. Functional imaging has higher specificity and has great value as a confirmatory exam, and also to evaluate the possibility of multifocal lesions in abdominal and extra-abdominal locations, as well as metastatic lesions. In pediatric patients a similar imaging algorithm is followed; however, MRI is preferred over CT due to lack of ionizing radiation, and ultrasound (US) may have a role as the initial imaging step for evaluation of the adrenal glands.

Imaging Modalities, Imaging Protocols, and Lesion Characteristics

The imaging modalities for identification and characterization of adrenal pheochromocytoma and paragangliomas can be divided in anatomical and functional as above. Anatomical modalities include computed tomography, magnetic resonance imaging, and ultrasound. Functional modalities include traditional gamma emission nuclear medicine exams such as metaiodobenzylguanidine (MIBG) labeled with ^{123}Iodine or ^{131}Iodine (^{123}I- and ^{131}I-MIBG), octreotide labeled with ^{111}Indium (^{111}In-Octreoscan), and positron-emission tomography (PET) exams using different PET tracers such as ^{18}Fluorine-flourodeoxyglucose (^{18}F-FDG) and ^{68}Gallium (^{68}Ga) DOTA agents.

Computed Tomography (CT)

Computed tomography is the anatomical imaging modality of choice for the localization of pheochromocytomas and paragangliomas. It is widely available, fast and has a relative lower cost compared with other imaging modalities such as MRI. The typical protocol used for CT imaging of the adrenal gland includes thin section images (3 mm or less), with a three-phase acquisition: initial non-contrast study, followed by an intravenous contrast-enhanced exam at the portal venous phase (usually about 70 s after intravenous contrast administration), and a 15-min delayed exam to evaluate the enhancement washout pattern of the adrenal lesion. The goal of the three-phase exam is to attempt characterization of other potential coincidental adrenal lesions such as adenomas, myelolipomas, and cysts. Each of the phases can be obtained in less than 1 min with the current multislice detector capabilities of CT. This markedly decreases potential respiratory motion artifact and allows for

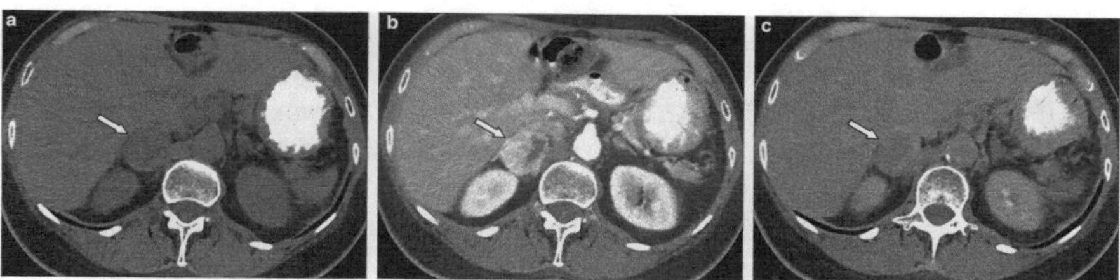

Fig. 7.1 Triphasic CT adrenal protocol. (**a**) Non-contrast axial image demonstrating a low attenuation mass in the right adrenal gland (arrow). (**b**) Post-contrast image demonstrating heterogeneous enhancement. (**c**) 15-min delayed phase image; the lesion "washes out" but not to the same degree expected for an adrenal adenoma. This was surgically removed with the pathologic diagnosis of pheochromocytoma

visualization and characterization of small lesions. CT images have the advantage of their excellent spatial resolution, and the ability of reconstructing the obtained axial images in different planes, facilitating surgical planning. However, it does involve ionizing radiation and includes the use of iodinated contrast, which can be detrimental to renal function and is not recommended for patients with renal insufficiency, especially on those with a glomerular filtration rate of less than 30 ml/min/1.73m^2. In patients with decreased renal function, a single-phase non-contrast exam can be obtained, with the goal of identifying an adrenal or extra-adrenal mass, with the aid of functional modalities for further characterization. There was a theoretical concern of eliciting a hypertensive crisis when giving CT ionic iodinated contrast to patients with pheochromocytoma. However, more recent studies have demonstrated safety of the current nonionic iodinated contrasts [4, 6, 7]. The use of oral contrast is not universal for the CT adrenal protocol; however, it may be helpful in differentiating an extra-adrenal lesion from unopacified bowel. Oral neutral contrast, such as low suspension barium (Volumen™), or regular barium may be used. The radiation dose for a three-phase CT exam of the abdomen will vary. Newer scanners use strategies such as modulation to adjust the radiation dose to the body part to be scanned and patient's body mass index (BMI) [8]. The effective radiation dose can be calculated by multiplying the dose length product (DLP), which is basically the radiation output of the scanner, by a conversion factor of 0.015 for the abdomen and pelvis. The average DLP for the three-phase adrenal CT protocol is of 1100 milligray cm (mGycm), or approximately 16.5 mSv effective dose (note 1 mGy = 1milisievert, or 1 mSv). For reference, the average effective radiation dose for a routine CT scan of the abdomen is of 10 mSv, and the effective radiation dose of a two-view chest X-ray (posterior-anterior and lateral) is of 0.06 mSv [9]. Background cosmic radiation at ground level is 0.06 μS.

On CT pheochromocytomas commonly present as a round, well-circumscribed, homogenous soft tissue mass, usually greater than 3 cm upon discovery [10]. The lesion usually has soft tissue attenuation greater than 10 Hounsfield units (Fig. 7.1). However, the appearance can vary widely, and lesions can contain macroscopic fat, a typical feature of adrenal myelolipomas, or can have enough intracellular lipid to mimic adenomas, with a non-contrast CT density of 10 or less HU. They can have cystic degeneration and calcification and can also hemorrhage [1], which are non-specific features and can be seen with adrenocorticocarcinomas and metastasis. They are usually unilateral and benign, but bilateral and malignant pheochromocytomas are found in up to 10% of the cases [2].

Following intravenous contrast they typically enhance avidly, but often heterogeneously, mostly due to areas of cystic degeneration. These degenerated areas show no enhancement although the associated thickened septae and wall do enhance (Fig. 7.1). The 15-min delayed CT exam, routinely used to characterize adrenal adenomatous versus non-adenomatous lesions due to their enhancement washout characteristics, is not always reliable as some pheochromocytomas may wash out to the same degree and therefore mimic adenoma [11, 12]. This was demonstrated in as many as 33% of the cases in some series [13, 14]. Therefore pheochromocytomas have nonspecific CT imaging characteristics [14], and their CT appearance overlaps with that of other adrenal lesions. So when looking for a pheochromocytoma, if an adrenal lesion with imaging characteristics of an adenoma or myelolipoma is identified, further imaging with functional characterization should be sought for confirmation [15].

Magnetic Resonance Imaging (MRI)

Magnetic resonance imaging has the advantage of no ionizing radiation for the acquisition of images. However, the acquisition is longer, and several different imaging series are required for an exam to be completed. Even with the current technology, most exams take 20 min or longer to be completed. The usual MRI adrenal protocol usually includes contrast media, which is gadolinium based, and not iodine based as is the case with CT exams. Gadolinium-based agents have the advantage of being safe in patients with allergy to the CT iodinated contrasts; however, some gadolinium based contrast agents may be unsafe in patients with renal failure, not due to toxic effects on the renal function, but due to the potential development of nephrogenic systemic sclerosis (NSF). Additionally, there have been reports of gadolinium deposition in the brain of patients who had undergone contrast enhanced MRI exams in the past.

A typical MRI protocol for adrenal imaging includes fat-saturated T1 weighted images with and without contrast, T2 weighted images with and without fat saturation, and in- and out-phase imaging. Acquisitions are usually performed on both the axial and coronal planes. Diffusion-weighted sequences are part of most protocols, predominantly in academic centers. MRI is more costly and involves several breath holds, which can be difficult to tolerate for some patients. The currently available MRI bore diameters can be claustrophobic to some patients. Open MRI scanners would not be recommended as their resolution can be significant lower, limiting the visualization of the adrenal glands. In general the spatial resolution of MRI is still lower than most CT exams; however, MRI has greater tissue resolution in MRI

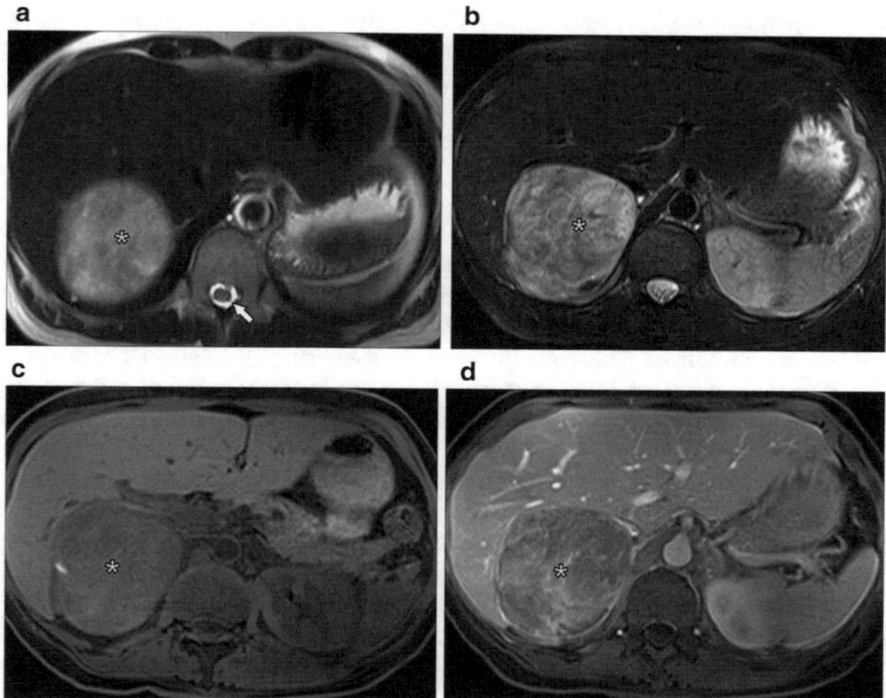

Fig. 7.2 MRI images of a typical pheochromocytoma. (**a**) T2WI images: a right adrenal pheochromocytoma (*) with high signal, similar to the fluid in the stomach (S) and cerebral spinal fluid (blue arrow). (**b**) T2WI with fat saturation: redemonstrating the high T2 signal of the pheochromocytoma. (**c**) T1WI with fat saturation: slightly heterogeneous low signal in the pheochromocytoma. (**d**) T1WI post-contrast fat-saturated image: the pheochromocytoma enhances heterogeneously

compared with CT (i.e., tissues of different quality such as the fluid and muscle, e.g., have a very different appearance), and this may help differentiate lesion patterns.

The typical MRI appearance of pheochromocytomas is always described as a well-circumscribed lesion with bright signal on T2 weighted images, with signal greater than fat and approximating fluid, and low signal, isointense to the muscle and hypointense to the liver in T1 weighted images [16]. Following contrast, the lesion avidly enhances, and this MRI appearance is also known as "light bulb." Unfortunately this so-called "light bulb" appearance is reported to be seen in 10–66% of the cases in some series [1, 4, 11, 16] (Fig. 7.2). Typically they are lipid poor and do not drop in signal (i.e., have a darker appearance) on the out-of-phase imaging compared with the in-phase imaging, which is a usual feature of lipid-rich adenomas. Occasionally, pheochromocytomas can have drop in signal when there is intralesional fat degeneration, but usually the observed drop in signal is minimal, unlike adenomas in which the drop in signal is more extensive and uniform. When the lesions have large areas of fat degeneration, these can be seen as macroscopic fat, a characteristic feature of myelolipomas, confusing the imaging diagnosis, as can happen on the CT exam [14]. MRI can demonstrate several prominent tumor vessels within pheochromocytomas, resulting in a salt and pepper appearance on T2 weighted images due to flow void effects.

Ultrasound (US)

Ultrasound is a portable imaging modality of low cost, without associated ionizing radiation. Ultrasonography is not a reliable imaging modality for the investigation of pheochromocytomas in adults, as often the adrenal glands and retroperitoneum are not well visualized. This modality is very dependent on the patient's body habitus, as well as the expertise of the technologist or physician performing the exam. When encountering a suprarenal lesion on ultrasound in adults, it can be difficult to ascertain its adrenal origin. When visible, the sonographic appearance of pheochromocytomas on US is usually a round and well-circumscribed lesion, isoechoic or hypoechoic to the adjacent renal parenchyma. As on CT and MRI, the lesion can vary widely in appearance. It can have cystic degeneration, which is seen as anechoic areas with or without low-level internal echoes; calcifications, which can be seen as echogenic areas with posterior acoustic shadowing; and hemorrhage, which is usually homogeneously or heterogeneously echogenic, but not shadowing. A single lesion may have a combination of these features. In children the modality can be very helpful as retroperitoneal masses such as those of adrenal origin are better detected given the patient's smaller body habitus. Contrast-enhanced ultrasound (CEUS) has been used in Europe and more recently approved for use in the United States; however, there has been little documentation on their value evaluating the adrenal glands. The currently available literature describes the potential value of adrenal lesion evaluation with CEUS in children with von Hippel-Lindau syndrome: an adrenal pheochromocytoma investigated with this modality demonstrated enhancement of the solid component of the lesion similar to the hepatic enhancement. Moreover, the benefits of US for the pediatric population include the advantage of not using ionizing radiation needed for the CT exams, nor requiring sedation, as usually necessary for MRI exams [17]. It may be a promising modality for the routine screening in syndromic patients.

Functional Imaging

Functional imaging aims to localize the lesion by focusing on the biochemical characteristics of the pheochromocytomas and paragangliomas. An intravenously injected radioactive tracer tailored to specific biochemical steps of the lesion will be uptaken by the primary tumor as well as the well-differentiated metastases. Tracers used in the functional imaging of pheochromocytomas and paragangliomas use the pathways of catecholamine synthesis, storage, and secretion for lesion detection. In the recent years, besides traditional nuclear medicine studies, there has been great progress in molecular imaging and positron-emission tomography (PET) with the increased knowledge of the specific biochemical characteristics of pheochromocytomas, especially those associated with syndromes [18]. With this knowledge, new radiotracers and radiopharmaceuticals have evolved for the localization and detection of these lesions. Gamma emitters ^{131}Iodine- and ^{123}Iodine-labeled metaiodobenzylguanidine (^{131}I-MIBG and ^{123}I-MIBG) and PET tracers ^{18}Fluorine-fluorodopamine (^{18}F-FDA), ^{18}Fluorine-fluorodihydroxyphenylalanine (^{18}F-FDOPA), and ^{11}C-hydroxyephedrine PET (HED PET) are radiotracers associated with the catecholamine production pathways. Somatostatin receptor binding mechanism agents include ^{111}Indium-pentetreotide as a gamma emitter and ^{68}Gallium-labeled somatostatin analog peptides (^{68}Ga-DOTA-TOC, ^{68}Ga-DOTA-NOC, ^{68}Ga-DOTA-TATE) as PET agents. The ^{68}Gallium agents have been available in Europe for almost a decade, and ^{68}Ga-DOTA-TATE has been FDA approved for clinical use in the United States in June 2016. A third category imaging agent is of ^{18}Fluorine-flourodeoxyglucose (^{18}F-FDG), which is a glucose analog and widely available [19].

Functional Imaging Approach

MIBG: MIBG scintigraphy has been the first line and most commonly used molecular imaging modality for paragangliomas for years [20]. It is a norepinephrine analog and useful to detect the tumors that arise from the embryologic precursors of the sympathetic nervous system, particularly the neural crest cells. It uses the cell membrane norepinephrine transporter (NET) to enter the cells. Once inside the cell, it is transported and stored in the presynaptic neurosecretory granules via the vesicular monoamine transporter 1 (VMAT1) [21].

The normal distribution of the MIBG includes the heart, salivary glands, spleen, and adrenal medulla. It is also uptaken by tumors containing adrenergic and neuroblastic tissues, due to rich adrenergic innervation. MIBG can be labeled with either ^{131}Iodine or ^{123}Iodine. The ^{123}I-labeled MIBG has lower radiation and higher image quality than the ^{131}I, with high sensitivity especially with the use of SPECT-SPECT/CT [22]. $^{123/131}$I-MIBG can be uptaken by the pheochromocytomas that arise in the chromaffin cells of the adrenal medulla (85% of the lesions) and by the 15% extra-adrenal tumors (paragangliomas), arising in chromaffin cells mainly along the aorta and in the neck. The sensitivity of MIBG may be lower in metastatic paragangliomas due to dedifferentiation of VMAT1 receptors in the metastatic tissue [23]. It has been also suggested that the sensitivity of MIBG is lower in the head and neck paragangliomas due to under-expression of VMAT1 receptors in these tumors [24].

The usual radiopharmaceutical doses for the MIBG exam are of 40–80 MBq (1.2–2.2 mCi) for ^{131}I-MIBG and 400 MBq (10.8 mCi) for ^{123}I-MIBG. After intravenous administration of the radiolabeled MIBG, whole-body imaging is usually obtained at 4–24 h and may be delayed up to 48 or 72 h (Fig. 7.3). The hybrid imag-

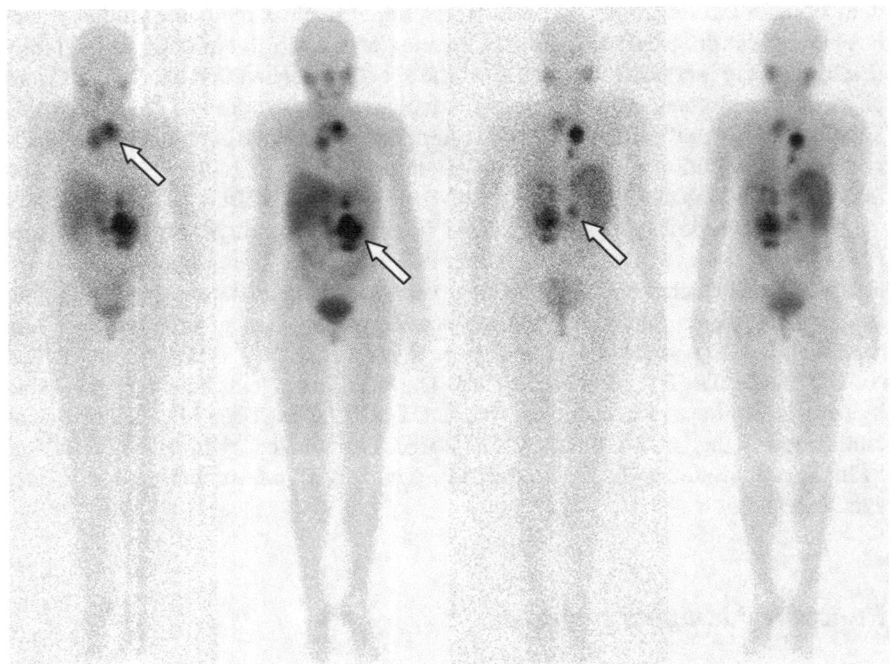

Fig. 7.3 ^{123}I-labeled MIBG imaging with 24 h and 48 h anterior and posterior views. There is physiologic accumulation of the radiotracer in the salivary glands, nasal mucosa, liver, gastrointestinal tract, and urinary bladder. However, there are multiple additional sites of abnormal tracer accumulation in the abdomen and chest, including a large focus in the left mid abdomen, consistent with metastatic pheochromocytoma (arrows)

ing with a single-photon emission computed tomography (SPECT) or SPECT/CT improves anatomical localization and increases the sensitivity, specificity, diagnostic accuracy, and reader agreement for the exam (Fig. 7.3). The sensitivity of MIBG ranges from 80% to 90% in the detection of pheochromocytomas, and the specificity ranges from 90% to 100% [2]. The one important point in the clinical practice is that MIBG has well-known drug interactions due to its cellular mechanism. Therefore a careful drug history should be obtained with specific attention to tricyclic antidepressant, cocaine, alpha- and beta-blocker labetalol, calcium channel blockers, and sympathomimetics, among others. Upon consultation with the referring physician, the interfering drugs should be withheld, if possible, for an adequate time prior imaging [25]. In addition, thyroid blockade with nonradioactive aqueous iodine, also known as Lugol's solution, or potassium iodide/perchlorate should be done prior to imaging.

MIBG imaging is commonly used for detection of pheochromocytoma but also detects neuroblastomas and several other tumors including carcinoid tumors and medullary thyroid carcinomas. Overall, based on the recommendations, ^{123}I-labeled MIBG is the first line of choice given the more favorable dosimetry and better image quality which allows an accurate anatomical localization by the use of SPECT/CT hybrid systems. The ^{131}I-MIBG is widely available and is preferred due to the possibility of obtaining delayed scans. In addition, ^{131}I-MIBG should be the choice if estimation of tumor uptake and retention measurement is required for MIBG therapy planning [25].

Octreoscan: ^{111}Indium-pentetreotide (Octreoscan) scintigraphy is another method to image pheochromocytomas and paragangliomas. It binds to somatostatin receptors (SSR), which are expressed in paragangliomas. There are five different SSR subtypes, and ^{111}In-pentetreotide binds to SSR types 2, 3, and 5, with the highest affinity to SSR2 and SSR5 [26]. In general practice ^{111}In-pentetreotide scintigraphy is less preferred method than ^{123}I-MIBG to detect adrenal paraganglioma due to lesser sensitivity. It has somewhat higher sensitivity to detect metastatic disease and head and neck paragangliomas than the primary adrenal lesions, most likely due to higher somatostatin receptor expression in the lesions. The imaging protocol is 5 mCi (185 MBq) of the radiopharmaceutical given intravenously and whole-body imaging performed at 4 and 24 h after the injection (Fig. 7.4). The Octreoscan sensitivity is of 75–90% for pheochromocytomas and paragangliomas.

Overall, MIBG and Octreoscan are complementary, as 50% of pheochromocytomas are seen with both agents, about 25% only with MIBG and 25% with octreotide [2].

PET imaging: There are several PET agents to image pheochromocytomas and paragangliomas. With recent tremendous developments of new agents for positron imaging, besides detection of the primary and metastatic tumors, there are very promising results for personalized radioisotope targeted treatment with peptide receptor radionuclide therapy (PRRT). The new tracers help to better understand the tumor characteristics as well as to predict and follow up the response to therapy. PET imaging has also several additional advantages including high spatial and temporal resolutions, relatively short half-life of the tracers, and quantitative measurements which may be helpful on follow-up and assessment of therapy response.

^{18}F-FDG (fluorine-18-2-fluoro-2-deoxy-D-glucose) is the most common PET tracer and has been successfully used in oncology, including in paragangliomas [27] (Fig. 7.5). It is a glucose analog and uses glucose transporters to enter the cells. The imaging is based on the fact that tumor cells have increased glucose metabolism than the most cells in the body and there is increased transporter activity in the tumor cells as well. Once inside the cell, it undergoes phosphorylation by hexokinase to become ^{18}F-FDG-6P and is then trapped in the cell. Overall, the high FDG avidity indicates high glucose metabolism and high aggressiveness. FDG avidity is greater for the malignant than for the benign pheochromocytomas. It has been suggested that FDG PET is especially useful in defining the distribution of those pheochromocytomas that fail to concentrate MIBG. ^{18}F-FDG PET is preferred for poorly differentiated neoplasms with loss of neuroendocrine features [27].

Somatostatin receptor (SSR) PET/CT imaging with ^{68}Gallium-DOTA peptides, more specifically ^{68}Gallium DOTATATE, is highly sensitive for imaging diagnosis and staging of neuroendocrine tumors [28] (Fig. 7.6). The synthesis of this tracer does not require an on-site cyclotron. ^{68}Gallium (^{68}Ga) has a physical half-life of

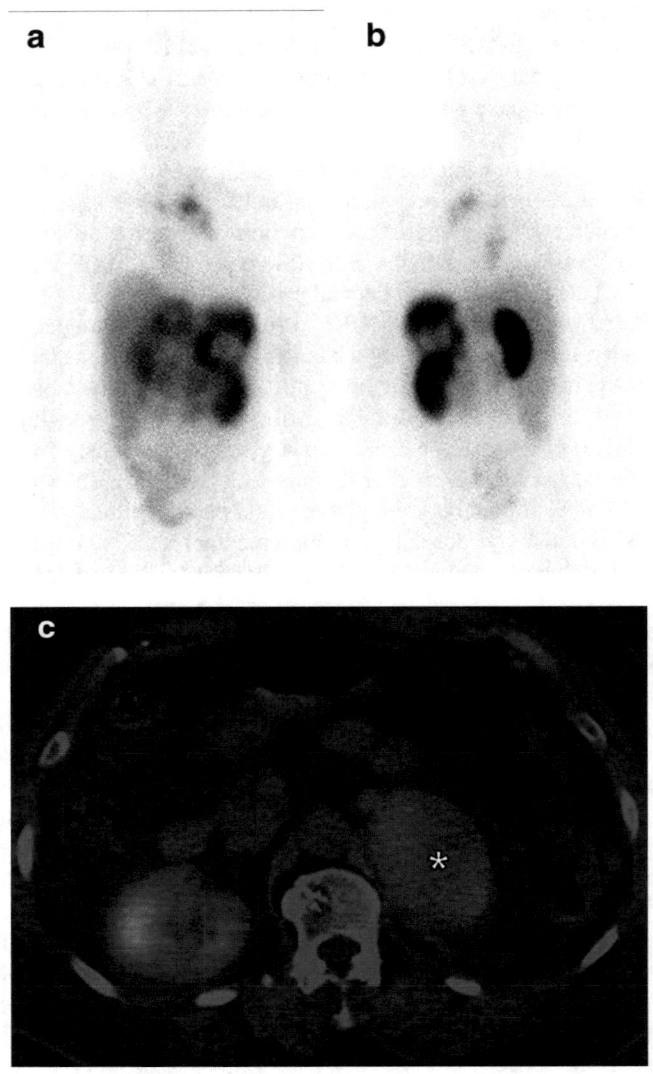

Fig. 7.4 (**a, b**) 24-h whole-body Octreoscan with anterior and posterior views. There is physiologic radiotracer in the kidneys, liver, bladder, and bowel. A large activity in the left adrenal gland and several small foci in the abdomen and mediastinum are due to metastatic pheochromocytoma. (**c**) An axial SPECT-CT fused image demonstrating tracer uptake localizing in the left adrenal pheochromocytoma (asterisk)

68.3 min and is eluted from an in-house ^{68}Ge-generator by electron capture with a physical half-life of 270.8 days [29]. It consists of the somatostatin analog tyrosine-3-octreotate (TATE) labeled with ^{68}Ga via the macrocyclic chelating agent dodecanetetraacetic acid (DOTA) conjugate. Although they use the same mechanism of

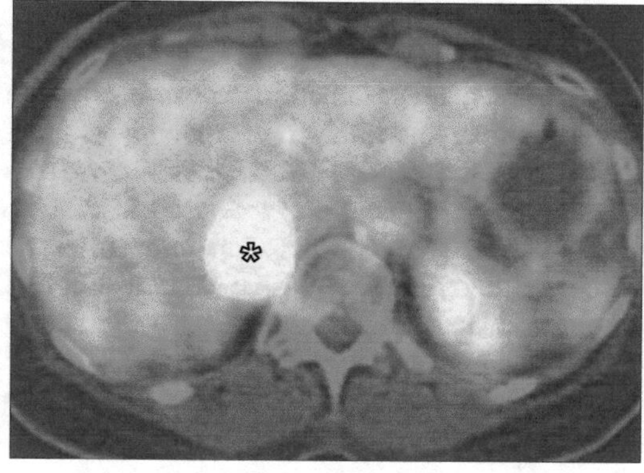

Fig. 7.5 ^{18}F-FDG PET/CT axial fused image demonstrating activity in the right adrenal pheochromocytoma (asterisk)

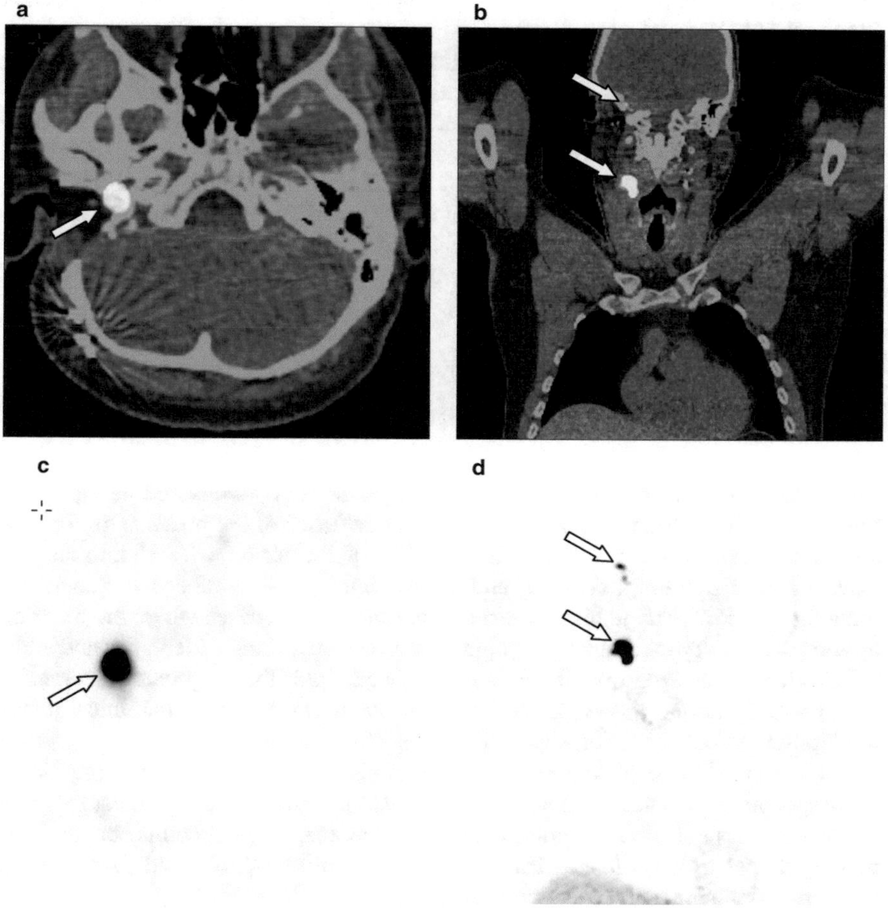

Fig. 7.6 ^{68}Ga DOTATATE PET/CT. (**a**) Axial and (**b**) coronal fused images; (**c**) axial and (**d**) coronal PET only images demonstrating radiotracer uptake (arrow) in the right neck and skull base near the jugular foramen, at areas of recurrent pheochromocytoma. (Image courtesy of Corina Millo, MD)

uptake, ^{68}Ga-DOTA PET imaging has several advantages over the ^{111}In-octreotide gamma imaging including higher sensitivity and specificity, detecting significantly more lesions, lower radiation exposure, and shorter image time with approximately 2 h as compared with 24 h of imaging with octreotide [30]. ^{68}Ga DOTATATE has higher sensitivity than F18 FDG, 96.2% vs 91.4% respectively.

Additional molecular agents used in PET imaging of pheochromocytomas and paragangliomas are ^{18}F-fluorodopamine (FDA) and ^{18}F-fluorodihydroxyphenylalanine (DOPA). In particular, ^{18}F-DOPA is a useful PET tracer for the imaging of paragangliomas, because these tumors have the ability to accumulate and decarboxylate biogenic amines such as levo-DOPA. Once taken into the cell by the amino acid transporter, it is decarboxylated into ^{18}F-DOPAmine and trapped intracellularly in storage granules by the vesicular monoamine transporter. Studies demonstrated that the ^{18}F-DOPA has larger percentage of accumulation in pheochromocytomas and paragangliomas than ^{18}F-FDG [31]. The sensitivity and specificity of ^{18}F-DOPA PET or PET/CT in patients with pheochromocytoma and paraganglioma range from 77% to 100% and 75% to 100%, respectively [32].

PET imaging can also be performed with ^{11}Carbon-hydroxyephedrine PET (HED PET). It is a catecholamine substrate analog with similar pathway to the neurotransmitter norepinephrine, which has higher sensitivity (91%) and specificity in detecting pheochromocytoma than MIBG scintigraphy [33]. Norepinephrine transporters selectively and rapidly transport it into sympathetic neuron, accumulating in organs with sympathetic innervation [34, 35]. Because of its short half-life of 20.4 min, ^{11}C requires an on-site cyclotron limiting the routine clinical use of ^{11}C-hydroxyephedrine PET imaging [31].

Conclusion

The imaging diagnosis and localization of pheochromocytomas and paragangliomas can be challenging. When there is clinical evidence of the presence of a pheochromocytoma, initial anatomical localization of the lesion with abdominal CT exam or MRI can be performed, and subsequently or simultaneously functional imaging could be obtained for confirmation, especially in cases where the imaging appearance overlaps with that of benign lesions such as adrenal adenomas and adrenal myelolipomas. Additionally, functional imaging aids the diagnosis of lesions in less typical locations, as well as evaluation of metastatic lesions. Anatomical imaging facilitates detailed lesion depiction for surgical planning.

As the knowledge of biochemical characteristics of these tumors progresses, more specific tracers are developed for functional imaging. While the most frequent incidental adrenal lesion is a nonfunctioning adenoma, when encountering an incidental adrenal lesion, biochemical correlation should be performed to exclude a hypofunctioning pheochromocytoma as a possible etiology.

References

1. Blake MA, Kalra MK, Maher MM, Sahani DV, Sweeney AT, Mueller PR, et al. Pheochromocytoma: an imaging chameleon. Radiographics Rev Publ Radiol Soc North Am Inc. 2004;24(Suppl 1):S87–99.
2. Mayo-Smith WW, Boland GW, Noto RB, Lee MJ. State-of-the-art adrenal imaging. Radiographics Rev Publ Radiol Soc North Am Inc. 2001;21(4):995–1012.
3. Choyke PL. ACR appropriateness criteria on incidentally discovered adrenal mass. J Am Coll Radiol JACR. 2006;3(7):498–504.
4. Miller JC, Blake MA, Boland GW, Copeland PM, Thrall JH, Lee SI. Adrenal masses. J Am Coll Radiol JACR. 2009;6(3):206–11.
5. Weber AL, Janower ML, Griscom T. Radiologic and clinical evaluation of Pheochromocytoma in children: report of 6 cases. Radiology. 1967;88(1):117–23.
6. Szolar DH, Korobkin M, Reittner P, Berghold A, Bauernhofer T, Trummer H, et al. Adrenocortical carcinomas and adrenal pheochromocytomas: mass and enhancement loss evaluation at delayed contrast-enhanced CT. Radiology. 2005;234(2):479–85.
7. Mukherjee JJ, Peppercorn PD, Reznek RH, Patel V, Kaltsas G, Besser M, et al. Pheochromocytoma: effect of nonionic contrast medium in CT on circulating catecholamine levels. Radiology. 1997;202(1):227–31.
8. McCollough CH, Primak AN, Braun N, Kofler J, Yu L, Christner J. Strategies for reducing radiation dose in CT. Radiol Clin N Am. 2009;47(1):27–40.
9. Mettler FA Jr, Huda W, Yoshizumi TT, Mahesh M. Effective doses in radiology and diagnostic nuclear medicine: a catalog. Radiology. 2008;248(1):254–63.
10. Lee TH, Slywotzky CM, Lavelle MT, Garcia RA. Best cases from the AFIP. Radiographics Rev Publ Radiol Soc North Am Inc. 2002;22(4):935–40.
11. Adam SZ, Nikolaidis P, Horowitz JM, Gabriel H, Hammond NA, Patel T, et al. Chemical shift MR imaging of the adrenal gland: principles, pitfalls, and applications. Radiographics Rev Publ Radiol Soc North Am Inc. 2016;36(2):414–32.
12. Yoon JK, Remer EM, Herts BR. Incidental pheochromocytoma mimicking adrenal adenoma because of rapid contrast enhancement loss. AJR Am J Roentgenol. 2006;187(5):1309–11.
13. Patel J, Davenport MS, Cohan RH, Caoili EM. Can established CT attenuation and washout criteria for adrenal adenoma accurately exclude pheochromocytoma? AJR Am J Roentgenol. 2013;201(1):122–7.
14. Shaaban AM, Rezvani M, Tubay M, Elsayes KM, Woodward PJ, Menias CO. Fat-containing retroperitoneal lesions: imaging characteristics, localization, and differential diagnosis. Radiographics Rev Publ Radiol Soc North Am Inc. 2016;36(3):710–34.
15. Goenka AH, Shah SN, Remer EM, Berber E. Adrenal imaging: a primer for oncosurgeons. J Surg Oncol. 2012;106(5):543–8.
16. Jacques AE, Sahdev A, Sandrasagara M, Goldstein R, Berney D, Rockall AG, et al. Adrenal phaeochromocytoma: correlation of MRI appearances with histology and function. Eur Radiol. 2008;18(12):2885–92.
17. Al Bunni F, Deganello A, Sellars ME, Schulte KM, Al-Adnani M, Sidhu PS. Contrast-enhanced ultrasound (CEUS) appearances of an adrenal phaeochromocytoma in a child with von Hippel-Lindau disease. J Ultrasound. 2014;17(4):307–11.
18. Mittendorf EA, Evans DB, Lee JE, Perrier ND. Pheochromocytoma: advances in genetics, diagnosis, localization, and treatment. Hematol Oncol Clin North Am. 2007;21(3):509–25. ix
19. Blanchet EM, Martucci V, Pacak K. Pheochromocytoma and paraganglioma: current functional and future molecular imaging. Front Oncol. 2011;1:58.
20. Sisson JC, Frager MS, Valk TW, Gross MD, Swanson DP, Wieland DM, et al. Scintigraphic localization of pheochromocytoma. N Engl J Med. 1981;305(1):12–7.
21. Huynh TT, Pacak K, Brouwers FM, Abu-Asab MS, Worrell RA, Walther MM, et al. Different expression of catecholamine transporters in phaeochromocytomas from patients with

von Hippel-Lindau syndrome and multiple endocrine neoplasia type 2. Eur J Endocrinol. 2005;153(4):551–63.
22. Shulkin BL, Shapiro B, Francis IR, Dorr R, Shen SW, Sisson JC. Primary extra-adrenal pheochromocytoma: positive I-123 MIBG imaging with negative I-131 MIBG imaging. Clin Nucl Med. 1986;11(12):851–4.
23. Timmers HJ, Chen CC, Carrasquillo JA, Whatley M, Ling A, Havekes B, et al. Comparison of 18F-fluoro-L-DOPA, 18F-fluoro-deoxyglucose, and 18F-fluorodopamine PET and 123I-MIBG scintigraphy in the localization of pheochromocytoma and paraganglioma. J Clin Endocrinol Metab. 2009;94(12):4757–67.
24. Fottner C, Helisch A, Anlauf M, Rossmann H, Musholt TJ, Kreft A, et al. 6-18F-fluoro-L-dihydroxyphenylalanine positron emission tomography is superior to 123I-metaiodobenzyl-guanidine scintigraphy in the detection of extraadrenal and hereditary pheochromocytomas and paragangliomas: correlation with vesicular monoamine transporter expression. J Clin Endocrinol Metab. 2010;95(6):2800–10.
25. Bombardieri E, Giammarile F, Aktolun C, Baum RP, Bischof Delaloye A, Maffioli L, et al. 131I/123I-metaiodobenzylguanidine (mIBG) scintigraphy: procedure guidelines for tumour imaging. Eur J Nucl Med Mol Imaging. 2010;37(12):2436–46.
26. de Herder WW, Lamberts SW. Somatostatin and somatostatin analogues: diagnostic and therapeutic uses. Curr Opin Oncol. 2002;14(1):53–7.
27. Shulkin BL, Thompson NW, Shapiro B, Francis IR, Sisson JC. Pheochromocytomas: imaging with 2-[fluorine-18]fluoro-2-deoxy-D-glucose PET. Radiology. 1999;212(1):35–41.
28. Hofman MS, Hicks RJ. Moving beyond "Lumpology": PET/CT imaging of Pheochromocytoma and Paraganglioma. Clin Cancer Res Off J Am Assoc Cancer Res. 2015;21(17):3815–7.
29. Maecke HR, Hofmann M, Haberkorn U. (68)Ga-labeled peptides in tumor imaging. J Nucl Med Off Publ Soc Nucl Med. 2005;46(Suppl 1):172s–8s.
30. Schreiter NF, Brenner W, Nogami M, Buchert R, Huppertz A, Pape UF, et al. Cost comparison of 111In-DTPA-octreotide scintigraphy and 68Ga-DOTATOC PET/CT for staging enteropancreatic neuroendocrine tumours. Eur J Nucl Med Mol Imaging. 2012;39(1):72–82.
31. Luster M, Karges W, Zeich K, Pauls S, Verburg FA, Dralle H, et al. Clinical value of 18F-fluorodihydroxyphenylalanine positron emission tomography/computed tomography (18F-DOPA PET/CT) for detecting pheochromocytoma. Eur J Nucl Med Mol Imaging. 2010;37(3):484–93.
32. Treglia G, Cocciolillo F, de Waure C, Di Nardo F, Gualano MR, Castaldi P, et al. Diagnostic performance of 18F-dihydroxyphenylalanine positron emission tomography in patients with paraganglioma: a meta-analysis. Eur J Nucl Med Mol Imaging. 2012;39(7):1144–53.
33. Mann GN, Link JM, Pham P, Pickett CA, Byrd DR, Kinahan PE, et al. [11C]metahydroxyephedrine and [18F]fluorodeoxyglucose positron emission tomography improve clinical decision making in suspected pheochromocytoma. Ann Surg Oncol. 2006;13(2):187–97.
34. Trampal C, Engler H, Juhlin C, Bergstrom M, Langstrom B. Pheochromocytomas: detection with 11C hydroxyephedrine PET. Radiology. 2004;230(2):423–8.
35. Yamamoto S, Hellman P, Wassberg C, Sundin A. 11C-hydroxyephedrine positron emission tomography imaging of pheochromocytoma: a single center experience over 11 years. J Clin Endocrinol Metab. 2012;97(7):2423–32.

Chapter 8 Medical Management of Pheochromocytoma

Daniel J. Toft and Mark E. Molitch

Introduction

Once a patient has been diagnosed with a catecholamine-secreting pheochromocytoma/paraganglioma, it is important to treat such a patient with the goals of (1) normalizing the blood pressure (BP) in those who are hypertensive, (2) controlling any tachyarrhythmias, and (3) readying the patient for surgery [1–3]. The untreated patient undergoing surgery is subject to severe BP elevations and arrhythmias during surgery as well as postoperative hypotension due to the sudden loss of the vasoconstrictive effect of the now reduced catecholamine levels. Although there are no true prospective, randomized controlled studies comparing treated vs. untreated/placebo-treated patients with respect to surgical outcomes [1, 4], it is the general consensus that such treatment lowers surgical morbidity/mortality [1–3]. α-Adrenergic receptor blockade forms the backbone of such therapy, and both non-selective blockers such as phenoxybenzamine and phentolamine and selective α_1 blockers have been used. There is less experience with calcium channel blockers for blood pressure reduction used either alone or as additional agents. β-Adrenergic blockers are often added after α-adrenergic blockade is achieved to control tachycardia and/or arrhythmias. Metyrosine, an inhibitor of catecholamine synthesis, has been used most often in cases refractory to conventional adrenergic blockade.

Occasional patients with pheochromocytomas and paragangliomas develop hypertensive emergencies, some spontaneously, and others in the setting of surgery performed for other reasons or during the pheochromocytoma/paraganglioma surgery itself. These hypertensive crises require emergent treatment with intravenous α-adrenergic blockade and other antihypertensive modalities. Fortunately, malignant

D. J. Toft · M. E. Molitch (✉)
Division of Endocrinology, Metabolism and Molecular Medicine,
Northwestern University Feinberg School of Medicine, Chicago, IL, USA
e-mail: djtoft@northwestern.edu; molitch@northwestern.edu

L. Landsberg (ed.), *Pheochromocytomas, Paragangliomas and Disorders of the Sympathoadrenal System*, Contemporary Endocrinology,
https://doi.org/10.1007/978-3-319-77048-2_8

tumors are rare but require specific treatment for the tumor itself as well as long-term control of the hyperadrenergic state.

Medications Used for the Treatment of Pheochromocytomas/Paragangliomas

Nonselective α-Adrenergic Receptor Blockade

Phenoxybenzamine binds to both α_1- and α_2-adrenergic receptors irreversibly and has a half-life of 24 h but is not available in all countries [4]. It is generally started at a dose of 10 mg twice daily and gradually increased over several days to achieve a target BP of <130/80 mmHg while seated with a drop on standing to no less than 90 mmHg systolic [1–3]. The usual dose needed is in the 40–60 mg/day range [2]. Although a maximum dose of 1 mg/kg has been suggested [1, 2], doses as high as 150 mg/day have been given [5]. Livingstone et al. reported a significant correlation of preoperative phenoxybenzamine dose and intraoperative stability, and their preoperative doses gradually increased from 59 mg/day to 106 mg/day over a 20-year period [5]. In some studies, the doses necessary to control the BP correlated with the degree of pretreatment catecholamine elevation [6, 7]. Adverse effects of phenoxybenzamine include postural hypotension with symptoms of tachycardia and lightheadedness, nasal stuffiness, mental "spaciness," lassitude, and inhibition of ejaculation [2], all of which are dose dependent. Once the BP goals have been achieved, the medication should be continued at this dose for 7–14 days prior to surgery to ensure cardiovascular stability during surgery [1–3]. Because of its long half-life, some clinicians give the last dose the evening prior to surgery in an effort to avoid postoperative hypotension, but others continue the medication up to the morning of surgery.

Although it is widely recognized that an increase in salt and fluid intake during these 7–14 days will restore diminished plasma volume and help to stabilize BP during surgery and to prevent postoperative hypotension [3], this latter effect has been questioned, and Lentschener et al. suggest that postoperative hypotension is more likely due to the prolonged effect of phenoxybenzamine [4]. Intra- and postoperative instability are more common in patients with higher catecholamine levels [6, 7].

Selective α_1-Adrenergic Receptor Blockade

To avoid the prolonged action of phenoxybenzamine, the selective α_1-adrenergic receptor blockers, doxazosin and prazosin, which have shorter half-lives, have been tried in patients with these tumors. Prys-Roberts and Farndon found that doxazosin, given in doses of 2–16 mg once daily, was as effective as phenoxybenzamine in controlling BP and heart rate during surgery but had fewer adverse effects before and during surgery [8]. The doses of doxazosin correlated with the pretreatment levels of urinary norepinephrine [8]. Similar results were found by others for doxazosin [9, 10], but a prospective study comparing phenoxybenzamine to prazosin found better control with phenoxybenzamine [11], while a retrospective study found no differences for outcomes in comparing all three drugs [12]. On the other hand, Kiernan et al. found a significantly higher number of intraoperative hypertensive episodes in patients who had been treated with selective α_1-adrenergic blockers, mostly doxazosin, compared to those treated with phenoxybenzamine [13], presumably since catecholamine surges could overcome the competitive blockade induced by doxazosin.

Metyrosine

Metyrosine (α-methyl-p-tyrosine) is an inhibitor of tyrosine hydroxylase, the rate-limiting step in catecholamine synthesis, reducing catecholamine production by these tumors. Although there have been no series reported in which metyrosine was used as monotherapy, it has been used in conjunction with phenoxybenzamine and prazosin with reported benefits of better intraoperative BP control and reduced cardiovascular complications when compared to patients receiving α-adrenergic receptor blockade alone [13–15]. Adverse effects include somnolence, bizarre dreams, visual hallucinations, confusion, and depression [14]. Metyrosine is not used as monotherapy [3]; however, some centers use metyrosine routinely along with phenoxybenzamine [16]. Metyrosine is not available in all countries and is costly.

Calcium Channel Blockers

Calcium channel blockers (CCB) have also been added to adrenergic receptor blocking agents to aid in BP control and tachyarrhythmias and have been used uncommonly as monotherapy if patients are intolerant of adrenergic receptor blockade [1–3]. In a retrospective analysis, Brunaud et al. found that patients treated with the CCB nicardipine as monotherapy had significantly higher preoperative BPs and greater intraoperative hypertension, but less intraoperative hypotension, compared to those treated with only α-adrenergic receptor blockade [17]. The starting dose of nicardipine is 30 mg twice daily; amlodipine (1–20 mg daily), nifedipine extended release (30–90 mg daily), and verapamil (180–540 mg daily) can also be used [18].

β-Adrenergic Receptor Blockade

β-Adrenergic receptor blockers are added to control tachycardia and anesthesia-related arrhythmias [3]. It is critical that α-blockade be fully established before starting a β-blocker to avoid unopposed α-adrenergic stimulation with vasoconstriction and an increase in BP [1–3]. Although labetalol has some α-adrenergic receptor blocking activity, its β-blocking activity is fivefold higher, so that it should not be used as monotherapy, and hypertensive crises have been reported with its use as a sole agent [3]. While carvedilol has superior α_1-receptor antagonism compared to labetalol, carvedilol is inferior to pure alpha receptor agents and also should not be used as monotherapy [19, 20]. Any β-blocker will suffice, and there is no preference for β_1-selective blockers [3]. Propranolol in modest doses usually suffices.

Volume Replacement

The prolonged vasoconstriction caused by the excessive catecholamines is thought to cause a state of volume contraction. Then when α-adrenergic receptor block is carried out with relaxation of the vessels, volume expansion is needed, and it is recommended that patients follow a high-salt diet and increase fluid intake [1–3]. This fluid replacement helps to minimize preoperative orthostatic hypotension and postoperative hypotension [1–3], as well as stabilizing the BP during surgery.

Special Cases

Normotensive Patients

Although there is some controversy as to whether normotensive patients with demonstrated hypersecreting pheochromocytomas/paragangliomas need the same medical treatment prior to surgery as do hypertensive patients, consensus is strong that all pheochromocytoma patients should be treated with adrenergic blockade. Shao et al. found no significant differences in intraoperative hemodynamics in 38 normotensive pheochromocytoma patients treated with doxazosin compared to 21 normotensive pheochromocytoma patients not treated with any medication [21]. Lafont et al. found hemodynamic instability to be similar in those pheochromocytoma patients with hypertension compared to those with normotension but did not find that hemodynamic instability differed in normotensive patients who received medical treatment with prazosin compared to those who did not, but the numbers were small [22]. Nonetheless, the Endocrine Society Guideline still recommends treatment of the normotensive patient with α-adrenergic receptor blockers and/or calcium channel blockers to prevent BP surges during surgery [3], and this seems to be a reasonable recommendation.

Patients with Catecholamine Cardiomyopathy

Acute and chronic myocardial damage can occur in patients with pheochromocytomas and paragangliomas [23]. This damage can occur from direct toxic effects of the catecholamines on the myocardium and from an outstripping of oxygen supply by oxygen demand because of catecholamine-induced coronary vasoconstriction or platelet aggregation [23]. As a result, patients may develop a severe left ventricular dysfunction and may have a Takotsubo-like contractile pattern (systolic ballooning of the apical and midportions of the left ventricle and severely depressed ejection fraction) [23]. Giavarini et al. found that 15 (11%) of the 140 newly diagnosed patients with pheochromocytomas/paragangliomas cared for between 2003 and 2012 experienced an acute episode of cardiorespiratory failure [24]. Of these 15, 12 presented in acute pulmonary edema with 10 progressing to cardiogenic shock. In the three patients without pulmonary edema, two had severe chest pain with stable hemodynamics and one had congestive heart failure. Twelve of the 15 were hypertensive and tachycardic and 3 were normotensive. Severe left ventricular systolic dysfunction was found in all 13 of those who had echocardiograms. Electrocardiograms were performed in 14 patients, with findings of acute ischemia/infarction in 7 and ST segment depression and/or diffuse T wave inversion in the other 7. Troponin values were high in 12 of the 13 in whom these were done. Despite these findings, coronary arteriography was normal in the 11 patients in whom this was performed. All 15 patients recovered clinically with institution of α_1-blockade with prazosin and β-blockade. In the 11 patients for whom echocardiography was performed before and after medical therapy before surgery, the left ventricular ejection fraction increased from 30% to 70%. When comparing those with and without cardiomyopathy, these investigators found no differences in sex, age, history of alcohol abuse, prevalence of adrenergic symptoms, other cardiovascular risk factors, tumor number and size, metanephrine and normetanephrine excretion, and the distribution of mutations. However, the acute cardiac episode was precipitated by nonadrenal surgery in five cases, by physical exercise in two patients, and by respiratory infections in two patients [24].

Patients with pheochromocytomas/paragangliomas who have any element of heart failure are at risk for progression to cardiogenic shock and therefore need emergent, aggressive management in an intensive care unit (ICU). In a systematic review, Batisse-Lignier et al. reported that patients who develop an acute cardiomyopathy have a 7.6% in-hospital mortality rate and a 51% cardiogenic shock rate at initial presentation [25]. Progressive α-adrenergic blockade with subsequent β-adrenergic blockade are important early therapeutic modalities along with standard aggressive supportive measures for such patients in an effort to restore normal cardiac function before proceeding to surgery [24, 26].

Patients with Exclusively Dopamine-Secreting Pheochromocytomas

Pheochromocytomas that secrete dopamine exclusively are very rare [27]. However, the diagnosis could be missed if routine catecholamine screening does not include dopamine. Although some of these patients present with more typical pheochromocytoma symptoms/signs, they may also be completely asymptomatic [27]. Almost all reported cases are malignant [27]. Dopamine has a vasodilatory action through dopamine receptors when the circulating levels are low but at higher levels releases NE from SNEs and directly stimulates adrenergic receptors thereby raising the BP. Administration of an α-adrenergic receptor blocking agent to such patients may cause hypotension and has even been reported to cause cardiovascular collapse [27]. Dopamine measurement should be a part of catecholamine screening for adrenal masses.

Patients with Acute Hypertensive Emergencies

The prevalence of pheochromocytoma crisis is unknown, but in case series of patients undergoing adrenalectomy for pheochromocytoma, the incidence of hypertensive emergency has been reported to be up to 15% [28, 29]. Hypertensive emergencies may occur spontaneously in patients with pheochromocytoma/paraganglioma, but catecholamine release leading to end-organ damage may also be provoked in patients with these tumors by adrenal biopsy, pregnancy, anesthesia for minor surgery, glucocorticoids or glucagon administration, or spontaneous tumor infarct [30–36]. Patients may first present with myocardial infarction or shock due to pheochromocytoma crisis; there are many case reports of new onset Takotsubo cardiomyopathy and heart failure in patients who are later found to harbor previously undiagnosed pheochromocytoma [37–40]. A summary of antihypertensive medications and typical starting doses are listed in Table 8.1.

There are no clinical trials to guide the management of pheochromocytoma hypertensive crisis, but there are expert guidelines based on case series to help the clinician [41, 42]. As with any patient with end-organ damage due to hypertension, treatment should take place in an ICU with continuous arterial pressure monitoring to allow for appropriate titration of short-acting intravenous medication. Phentolamine is preferred for its nonselective competitive alpha receptor blockade. The half-life of phentolamine is approximately 19 min; a starting dose of 1 mg/hr is typical; however, required doses of up to 40 mg/hr have been reported [43, 44]. The short-acting selective α1 blocker prazosin may be used as well. In Europe, urapidil, which possesses α_1-receptor antagonist, $5HT_{1A}$-receptor agonist, and weak β_1-receptor antagonist activity, has been used to successfully prepare patients with pheochromocytoma for surgery [45, 46]. Both oral and intravenous formulations of urapidil exist; however, urapidil is not available for use in the United States. Calcium

Table 8.1 Antihypertensive medications used for the treatment of pheochromocytoma/paraganglioma

	Mechanism of action	Starting dose	Approximate cost[a]
Phenoxybenzamine	α_1- and α_2-adrenergic receptor noncompetitive inhibition	10 mg twice daily	$7000/30 tablets
Doxazosin	α_1-adrenergic receptor competitive inhibition	2 mg daily	$20/30 tablets
Prazosin		2 mg twice daily	$40/60 tablets
Metyrosine	Tyrosine hydroxylase inhibition	250 mg every 6 h	$20,000/60 tablets
Nicardipine	Calcium channel blocker	30 mg twice daily	$140/60 tablets
Nifedipine		30 mg daily	$20/30 tablets
Amlodipine		10 mg daily	$10/30 tablets
Verapamil		180 mg daily	$30/30 tablets
Urapidil	α_1-receptor competitive antagonist, $5HT_{1A}$-receptor agonist, and weak β_1-receptor antagonist	25 mg IVPB or 10 mg/h IV infusion	NA
Phentolamine	Nonselective competitive α-receptor inhibition	1 mg/h IV infusion	$510/5 mg
Nicardipine	Calcium channel blocker	5 mg/h IV infusion	$114/20 mg
Magnesium sulfate	Calcium receptor antagonist	2 g IVPB followed by 1 g/h IV infusion	$7/20 g

[a]US dollar. Lexi-Drugs. Lexicomp Online. Hudson, OH: Wolters Kluwer Health, Inc. 1978–2017. Accessed February 25, 2017

channel blockers such as nicardipine have been used to manage hypertensive emergency in pheochromocytoma patients; lowering systemic vascular resistance, rather than inhibition of calcium-dependent catecholamine release, is the main mode of action [47, 48]. Magnesium sulfate has been used to block calcium signaling both in the peripheral vascular system and in the pheochromocytoma itself to limit catecholamine release and, in some case reports, has been an effective adjunct therapy when other agents have failed [49]. Magnesium sulfate is given as a 2–4 g IV bolus followed by 1 g/h infusion. Fluid resuscitation to correct the invariable intravascular depletion caused by catecholamine excess is essential, and when shock is present, volume resuscitation should of course precede the initiation of vasoconstrictive agents. Once stabilized, patients should undergo surgery in a timely fashion, as recurrent pheochromocytoma crisis may occur – in one retrospective case series of 25 patients, the rate of recurrence was 25% [50].

Patients with Malignant Pheochromocytomas/Paragangliomas

Catecholamine-producing tumors found outside the location of the normal sympathetic nervous system are defined to be metastatic. Common malignant pheochromocytoma/paraganglioma metastatic sites include the lung, liver, lymphatic system, and bone. Surgical excision is the preferred treatment when possible. When not curative, surgery may still be appropriate for enlarging lesions threatening vital structures or to lower tumor burden. Off-label use of cyclophosphamide, vincristine, and dacarbazine (CVD) chemotherapy has been the mainstay for palliative treatment of unresectable disease [51]. In meta-analysis of 4 trials including 50 patients, partial tumor response was seen in 37% of patients, with 40% seeing partial improvement in catecholamine levels [52]. Reported side effects of CVD treatment include neuropathy, myelosuppression, nausea and vomiting, and hypotension [53]. In the limited retrospective cohort data available, no survival advantage from CVD therapy has been documented [54, 55].

As an alternative to dacarbazine, the orally administered alkylating agent temozolomide has been used off-label to treat metastatic pheochromocytoma. In a phase II study examining the efficacy of the combination of temozolomide and thalidomide in patients with metastatic neuroendocrine tumors, one of three patients with pheochromocytoma was reported to have a partial response to treatment [56]. In a retrospective case series of 15 patients with metastatic pheochromocytoma/paraganglioma treated with temozolomide, 5 partial responses and 7 stable disease outcomes were reported [57]. The progression-free survival was 13.3 months. Of note, the patients with partial response all had tumors that harbored SDHB mutations.

Radiolabeled metaiodobenzylguanidine (MIBG) has been used to target ^{131}I to adrenal medullary tissue. MIBG is actively transported by noradrenaline receptors and concentrated in secretory granules, resulting in tumor targeting, but also in uptake by the normal salivary gland, liver, and spleen [58]. Each treatment typically administers between 100 and 300 mCi ^{131}I, and patients are typically given multiple doses resulting in cumulative doses as high as 3191 mCi [59, 60]. Early reports demonstrated partial tumor response in 33–58%, with subsequent larger combined case series seeing more modest 30% tumor response and 45% hormonal response in treated patients [59, 61–63]. A 2014 meta-analysis of 17 studies involving a total of 243 patients reported pooled proportions of complete or partial response of 3% and 27% using data from 12 studies (n not reported); stable disease pooled proportion was 52% using data from 11 studies (n not reported) [64]. In a phase II trial involving 30 patients, complete response, partial response, or stable disease was seen in 67% [65]. In a separate phase II trial evaluating 49 patients, 65% had either complete response, partial response, or stable disease at 1 year [60]. Side effects of ^{131}I-MIBG include myelosuppression which may be fatal, GI toxicity, liver toxicity when hepatic metastasis is present, oral mucositis, hypogonadism, and myelodysplastic syndrome. Limited long-term follow-up data is available; in case series with patient size of 14, 22, and 33 patients, the 5-year survival was reported to be 68%, 68%, and 45%, respectively [66–68]. In the aforementioned phase II trials, the estimated 5-year survival rates were 75% ($n = 30$) and 64% ($n = 49$) [65, 60].

Pheochromocytomas and paragangliomas frequently express somatostatin receptors, and although octreotide treatment does not regulate catecholamine release, octreotide analogues have been used to image and treat metastatic disease [69, 70]. [DOTA-Tyr(3)]-octreotide (DOTATOC) radiolabeled with yttrium or lutetium has been described in small case series, with partial response rates from 2% to 57% reported [71–74]. While the limited data cited in the reports above and as summarized in more comprehensive reviews of peptide-based therapy is encouraging, prospective trials are lacking [75, 76].

The mTor inhibitor everolimus, currently FDA approved for the prevention of organ transplant rejection and the treatment of kidney and breast cancer as well as GI, lung, and pancreatic neuroendocrine tumors, has been used off-label to treat patients with metastatic pheochromocytoma/paraganglioma [77]. In a phase II trial that included seven patients with metastatic pheochromocytoma/paraganglioma, five out of seven showed initially stable disease with a progression-free survival of 4.2 months [78]. Common side effects included bone marrow suppression, hyperglycemia, and stomatitis. The efficacy of everolimus for these tumors remains to be demonstrated as their intrinsic tendency for progression is variable; prospective trials are needed.

Tumor-directed radiofrequency, cryoablation, and ethanol ablation have been used successfully to treat metastatic pheochromocytoma, with a reported progression-free survival of 7.2 months in one retrospective series of 10 patients [79–81]. Not surprisingly, intra- and post-procedural hypertension is reported to be common despite pre-procedural blood pressure optimization with alpha blockade.

The small molecule multikinase inhibitor sunitinib is approved to treat gastrointestinal stromal cell tumors, pancreatic neuroendocrine tumors, and renal cell carcinoma; it has been used off-label in patients with metastatic pheochromocytoma. A retrospective case series of 17 patients treated at a single institution reported partial response or stable disease in 47% and improvement in hypertension in 43%. The progression-free survival was 4.1 months [82]. There are two ongoing studies listed at clinicaltrials.gov that are actively recruiting patients to assess the efficacy of sunitinib prospectively.

There are currently 29 open clinical trials listed at clinicaltrials.gov available to patients with pheochromocytoma. In addition to trials testing MIBG, sunitinib, and temozolomide, the multikinase inhibitors cabozantinib and lenvatinib as well as the immune checkpoint regulators nivolumab, ipilimumab, and pembrolizumab are all offered in trials designed to treat rare tumors. Of note, there is no published preclinical data to support the activity of these novel agents to treat metastatic pheochromocytoma/paraganglioma. The investigational small molecule ONC201, initially identified in a screen to identify agents capable of inducing expression of tumor necrosis factor-related apoptosis-inducing ligand (TRAIL), has been shown to antagonize dopamine receptor D_2 [83, 84]. Due to high expression of dopamine receptor D2 on pheochromocytoma, a phase II study assessing the efficacy of ONC201 in treating metastatic pheochromocytoma/paraganglioma will soon begin enrollment [85].

References

1. Challis BG, Casey RT, Simpson HL, Gurnell M. Is there an optimal preoperative management strategy for phaeochromocytoma/paraganglioma? Clin Endocrinol. 2017;86(2):163–7. https://doi.org/10.1111/cen.13252.
2. Gunawardane PT, Grossman A. Phaeochromocytoma and Paraganglioma. Adv Exp Med Biol. 2016. https://doi.org/10.1007/5584_2016_76.
3. Lenders JW, Duh QY, Eisenhofer G, Gimenez-Roqueplo AP, Grebe SK, Murad MH, Naruse M, Pacak K, Young WF Jr, Endocrine S. Pheochromocytoma and paraganglioma: an endocrine society clinical practice guideline. J Clin Endocrinol Metab. 2014;99(6):1915–42. https://doi.org/10.1210/jc.2014-1498.
4. Lentschener C, Gaujoux S, Tesniere A, Dousset B. Point of controversy: perioperative care of patients undergoing pheochromocytoma removal-time for a reappraisal? Eur J Endocrinol. 2011;165(3):365–73. https://doi.org/10.1530/EJE-11-0162.
5. Livingstone M, Duttchen K, Thompson J, Sunderani Z, Hawboldt G, Sarah Rose M, Pasieka J. Hemodynamic Stability During Pheochromocytoma Resection: Lessons Learned Over the Last Two Decades. Ann Surg Oncol. 2015;22(13):4175–80. https://doi.org/10.1245/s10434-015-4519-y.
6. Chang RY, Lang BH, Wong KP, Lo CY. High pre-operative urinary norepinephrine is an independent determinant of peri-operative hemodynamic instability in unilateral pheochromocytoma/paraganglioma removal. World J Surg. 2014;38(9):2317–23. https://doi.org/10.1007/s00268-014-2597-9.
7. Weingarten TN, Welch TL, Moore TL, Walters GF, Whipple JL, Cavalcante A, Bancos I, Young WF Jr, Gruber LM, Shah MZ, McKenzie TJ, Schroeder DR, Sprung J. Preoperative Levels of Catecholamines and Metanephrines and Intraoperative Hemodynamics of Patients Undergoing Pheochromocytoma and Paraganglioma Resection. Urology. 2017;100:131–8. https://doi.org/10.1016/j.urology.2016.10.012.
8. Prys-Roberts C, Farndon JR. Efficacy and safety of doxazosin for perioperative management of patients with pheochromocytoma. World J Surg. 2002;26(8):1037–42. https://doi.org/10.1007/s00268-002-6667-z.
9. Li J, Yang CH. Improvement of preoperative management in patients with adrenal pheochromocytoma. Int J Clin Exp Med. 2014;7(12):5541–6.
10. Zhu Y, He HC, Su TW, Wu YX, Wang WQ, Zhao JP, Shen Z, Zhang CY, Rui WB, Zhou WL, Sun FK, Ning G. Selective alpha1-adrenoceptor antagonist (controlled release tablets) in preoperative management of pheochromocytoma. Endocrine. 2010;38(2):254–9. https://doi.org/10.1007/s12020-010-9381-x.
11. Agrawal R, Mishra SK, Bhatia E, Mishra A, Chand G, Agarwal G, Agarwal A, Verma AK. Prospective study to compare peri-operative hemodynamic alterations following preparation for pheochromocytoma surgery by phenoxybenzamine or prazosin. World J Surg. 2014;38(3):716–23. https://doi.org/10.1007/s00268-013-2325-x.
12. Kocak S, Aydintug S, Canakci N. Alpha blockade in preoperative preparation of patients with pheochromocytomas. Int Surg. 2002;87(3):191–4.
13. Kiernan CM, Du L, Chen X, Broome JT, Shi C, Peters MF, Solorzano CC. Predictors of hemodynamic instability during surgery for pheochromocytoma. Ann Surg Oncol. 2014;21(12):3865–71. https://doi.org/10.1245/s10434-014-3847-7.
14. Steinsapir J, Carr AA, Prisant LM, Bransome ED Jr. Metyrosine and pheochromocytoma. Arch Intern Med. 1997;157(8):901–6.
15. Wachtel H, Kennedy EH, Zaheer S, Bartlett EK, Fishbein L, Roses RE, Fraker DL, Cohen DL. Preoperative Metyrosine Improves Cardiovascular Outcomes for Patients Undergoing Surgery for Pheochromocytoma and Paraganglioma. Ann Surg Oncol. 2015;22(Suppl 3):S646–54. https://doi.org/10.1245/s10434-015-4862-z.
16. Fishbein L, Orlowski R, Cohen D. Pheochromocytoma/Paraganglioma: Review of perioperative management of blood pressure and update on genetic mutations associated with pheo-

chromocytoma. J Clin Hypertens (Greenwich). 2013;15(6):428–34. https://doi.org/10.1111/jch.12084.

17. Brunaud L, Boutami M, Nguyen-Thi PL, Finnerty B, Germain A, Weryha G, Fahey TJ 3rd, Mirallie E, Bresler L, Zarnegar R. Both preoperative alpha and calcium channel blockade impact intraoperative hemodynamic stability similarly in the management of pheochromocytoma. Surgery. 2014;156(6):1410–7. discussion1417-1418. https://doi.org/10.1016/j.surg.2014.08.022.
18. Mazza A, Armigliato M, Marzola MC, Schiavon L, Montemurro D, Vescovo G, Zuin M, Chondrogiannis S, Ravenni R, Opocher G, Colletti PM, Rubello D. Anti-hypertensive treatment in pheochromocytoma and paraganglioma: current management and therapeutic features. Endocrine. 2014;45(3):469–78. https://doi.org/10.1007/s12020-013-0007-y.
19. Cubeddu LX, Fuenmayor N, Varin F, Villagra VG, Colindres RE, Powell JR. Mechanism of the vasodilatory effect of carvedilol in normal volunteers: a comparison with labetalol. J Cardiovasc Pharmacol. 1987;10(Suppl 11):S81–4.
20. Giannattasio C, Cattaneo BM, Seravalle G, Carugo S, Mangoni AA, Grassi G, Zanchetti A, Mancia G. Alpha 1-blocking properties of carvedilol during acute and chronic administration. J Cardiovasc Pharmacol. 1992;19(Suppl 1):S18–22.
21. Shao Y, Chen R, Shen ZJ, Teng Y, Huang P, Rui WB, Xie X, Zhou WL. Preoperative alpha blockade for normotensive pheochromocytoma: is it necessary? J Hypertens. 2011;29(12):2429–32. https://doi.org/10.1097/HJH.0b013e32834d24d9.
22. Lafont M, Fagour C, Haissaguerre M, Darancette G, Wagner T, Corcuff JB, Tabarin A. Per-operative hemodynamic instability in normotensive patients with incidentally discovered pheochromocytomas. J Clin Endocrinol Metab. 2015;100(2):417–21. https://doi.org/10.1210/jc.2014-2998.
23. Prejbisz A, Lenders JW, Eisenhofer G, Januszewicz A. Cardiovascular manifestations of phaeochromocytoma. J Hypertens. 2011;29(11):2049–60. https://doi.org/10.1097/HJH.0b013e32834a4ce9.
24. Giavarini A, Chedid A, Bobrie G, Plouin PF, Hagege A, Amar L. Acute catecholamine cardiomyopathy in patients with phaeochromocytoma or functional paraganglioma. Heart. 2013;99(19):1438–44. https://doi.org/10.1136/heartjnl-2013-304073.
25. Batisse-Lignier M, Pereira B, Motreff P, Pierrard R, Burnot C, Vorilhon C, Maqdasy S, Roche B, Desbiez F, Clerfond G, Citron B, Lusson JR, Tauveron I, Eschalier R. Acute and Chronic Pheochromocytoma-Induced Cardiomyopathies: Different Prognoses?: A Systematic Analytical Review. Medicine (Baltimore). 2015;94(50):e2198. https://doi.org/10.1097/MD.0000000000002198.
26. Kassim TA, Clarke DD, Mai VQ, Clyde PW, Mohamed Shakir KM. Catecholamine-induced cardiomyopathy. Endocr Pract. 2008;14(9):1137–49. https://doi.org/10.4158/EP.14.9.1137.
27. Poirier E, Thauvette D, Hogue JC. Management of exclusively dopamine-secreting abdominal pheochromocytomas. J Am Coll Surg. 2013;216(2):340–6. https://doi.org/10.1016/j.jamcollsurg.2012.10.002.
28. Conzo G, Musella M, Corcione F, De Palma M, Ferraro F, Palazzo A, Napolitano S, Milone M, Pasquali D, Sinisi AA, Colantuoni V, Santini L. Laparoscopic adrenalectomy, a safe procedure for pheochromocytoma. A retrospective review of clinical series. Int J Surg. 2013;11(2):152–6. https://doi.org/10.1016/j.ijsu.2012.12.007.
29. Riester A, Weismann D, Quinkler M, Lichtenauer UD, Sommerey S, Halbritter R, Penning R, Spitzweg C, Schopohl J, Beuschlein F, Reincke M. Life-threatening events in patients with pheochromocytoma. Eur J Endocrinol. 2015;173(6):757–64. https://doi.org/10.1530/EJE-15-0483.
30. Mohamed HA, Aldakar MO, Habib N. Cardiogenic shock due to acute hemorrhagic necrosis of a pheochromocytoma: a case report and review of the literature. Can J Cardiol. 2003;19(5):573–6.
31. Hosseinnezhad A, Black RM, Aeddula NR, Adhikari D, Trivedi N. Glucagon-induced pheochromocytoma crisis. Endocr Pract. 2011;17(3):e51–4. https://doi.org/10.4158/EP10388.CR.

32. Preuss J, Woenckhaus C, Schwesinger G, Madea B. Non-diagnosed pheochromocytoma as a cause of sudden death in a 49-year-old man: a case report with medico-legal implications. Forensic Sci Int. 2006;156(2–3):223–8. https://doi.org/10.1016/j.forsciint.2005.05.025.
33. Rosas AL, Kasperlik-Zaluska AA, Papierska L, Bass BL, Pacak K, Eisenhofer G. Pheochromocytoma crisis induced by glucocorticoids: a report of four cases and review of the literature. Eur J Endocrinol. 2008;158(3):423–9. https://doi.org/10.1530/EJE-07-0778.
34. Hemmady P, Snyder RW, Klink M. A hypertensive emergency following cataract extraction and cornea transplantation. Ophthalmic Surg. 1989;20(9):647–9. Discussion, 650
35. Pineda Pompa LR, Barrera-Ramirez CF, Martinez-Valdez J, Rodriguez PD, Guzman CE. Pheochromocytoma-induced acute pulmonary edema and reversible catecholamine cardiomyopathy mimicking acute myocardial infarction. Rev Port Cardiol. 2004;23(4):561–8.
36. Casola G, Nicolet V, vanSonnenberg E, Withers C, Bretagnolle M, Saba RM, Bret PM. Unsuspected pheochromocytoma: risk of blood-pressure alterations during percutaneous adrenal biopsy. Radiology. 1986;159(3):733–5. https://doi.org/10.1148/radiology.159.3.3517958.
37. Iio K, Sakurai S, Kato T, Nishiyama S, Hata T, Mawatari E, Suzuki C, Takekoshi K, Higuchi K, Aizawa T, Ikeda U. Endomyocardial biopsy in a patient with hemorrhagic pheochromocytoma presenting as inverted Takotsubo cardiomyopathy. Heart Vessel. 2013;28(2):255–63. https://doi.org/10.1007/s00380-012-0247-4.
38. Kim S, Yu A, Filippone LA, Kolansky DM, Raina A. Inverted-Takotsubo pattern cardiomyopathy secondary to pheochromocytoma: a clinical case and literature review. Clin Cardiol. 2010;33(4):200–5. https://doi.org/10.1002/clc.20680.
39. Sanchez-Recalde A, Costero O, Oliver JM, Iborra C, Ruiz E, Sobrino JA. Images in cardiovascular medicine. Pheochromocytoma-related cardiomyopathy: inverted Takotsubo contractile pattern. Circulation. 2006;113(17):e738–9. https://doi.org/10.1161/CIRCULATIONAHA.105.581108.
40. Subramanyam S, Kreisberg RA. Pheochromocytoma: a cause of ST-segment elevation myocardial infarction, transient left ventricular dysfunction, and takotsubo cardiomyopathy. Endocr Pract. 2012;18(4):e77–80. https://doi.org/10.4158/EP11346.CR.
41. Brouwers FM, Eisenhofer G, Lenders JW, Pacak K. Emergencies caused by pheochromocytoma, neuroblastoma, or ganglioneuroma. Endocrinol Metab Clin N Am. 2006;35(4):699–724., viii. https://doi.org/10.1016/j.ecl.2006.09.014.
42. Whitelaw BC, Prague JK, Mustafa OG, Schulte KM, Hopkins PA, Gilbert JA, McGregor AM, Aylwin SJ. Phaeochromocytoma [corrected] crisis. Clin Endocrinol. 2014;80(1):13–22. https://doi.org/10.1111/cen.12324.
43. Gabrielson GV, Guffin AV, Kaplan JA, Pertsemlidis D, Iberti TJ. Continuous intravenous infusions of phentolamine and esmolol for preoperative and intraoperative adrenergic blockade in patients with pheochromocytoma. J Cardiothorac Anesth. 1987;1(6):554–8.
44. McMillian WD, Trombley BJ, Charash WE, Christian RC. Phentolamine continuous infusion in a patient with pheochromocytoma. Am J Health Syst Pharm. 2011;68(2):130–4. https://doi.org/10.2146/ajhp090619.
45. Habbe N, Ruger F, Bojunga J, Bechstein WO, Holzer K. Urapidil in the preoperative treatment of pheochromocytomas: a safe and cost-effective method. World J Surg. 2013;37(5):1141–6. https://doi.org/10.1007/s00268-013-1933-9.
46. Miura Y, Yoshinaga K, Fukuchi S, Kikawada R, Kuramoto K, Takeuchi T, Satoh T. Antihypertensive efficacy and safety of urapidil, alone or in combination with beta-blockers, in patients with phaeochromocytoma. J Hypertens Suppl. 1988;6(2):S59–62.
47. Arai T, Hatano Y, Ishida H, Mori K. Use of nicardipine in the anesthetic management of pheochromocytoma. Anesth Analg. 1986;65(6):706–8.
48. Proye C, Thevenin D, Cecat P, Petillot P, Carnaille B, Verin P, Sautier M, Racadot N. Exclusive use of calcium channel blockers in preoperative and intraoperative control of pheochromocytomas: hemodynamics and free catecholamine assays in ten consecutive patients. Surgery. 1989;106(6):1149–54.

49. James MF, Cronje L. Pheochromocytoma crisis: the use of magnesium sulfate. Anesth Analg. 2004;99(3):680–6., table of contents. https://doi.org/10.1213/01.ane.0000133136.01381.52.
50. Scholten A, Cisco RM, Vriens MR, Cohen JK, Mitmaker EJ, Liu C, Tyrrell JB, Shen WT, Duh QY. Pheochromocytoma crisis is not a surgical emergency. J Clin Endocrinol Metab. 2013;98(2):581–91. https://doi.org/10.1210/jc.2012-3020.
51. Keiser HR, Goldstein DS, Wade JL, Douglas FL, Averbuch SD. Treatment of malignant pheochromocytoma with combination chemotherapy. Hypertension. 1985;7(3 Pt 2):I18–24.
52. Niemeijer ND, Alblas G, van Hulsteijn LT, Dekkers OM, Corssmit EP. Chemotherapy with cyclophosphamide, vincristine and dacarbazine for malignant paraganglioma and pheochromocytoma: systematic review and meta-analysis. Clin Endocrinol. 2014;81(5):642–51. https://doi.org/10.1111/cen.12542.
53. Huang H, Abraham J, Hung E, Averbuch S, Merino M, Steinberg SM, Pacak K, Fojo T. Treatment of malignant pheochromocytoma/paraganglioma with cyclophosphamide, vincristine, and dacarbazine: recommendation from a 22-year follow-up of 18 patients. Cancer. 2008;113(8):2020–8. https://doi.org/10.1002/cncr.23812.
54. Asai S, Katabami T, Tsuiki M, Tanaka Y, Naruse M. Controlling tumor progression with cyclophosphamide, vincristine, and dacarbazine treatment improves survival in patients with metastatic and unresectable malignant pheochromocytomas/paragangliomas. Horm Cancer. 2017. https://doi.org/10.1007/s12672-017-0284-7.
55. Nomura K, Kimura H, Shimizu S, Kodama H, Okamoto T, Obara T, Takano K. Survival of patients with metastatic malignant pheochromocytoma and efficacy of combined cyclophosphamide, vincristine, and dacarbazine chemotherapy. J Clin Endocrinol Metab. 2009;94(8):2850–6. https://doi.org/10.1210/jc.2008-2697.
56. Kulke MH, Stuart K, Enzinger PC, Ryan DP, Clark JW, Muzikansky A, Vincitore M, Michelini A, Fuchs CS. Phase II study of temozolomide and thalidomide in patients with metastatic neuroendocrine tumors. J Clin Oncol. 2006;24(3):401–6. https://doi.org/10.1200/JCO.2005.03.6046.
57. Hadoux J, Favier J, Scoazec JY, Leboulleux S, Al Ghuzlan A, Caramella C, Deandreis D, Borget I, Loriot C, Chougnet C, Letouze E, Young J, Amar L, Bertherat J, Libe R, Dumont F, Deschamps F, Schlumberger M, Gimenez-Roqueplo AP, Baudin E. SDHB mutations are associated with response to temozolomide in patients with metastatic pheochromocytoma or paraganglioma. Int J Cancer. 2014;135(11):2711–20. https://doi.org/10.1002/ijc.28913.
58. Nakajo M, Shapiro B, Copp J, Kalff V, Gross MD, Sisson JC, Beierwaltes WH. The normal and abnormal distribution of the adrenomedullary imaging agent m-[I-131]iodobenzylguanidine (I-131 MIBG) in man: evaluation by scintigraphy. J Nucl Med. 1983;24(8):672–82.
59. Kaltsas GA, Mukherjee JJ, Foley R, Britton KE, Grossman AB. Treatment of Metastatic Pheochromocytoma and Paraganglioma With 131I-Meta-Iodobenzylguanidine (MIBG). Endocrinologist. 2003;13(4):321–33.
60. Gonias S, Goldsby R, Matthay KK, Hawkins R, Price D, Huberty J, Damon L, Linker C, Sznewajs A, Shiboski S, Fitzgerald P. Phase II study of high-dose [131I]metaiodobenzylguanidine therapy for patients with metastatic pheochromocytoma and paraganglioma. J Clin Oncol. 2009;27(25):4162–8. https://doi.org/10.1200/JCO.2008.21.3496.
61. Krempf M, Lumbroso J, Mornex R, Brendel AJ, Wemeau JL, Delisle MJ, Aubert B, Carpentier P, Fleury-Goyon MC, Gibold C, et al. Treatment of malignant pheochromocytoma with [131I] metaiodobenzylguanidine: a French multicenter study. J Nucl Biol Med (Turin Italy: 1991). 1991;35(4):284–7.
62. Loh KC, Fitzgerald PA, Matthay KK, Yeo PP, Price DC. The treatment of malignant pheochromocytoma with iodine-131 metaiodobenzylguanidine (131I-MIBG): a comprehensive review of 116 reported patients. J Endocrinol Investig. 1997;20(11):648–58.
63. Troncone L, Rufini V, Daidone MS, De Santis M, Luzi S. [131I]metaiodobenzylguanidine treatment of malignant pheochromocytoma: experience of the Rome group. J Nucl Biol Med (Turin Italy: 1991). 1991;35(4):295–9.

64. van Hulsteijn LT, Niemeijer ND, Dekkers OM, Corssmit EP. (131)I-MIBG therapy for malignant paraganglioma and phaeochromocytoma: systematic review and meta-analysis. Clin Endocrinol. 2014;80(4):487–501. https://doi.org/10.1111/cen.12341.
65. Fitzgerald PA, Goldsby RE, Huberty JP, Price DC, Hawkins RA, Veatch JJ, Dela Cruz F, Jahan TM, Linker CA, Damon L, Matthay KK. Malignant pheochromocytomas and paragangliomas: a phase II study of therapy with high-dose 131I-metaiodobenzylguanidine (131I-MIBG). Ann N Y Acad Sci. 2006;1073:465–90. https://doi.org/10.1196/annals.1353.050.
66. Sze WC, Grossman AB, Goddard I, Amendra D, Shieh SC, Plowman PN, Drake WM, Akker SA, Druce MR. Sequelae and survivorship in patients treated with (131)I-MIBG therapy. Br J Cancer. 2013;109(3):565–72. https://doi.org/10.1038/bjc.2013.365.
67. Rutherford MA, Rankin AJ, Yates TM, Mark PB, Perry CG, Reed NS, Freel EM. Management of metastatic phaeochromocytoma and paraganglioma: use of iodine-131-meta-iodobenzylguanidine therapy in a tertiary referral centre. QJM. 2015;108(5):361–8. https://doi.org/10.1093/qjmed/hcu208.
68. Safford SD, Coleman RE, Gockerman JP, Moore J, Feldman JM, Leight GS Jr, Tyler DS, Olson JA Jr. Iodine −131 metaiodobenzylguanidine is an effective treatment for malignant pheochromocytoma and paraganglioma. Surgery. 2003;134(6):956–62.; discussion 962-953. https://doi.org/10.1016/S0039.
69. Reubi JC, Waser B, Khosla S, Kvols L, Goellner JR, Krenning E, Lamberts S. In vitro and in vivo detection of somatostatin receptors in pheochromocytomas and paragangliomas. J Clin Endocrinol Metab. 1992;74(5):1082–9. https://doi.org/10.1210/jcem.74.5.1349024.
70. Plouin PF, Bertherat J, Chatellier G, Billaud E, Azizi M, Grouzmann E, Epelbaum J. Short-term effects of octreotide on blood pressure and plasma catecholamines and neuropeptide Y levels in patients with phaeochromocytoma: a placebo-controlled trial. Clin Endocrinol. 1995;42(3):289–94.
71. Forrer F, Riedweg I, Maecke HR, Mueller-Brand J. Radiolabeled DOTATOC in patients with advanced paraganglioma and pheochromocytoma. Q J Nucl Med Mol Imaging. 2008;52(4):334–40.
72. Medina-Ornelas SS, Garcia-Perez FO. Effectiveness of radiolabelled somatostatin analogues (90Y-DOTATOC and 177Lu-DOTATATE) in patients with metastatic neuroendocrine tumours: a single centre experience in Mexico. Rev Esp Med Nucl Imagen Mol. 2016. https://doi.org/10.1016/j.remn.2016.09.005.
73. Zovato S, Kumanova A, Dematte S, Sansovini M, Bodei L, Di Sarra D, Casagranda E, Severi S, Ambrosetti A, Schiavi F, Opocher G, Paganelli G. Peptide receptor radionuclide therapy (PRRT) with 177Lu-DOTATATE in individuals with neck or mediastinal paraganglioma (PGL). Horm Metab Res. 2012;44(5):411–4. https://doi.org/10.1055/s-0032-1311637.
74. Puranik AD, Kulkarni HR, Singh A, Baum RP. Peptide receptor radionuclide therapy with (90)Y/ (177)Lu-labelled peptides for inoperable head and neck paragangliomas (glomus tumours). Eur J Nucl Med Mol Imaging. 2015;42(8):1223–30. https://doi.org/10.1007/s00259-015-3029-2.
75. Gulenchyn KY, Yao X, Asa SL, Singh S, Law C. Radionuclide therapy in neuroendocrine tumours: a systematic review. Clin Oncol (R Coll Radiol). 2012;24(4):294–308. https://doi.org/10.1016/j.clon.2011.12.003.
76. Castinetti F, Kroiss A, Kumar R, Pacak K, Taieb D. 15 YEARS OF PARAGANGLIOMA: Imaging and imaging-based treatment of pheochromocytoma and paraganglioma. Endocr Relat Cancer. 2015;22(4):T135–45. https://doi.org/10.1530/ERC-15-0175.
77. Druce MR, Kaltsas GA, Fraenkel M, Gross DJ, Grossman AB. Novel and evolving therapies in the treatment of malignant phaeochromocytoma: experience with the mTOR inhibitor everolimus (RAD001). Horm Metab Res. 2009;41(9):697–702. https://doi.org/10.1055/s-0029-1220687.
78. Oh DY, Kim TW, Park YS, Shin SJ, Shin SH, Song EK, Lee HJ, Lee KW, Bang YJ. Phase 2 study of everolimus monotherapy in patients with nonfunctioning neuroendocrine tumors

or pheochromocytomas/paragangliomas. Cancer. 2012;118(24):6162–70. https://doi.org/10.1002/cncr.27675.

79. McBride JF, Atwell TD, Charboneau WJ, Young WF Jr, Wass TC, Callstrom MR. Minimally invasive treatment of metastatic pheochromocytoma and paraganglioma: efficacy and safety of radiofrequency ablation and cryoablation therapy. J Vasc Interv Radiol. 2011;22(9):1263–70. https://doi.org/10.1016/j.jvir.2011.06.016.
80. Venkatesan AM, Locklin J, Lai EW, Adams KT, Fojo AT, Pacak K, Wood BJ. Radiofrequency ablation of metastatic pheochromocytoma. J Vasc Interv Radiol. 2009;20(11):1483–90. https://doi.org/10.1016/j.jvir.2009.07.031.
81. Pacak K, Fojo T, Goldstein DS, Eisenhofer G, Walther MM, Linehan WM, Bachenheimer L, Abraham J, Wood BJ. Radiofrequency ablation: a novel approach for treatment of metastatic pheochromocytoma. J Natl Cancer Inst. 2001;93(8):648–9.
82. Ayala-Ramirez M, Chougnet CN, Habra MA, Palmer JL, Leboulleux S, Cabanillas ME, Caramella C, Anderson P, Al Ghuzlan A, Waguespack SG, Deandreis D, Baudin E, Jimenez C. Treatment with sunitinib for patients with progressive metastatic pheochromocytomas and sympathetic paragangliomas. J Clin Endocrinol Metab. 2012;97(11):4040–50. https://doi.org/10.1210/jc.2012-2356.
83. Madhukar NS, Elemento O, Benes CH, Garnett MJ, Stein M, Bertino JR, Kaufman HL, Arrillaga-Romany I, Batchelor TT, Schalop L, Oster W, Stogniew M, Andreeff M, El-Deiry WS, Allen JE. Abstract LB-209: D2-like dopamine receptor antagonism by ONC201 identified by confluence of computational, receptor binding, and clinical studies. Cancer Res. 2016;76(14 Supplement):LB-209-LB-209. https://doi.org/10.1158/1538-7445.am2016-lb-209.
84. Allen JE, Krigsfeld G, Mayes PA, Patel L, Dicker DT, Patel AS, Dolloff NG, Messaris E, Scata KA, Wang W, Zhou JY, Wu GS, El-Deiry WS. Dual inactivation of Akt and ERK by TIC10 signals Foxo3a nuclear translocation, TRAIL gene induction, and potent antitumor effects. Sci Transl Med. 2013;5(171):171ra117. https://doi.org/10.1126/scitranslmed.3004828.
85. Saveanu A, Sebag F, Guillet B, Archange C, Essamet W, Barlier A, Palazzo FF, Taieb D. Targeting dopamine receptors subtype 2 (D2DR) in pheochromocytomas: head-to-head comparison between in vitro and in vivo findings. J Clin Endocrinol Metab. 2013;98(12):E1951–5. https://doi.org/10.1210/jc.2013-2269.

Chapter 9
Anesthetic Management of Pheochromocytoma and Paraganglioma

Ljuba Stojiljkovic

Introduction

Pheochromocytoma (PH) and paraganglioma (PG) are rare tumors that secrete catecholamines. Incidence of pheochromocytoma is 2–8 diagnoses per million people in a whole population per year. In patients with hypertension, prevalence is 0.2–0.6% [1]. Common clinical symptoms are hypertension, headaches, sweating, palpitations, tachycardia, and anxiety or panic attacks. Hypertension episodes are usually paroxysmal and severe and can lead to significant morbidity and life-threatening emergencies, such as hypertensive emergencies, myocardial infarction, and stroke [2].

PH originates from the adrenal gland, and PG originates from parasympathetic or sympathetic ganglia. PG can be further divided to ones present in the head and neck, which are from parasympathetic ganglia (usually nonsecreting), and those outside of the head and neck, which develop from sympathetic ganglia and secrete catecholamines [3].

PH and PG have a relatively high prevalence (32–41%) of germline mutations in ten known susceptibility genes [4]. This is especially true when they present as a part of family syndromes or when they are malignant [4]. Three most known family syndromes associated with PH and PG are neurofibromatosis type 1, von Hippel-Lindau syndrome, and multiple endocrine neoplasia type 2 [3].

PH and PG can produce and secrete various combinations of catecholamines. Most commonly they produce and secrete norepinephrine (NE) and epinephrine (E) [5]. In one study, NE was secreted by 32% of the tumors, while combination of NE and E was secreted by additional 27% of the tumors [5]. Only 5.7% of the tumors were nonsecreting.

L. Stojiljkovic (✉)
Department of Anesthesiology, Northwestern University, Feinberg School of Medicine, Northwestern Medical Group, Chicago, IL, USA
e-mail: l-stojiljkovic@northwestern.edu; lstojilj@nm.org

L. Landsberg (ed.), *Pheochromocytomas, Paragangliomas and Disorders of the Sympathoadrenal System*, Contemporary Endocrinology,
https://doi.org/10.1007/978-3-319-77048-2_9

Preoperative Preparation

The treatment of PH and PG tumors is surgical removal. Induction of anesthesia and surgical manipulation of the tumor can cause excessive catecholamine release which can lead to significant intraoperative hemodynamic instability. Because of the high incidence of intraoperative hypertensive crises, malignant arrhythmias, myocardial infarctions, and strokes, historically reported perioperative mortality was as high as 20–50% [6]. With improvements in preoperative medical management, new surgical techniques, and advancements in anesthesia techniques, perioperative mortality has decreased to 0–2.9% [5, 7].

(a) *Laboratory Tests*

Preoperative catecholamine levels in urine predict intraoperative hemodynamic instability and postoperative hypotension requiring pressor support, despite adequate preoperative preparation with α- and β-blockade [8–10]. Therefore, it is important for anesthesiologists to obtain detailed information about 24-h urinary catecholamine and metanephrine levels, to identify and prepare for the patients who are at increased risk for intraoperative and postoperative hemodynamic instability.

Preoperative laboratory tests should also include complete blood cell count and basic metabolic profile [11].

(b) *Cardiac Tests*

A 12-lead ECG is mandatory in all PH and PG patients to evaluate for ischemia, arrhythmia, conduction abnormalities, ST-segment/T wave changes, and left ventricular hypertrophy.

Echocardiography (ECHO) is performed to evaluate bi-ventricular function and to look for the presence of congestive heart failure and cardiomyopathy. It is also useful to gain insights to volume status and to prepare for perioperative fluid management.

(c) *Medical Optimization*

Avoidance of intraoperative hemodynamic instability is the most important anesthetic goal. Preoperative medical management is a cornerstone of preparation for surgery and anesthesia. Alpha-blockade has been the gold standard for preoperative preparation of these patients. The noncompetitive, nonselective α1 and α2-blocker phenoxybenzamine is most widely used. Selective α1-receptor antagonists, prazosin or doxazosin, have also been used. It has been reported that selective α1 antagonists induce less perioperative and postoperative hypotension because of their shorter half-lives [12]. The β-blockade is initiated after the α-blockade is established to prevent reflex tachycardia and arrhythmias. In addition, calcium channel blockers, which block catecholamine-induced calcium release in vascular smooth muscle cells, have been used as either main therapy or as an adjunct in preoperative medical optimization [5, 13]. Metyrosine, inhibitor of tyrosine hydroxylase, the rate-limiting enzyme in catecholamine synthesis, inhibits production of catecholamines. It is rarely used because of its numerous side-effects. Recent retrospective analysis has showed improved perioperative hemodynamics in patients where metyrosine was added to phenoxybenzamine but without any difference in overall outcome [14].

The goals of preoperative medical management are to normalize blood pressure and heart rate and to restore intravascular volume. The duration of the preoperative preparation is at least 7–14 days, and in most centers preparation takes between 2 and 6 weeks [12]. Most centers use Roizen criteria for adequacy of preoperative alpha-blockade [15]:

1. No blood pressure > 160/90 mmHg on four or more measurements within 24 h
2. Systolic blood pressure decrease of at least 15% from supine to standing and >80/45 mmHg while standing
3. No ST-segment or T wave changes on ECG for 2 weeks
4. No more than five premature ventricular beats per minute

Anesthetic Considerations

All patients should have adequate preoperative fasting prior to surgery. A light meal is allowed up to 6 h prior to surgery, and clear liquids are allowed up to 2 h prior to induction of general anesthesia [16]. An additional fasting time of up to 8 h may be required if a patient ingested a fatty meal or in patients with comorbidities (i.e., diabetes or gastroparesis) since it increases their risk for aspiration during induction of anesthesia [16].

(a) *Monitoring*

In addition to standard American Society of Anesthesiologists monitors which include pulse oximetry, ECG, noninvasive blood pressure monitor, capnography, and temperature monitors [17], all patients undergoing PH and PG surgery should have preinduction arterial line placement. The arterial line allows for beat-to-beat arterial pressure monitoring during anesthesia and surgery. Peripheral intravenous access is always obtained with a large-bore intravenous catheter. Central venous access is also obtained. The choice of central line catheter primarily depends on the presence or absence of heart failure. In patients with preserved ejection fraction, we choose to place the 7Fr triple lumen catheter (TLC). The TLC allows for infusion of vasodilators and vasopressors, which are needed in most of these surgeries, and for measurements of central venous pressure. In the presence of significant left ventricular dysfunction, or valvular abnormalities, large-bore central venous catheters, either 8.5 Fr cordis or 9 Fr multi-access catheter, should be considered, as they can be used as introducers for the pulmonary artery catheter (PAC). The PAC is used for monitoring cardiac output, pulmonary artery occlusion pressures, and systemic vascular resistance. These parameters may help guide fluid management and pressor/inotrope support in patients with severe cardiac dysfunction. In addition, large-bore central venous catheters are chosen in patients who are at high risk for significant blood loss, as they can be attached to rapid infusers for volume and blood resuscitation.

A urinary catheter should be placed for monitoring renal function and urine output.

A transesophageal echocardiogram (TEE) is reserved for intraoperative monitoring of high-risk patients with severe catecholamine-induced cardiomyopathy and significantly reduced bi-ventricular function. In these cases, TEE helps to guide pressor and inotrope support and provides information about fluid resuscitation and management. The main limitation of TEE is that data interpretation requires special expertise and training.

(b) *Choice of Anesthesia*

Induction of anesthesia in patients with PH poses significant challenges to the anesthesiologist, since it may precipitate hypertensive crisis and induce significant arrhythmia, followed by hemodynamic instability and hypotension. Acute cardiac decompensation and pulmonary edema may follow. This is one of the most critical moments in perioperative management of these patients. Careful preoperative preparation as outlined above and meticulous attention to details are of top importance. It includes anxiolytic and narcotic administration in preparation for preinduction invasive procedures (arterial and central line placements) and careful titration of hypnotic and paralytic agents during induction of general anesthesia. Patients should receive an intravenous anxiolytic prior to transfer to the operating room. Our agent of choice is midazolam, since it has quick onset, and it is well tolerated. Upon arrival to the operating room, a short-acting opioid fentanyl is titrated to avoid excessive hypertension during arterial line placement. Once the arterial line is placed, a slow, controlled induction with intravenous anesthetic is achieved. It is our practice to administer intravenous lidocaine of up to 1.5 mg/kg prior to induction. Intravenous lidocaine has long been used as an adjuvant during induction of anesthesia to attenuate hemodynamic responses to laryngoscopy and tracheal intubation [18], and in PH patients it may also serve as an antiarrhythmic agent [19]. In patients with preserved cardiac function propofol is titrated in incremental doses every 10 s until onset of anesthesia is achieved (Table 9.1). Propofol prevents hypertensive response to laryngoscopy and intubation by inhibiting sympathetic activity and attenuates an increase in heart rate via inhibition of sympathetic baroreceptors [20]. These effects make propofol probably the best hypnotic agent for the induction of anesthesia in PH patients. However, in patients with significantly diminished cardiac reserve and severely depressed ejection fraction, propofol may induce significant hypotension and circulatory collapse, especially if patients are volume depleted. In these patients, etomidate may provide more hemodynamic stability by preserving sympathetic outflow and autonomic reflexes [20].

After bag-mask ventilation is confirmed, a muscle relaxant is then administered to facilitate tracheal intubation. The muscle relaxant of choice should not have a vagolytic effect, since it can trigger tachycardia and hypertension in these patients, or propensity for histamine release, as histamine may trigger catecholamine-induced hemodynamic instability. Non-depolarizing muscle relaxants rocuronium and vecuronium are the most commonly used agents in PH patients (Table 9.1). They do

Table 9.1 Anesthesia induction agents

Name	Intravenous dose	Onset of action	Duration of action
Anxiolytics			
Midazolam	1–5 mg	1.5–5 min	2–6 h
Narcotics			
Fentanyl	1–3 mcg/kg	3–5 min	20–60 min (dose-related)
Hydromorphone	0.015–0.03 mg/kg	15 min	2–4 h
Hypnotics			
Propofol	1.5–2.5 mg/kg	40 s	3–5 min
Etomidate	0.3 mg/kg	< 1 min	3–5 min
Muscle relaxants			
Rocuronium	0.45–0.6 mg/kg (intubation) 0.1 mg/kg (maintenance)	2–3 min	33–50 min after intubation dose to first twitch appearance
Vecuronium	80–100 mcg/kg (intubation) 10–15 mcg/kg (maintenance)	2–3 min	31–60 min after intubation dose to first twitch appearance
Cisatracurium	0.15–0.2 mg/kg (intubation) 0.03 mg/kg (maintenance)	3–4 min	50–60 min to first twitch appearance
Succinylcholine	0.5–1 mg/kg	30–60 s	3–5 min (all four twitches)

not have a vagolytic effect of pancuronium and do not cause significant histamine release. The onset of action in doses given for endotracheal intubation is 2–5 min. If rapid sequence induction is chosen, a larger initial dose of rocuronium of 1.2 mg/kg will achieve intubating conditions within a minute. Cisatracurium is chosen in patients with significant hepatic and renal impairment, as it is primarily eliminated by nonenzymatic hydrolysis in the blood (Hoffman elimination). The only depolarizing agent available in the USA is succinylcholine. Historically, arrhythmias have been reported with use of succinylcholine during the induction of anesthesia with halothane [21]. However, succinylcholine has been safely used during induction of general anesthesia in the absence of halothane, and should be considered, especially in patients who are at risk for aspiration and in whom a rapid sequence induction is indicated, such as in pregnancy [22].

The short-acting β-blocker esmolol and potent vasodilators such as nitroglycerin, nicardipine, or sodium nitroprusside should be readily available since hemodynamic instability is quite common during induction of anesthesia. Hypotension should be avoided by careful titration of anesthetic agents. If supraventricular and ventricular tachyarrhythmia arise, amiodarone can be used for treatment (Table 9.2C). Electrical cardioversion should be considered early in unstable patients.

Epidural anesthesia has been used in combination with general anesthesia for open and laparoscopic surgeries for PH and PG [23–25]. However, an increased risk

Table 9.2 Vasoactive drugs for intraoperative management of hemodynamic instability during pheochromocytoma and paraganglioma surgery

A. *Vasodilators*

Name	Mechanism of action	IV loading dose	IV infusion dose	Onset of action	Duration of action	Limitations
Nicardipine	Second-generation dihydropyridine calcium channel blocker	2–8 mg	5–15 mg/hr	5–15 min	15–30 min	
Esmolol	Selective β1 antagonist	Up to 500 mcg/kg	25–300 mcg/kg/min	1–2 min	18–30 min	
Nitroglycerine	NO donor		5–100 mcg/min	2–5 min	5–10 min	Tolerance
Sodium nitroprusside	NO donor		1.5–10 mcg/kg/min	Immediate	1–2 min	Cyanide toxicity
Magnesium sulfate	Modulatory effect on Na and K current (affects transmembrane potential)	40–60 mg/kg	1–2 g/hr	Immediate	30 min	Increased duration of neuromuscular blockade

B. *Vasopressors*

Name	Mechanism of action	IV loading dose	IV infusion dose	Onset of action	Duration of action	Limitations
Phenylephrine	α-receptor agonist	0.1–0.5 mg	0.5–6 mcg/kg/min	Immediately	15–20 min	Reflex bradycardia
Norepinephrine	α- and β1-receptor agonist		2–30 mcg/min	Immediately	1–2 min	
Vasopressin	V1-receptor agonist		0.01–0.07 units/min	Within minutes	4–20 min	

C. *Antiarrhythmics*

Name	Classification	IV loading dose	IV infusion dose	Clinical use	Limitations
Amiodarone	Class III antiarrhythmic	150 mg (A-Fib, stable VT) 300 mg (pulseless VT, VF)	1 mg/min for 6 hr. 0.5 mg/min thereafter	A-Fib, VT, VF	Bradycardia and hypotension
Lidocaine	Class Ib antiarrhythmic	0.5–1.5 mg/kg	1–4 mg/min	VT	

Abbreviations: *NO* nitric oxide, *V1* vasopressin 1 receptor, *A-Fib* atrial fibrillation, *VT* ventricular tachycardia, *VF* ventricular fibrillation for exacerbated hypotension after tumor resection and increased fluid resuscitation requirements limit its usefulness, and it is not advisable in laparoscopic resections [26].

(c) *Positioning*

Laparoscopic adrenalectomies are performed in lateral decubitus position, usually using additional flexing of the operating room table. Repositioning of patients from a supine to a lateral decubitus position should not be attempted before adequate depth of anesthesia is achieved and all lines are secured and sutured in place, since change in position may cause line disconnections, displacements, and malfunction and it may precipitate hypertension and arrhythmia. Additionally, all pressure points should be carefully padded to decrease the risk of postoperative nerve damage and rhabdomyolysis.

(d) *Maintenance of Anesthesia*

Anesthesia is maintained with volatile anesthetics. Halothane, which is not available in the USA, sensitizes the heart to catecholamines, and it is contraindicated in these surgeries [1]. Desflurane, a short-acting volatile anesthetic with a very low blood-gas partition coefficient, should also be avoided since it has been shown to induce profound and sustained sympathetic stimulation even when it is slowly titrated after induction of anesthesia [27]. Isoflurane, the older, structurally similar volatile anesthetic to desflurane, does not produce a similar sympathetic response and can be safely used in PH patients. Sevoflurane does not have arrhythmogenicity potential like halothane, and it does not stimulate sympathetic response like desflurane. In addition, it has a more favorable blood-gas partition coefficient, and it is less irritable to the airway than isoflurane. These characteristics make sevoflurane the volatile anesthetic of choice in PH and PG surgery. Sevoflurane is used in mixture with oxygen and air. In our institution we do not use nitrous oxide, since it has the potential to cause bowel distension [28], and it increases the risk of postoperative nausea and vomiting [29].

The short-acting synthetic opioid remifentanil has been advocated to inhibit sympathetic activation during induction of anesthesia and laryngoscopy. However, its administration was associated with bradycardia and hypotension in patients who were α-blocked preoperatively and was not able to prevent hypertensive responses to tumor manipulation [30]. Therefore, it should be used with caution, if at all, in PH and PG surgery. Dexmedetomidine, an α2-receptor agonist with sympatholytic properties, has also been tried in PH surgery. Unfortunately, it was inadequate in preventing hemodynamic instability during induction of anesthesia and tumor manipulation [31], and it is not recommended for routine use.

(e) *Intraoperative Fluid Management*

Even though preoperative preparation of these patients includes oral fluid expansion, which is achieved over 2–6 weeks together with adequate α- and β-blockade, not all patients reach intravascular euvolemia. Fluid management is therefore one of the important aspects of intraoperative anesthetic care. Historically, central venous pressure (CVP) and pulmonary artery pressures were used to assess fluid status during complex surgeries [32, 33]. However, recent analyses have shown that CVP does not correlate with fluid responsiveness [34, 35]. Dynamic parameters of fluid status, such as arterial waveform analysis, or flow-guided measurements obtained by an esophageal Doppler probe, provide more accurate measurements of fluid status [36]. Esophageal Doppler-guided fluid management has been described in anesthetic management of pediatric patients undergoing PH resection [37]. As PH and PG patients need meticulous intraoperative fluid management, and often require fluid expansion after resection of the tumor, it is prudent to consider the use of Doppler-guided fluid management. The downside of this monitor is that it is usually removed after surgery, before tracheal extubation, and hence does not help in the postoperative fluid management.

Choice of Intravenous Fluids Intraoperatively, the choice of fluids includes crystalloid solutions and colloids. Blood products should be reserved for patients who experience severe, uncontrolled blood loss. Crystalloid solutions are administered for regular fluid maintenance and for volume expansion after tumor resection. Lactated Ringer's solution is the most commonly administered crystalloid intraoperatively. Excessive use of normal saline is discouraged, since it leads to hyperchloremic metabolic acidosis. Plasmalyte, a balanced salt solution with an adjusted pH of 7.4, is also available for intraoperative fluid replacement. We administer Plasmalyte in patients who present with metabolic acidosis and liver dysfunction. Additional benefit of Plasmalyte is that it can be safely mixed with packed red blood cells, where lactated Ringer's solution is contraindicated. Colloid solutions include 5% human albumin and colloids derived from starch. We administer colloids rarely, since studies have not shown improved outcomes as compared to crystalloid infusions.

(f) *Management of Intraoperative Hypertension and Arrhythmia*

Intraoperative hemodynamic instability with severe hypertension and arrhythmia arises from two different pathophysiological mechanisms [38]. One is enhanced reactivity of the sympathetic nervous system. The sympathetic nervous system response to stimuli is markedly increased in these patients due to several mechanisms: increased catecholamine neuronal vesicle load, increased impulse frequency, and presynaptic α-2 receptor desensitization [39]. Any stimulus that causes sympathetic system activation may induce severe hypertensive crisis and arrhythmia in these patients. In the perioperative period, preoperative anxiety, induction of anesthesia, tracheal intubation, hypoxia, hypercarbia, and surgical incision are some examples. The best prevention of exacerbated sympathetic response is achievement of a deep plain of anesthesia prior to the stimulation. The other reason for hemodynamic instability in these patients is induced by direct catecholamine release from the tumor, either by creating pneumoperitoneum or by direct tumor manipulation. The hemodynamic consequences may be severe life-threatening hypertension crisis from NE release or arrhythmia from E release. The most important first intervention is timely communication with a surgeon to either desufflate the pneumoperitoneum and/or stop tumor manipulation until hemodynamic control is achieved with infusion of rapid-acting, potent vasodilator agents.

In our institution, we prepare IV infusions of calcium channel blocker nicardipine and beta-blocker esmolol (Table 9.2A). In our experience, nicardipine is very effective as a first-line agent in patients who are already α-blocked with phenoxybenzamine. It prevents catecholamine-induced calcium release downstream of adrenergic receptors and catecholamine-induced coronary spasm and attenuates hypertensive response to stimuli that activate the sympathetic nervous system, such as tracheal intubation and surgical incision. The short-acting β-blocker esmolol is used to control tachycardia and arrhythmia that can ensue from E release (Table 9.2A).

Sodium nitroprusside has also been used successfully for control of hypertensive crises in PH surgery [38, 39]. Sodium nitroprusside is a potent arterial vasodilator that acts via nitric oxide (NO) pathway and inhibits intracellular calcium release in smooth muscle cells. It has a rapid onset and offset of action and it is easily titrated (Table 9.2A). However, sodium nitroprusside has a potential for inducing methemoglobinemia and cyanide toxicity, which limits its use, especially in higher doses and for longer periods of time [40]. Intravenous infusion of nitroglycerine (NTG) is also commonly used in PH surgery. NTG is an organic nitrate which is converted into NO and increases the level of cGMP in vascular smooth muscle cells [41]. It causes an increase in the venous capacitance system and a decrease in preload. This effect is especially important in PH patients with cardiomyopathy and heart failure. NTG has a quick onset, it is easily titrated, and it has a short half-life (Table 9.2A). The downside is a development of tolerance.

Magnesium sulfate has been shown to be effective in management of hypertension during PH resection in pregnancy [42]. Magnesium prevents catecholamine release, inhibits catecholamine receptors, and is a calcium antagonist. It also has a stabilizing effect on cardiac conduction and can help in controlling catecholamine-induced arrhythmias. It has been proposed that intravenous magnesium sulfate should be used as the vasodilating agent of choice in PH surgery during pregnancy [42].

(g) *Management of Hypotension Following Tumor Resection*

Hypotension after tumor resection is common, and it is caused by a sudden decrease of circulating catecholamines that follows tumor resection. Residual α-blockade with the long-acting irreversible inhibitor phenoxybenzamine and α-receptor downregulation are additional contributing factors. Hypotension is more severe if euvolemia is not achieved. Therefore, it is important to anticipate and prepare for the time of surgical resection. Communication with the surgical team is of paramount importance, and a surgeon should communicate their plan for clamping the venous drainage of the tumor. At that point, all vasodilators should be discontinued and fluid bolus should be administered. Fluid resuscitation is best guided by dynamic parameters as described above, to ensure euvolemia. If hypotension still occurs despite adequate volume resuscitation, which is not uncommon, infusion of vasopressors is started.

In our institution, phenylephrine and NE IV infusions are always prepared ahead of time and are connected to the central line prior to tumor resection. If hypotension does not respond to escalating doses of phenylephrine, NE is started and titrated to effect (Table 9.2B). Clinical variables that have been identified to predict prolonged post-resection hypotension are tumor size greater than 60 mm and a high level of preoperative urinary NE and E [10]. Patients with high NE and dopamine-secreting tumors are particularly prone to persistent post-resection hypotension [43]. In addition, open procedures were associated with prolonged need for vasopressor support [44]. In cases of refractory hypotension, not responding to NE infusion, vasopressin should be added (Table 9.2B). Vasopressin acts via vasopressin V1 receptors on vascular smooth muscle cells and induces vasoconstriction and improves hemodynamics in catecholamine-resistant hypotension [45]. It has been successfully used in refractory hypotension after PH resection [42, 46, 47]. If hypotension persists, methylene blue, which has been used in treatment of vasoplegia after cardiopulmonary bypass surgery, has been proposed as a rescue therapy for refractory hypotension following PH resection [42].

Most patients are safely extubated in the operating room following emergence from general anesthesia. Pain control is achieved with fentanyl or hydromorphone, administered prior to emergence. Morphine can cause histamine release and should be avoided. Intravenous acetaminophen administration 15–30 min prior to emergence will decrease postoperative narcotic requirements. The nonsteroidal analgesic ketorolac may be given to patients with preserved renal function and who are at low risk for bleeding complications.

Postoperatively, all patients are recovered in the intensive care unit (ICU). The ICU allows for the highest level of monitoring, including invasive monitoring of blood pressure and CVP. In addition, many patients require at least a short duration of vasopressor support postoperatively, which is effectively managed in an ICU setting. It has been reported that the incidence of postoperative morbidity is 22–36% and risk factors are history of coronary artery disease, female gender, and intraoperative hypertensive episodes with systolic blood pressure ≥ 200 mmHg and mean arterial pressure < 60 mmHg [48].

Glucose levels should be followed closely postoperatively, since impairment of glucose control is common after tumor resection.

Special Anesthetic Considerations

(a) *Anesthetic Management of PH in Elderly Patients*

With advances in imaging and biochemical techniques, PH is now diagnosed more often in the elderly population. As the elderly have multiple comorbidities, their anesthetic management may pose a significant challenge in the perioperative period. Recent retrospective comparative analysis showed that elderly patients have not suffered more hemodynamic instability during anesthesia and surgery; however, they had a significantly increased rate of postoperative complications, including a six times higher risk of receiving vasopressor support postoperatively, and had longer ICU and hospital stays as compared to younger patients [49]. Despite a higher rate of complications and slower recovery, there was no increase in mortality [49].

(b) *Anesthetic Management of PH in Pregnancy*

PH is a rare cause of hypertension in pregnancy, and the incidence is <0.2 per 10,000 pregnancies [50]. Unfortunately, especially if it is not diagnosed antepartum, it leads to severe consequences, with a high maternal (17–48%) and fetal (26–55%) mortality rate [26]. With proper antepartum diagnosis, maternal mortality drops to nearly 0% and fetal loss is 15% [50]. When PH is diagnosed early in pregnancy, the treatment is controversial, and it may include surgical removal of the tumor, termination of pregnancy, or medical management until the fetus is viable [42]. Alpha-blockade and subsequent β-blockade are initiated until blood pressure and arrhythmia are controlled. In the third trimester of pregnancy, simultaneous Cesarean section with tumor resection is advocated [50, 51]. A multidisciplinary approach with an endocrinologist, obstetrician, surgeon, and anesthesiologist is recommended in preparation for these surgeries. Anesthetic management is especially challenging because there are two patients involved, a parturient and a fetus. Many of the anesthetic agents cross into fetal circulation and should be used with caution. Regional anesthesia with spinal or epidural neuraxial block is the most common anesthesia for regular Cesarean sections. However, in parturients with PH, spinal anesthesia is contraindicated because it may induce profound hypotension [26]. Lumbar epidural anesthesia has been used successfully in PH parturients [26]. General anesthesia is most commonly used if combined Cesarean section and the tumor removal are planned. Special consideration should be given to hemodynamic control during induction of anesthesia and tracheal intubation. Parturients should be placed in the left uterine displacement position prior to induction of anesthesia. All monitors that are described for PH surgery should be used in these cases as well. All parturients are at risk for aspiration, which must be weighed against the risk of severe hypertension if rapid sequence induction is chosen. Succinylcholine has been used in parturients since it is as fast-acting muscle relaxant with a short duration of action [50, 51]. A high dose of rocuronium (1.2 mg/kg) may be a suitable alternative, especially if patients are at risk for tachyarrhythmia (high E-secreting tumors). If rocuronium is chosen, the rapid reversal agent sugammadex should be readily available in the case that intubation becomes difficult. High doses of volatile agents (sevoflurane or isoflurane) are discouraged, because they may lead to uterine atony and excessive hemorrhage after delivery. Nitrous oxide could be used as an adjunct to the volatile agent for maintenance of anesthesia in these cases. Magnesium sulfate is the first agent of choice for hypertension control during anesthesia and surgery, since it has a long history of safety in parturients and it has been used successfully in these cases [42].

References

1. Ramakrishna H. Pheochromocytoma resection: current concepts in anesthetic management. J Anaesthesiol Clin Pharmacol. 2015;31(3):317–23. PubMed PMID: 26330708. Pubmed Central PMCID: PMC4541176. Epub 2015/09/04. Eng
2. Lenders JW, Eisenhofer G, Mannelli M, Pacak K. Phaeochromocytoma. Lancet (London, England). 2005;366(9486):665–75. PubMed PMID: 16112304. Epub 2005/08/23. eng
3. Fishbein L, Orlowski R, Cohen D. Pheochromocytoma/Paraganglioma: review of perioperative management of blood pressure and update on genetic mutations associated with pheochromocytoma. J Clin Hypertens (Greenwich). 2013;15(6):428–34. PubMed PMID: 23730992. Pubmed Central PMCID: PMC4581847. Epub 2013/06/05. eng
4. Fishbein L, Merrill S, Fraker DL, Cohen DL, Nathanson KL. Inherited mutations in pheochromocytoma and paraganglioma: why all patients should be offered genetic testing. Ann Surg Oncol. 2013;20(5):1444–50. PubMed PMID: 23512077. Pubmed Central PMCID: PMC4291281. Epub 2013/03/21. eng
5. Lebuffe G, Dosseh ED, Tek G, Tytgat H, Moreno S, Tavernier B, et al. The effect of calcium channel blockers on outcome following the surgical treatment of phaeochromocytomas and paragangliomas. Anaesthesia. 2005;60(5):439–44. PubMed PMID: 15819762. Epub 2005/04/12. eng
6. Apgar V, Papper EM. Pheochromocytoma. Anesthetic management during surgical treatment. AMA Arch Surg. 1951;62(5):634–48. PubMed PMID: 14818537. Epub 1951/05/01. eng
7. Kinney MA, Warner ME, van Heerden JA, Horlocker TT, Young WF Jr, Schroeder DR, et al. Perianesthetic risks and outcomes of pheochromocytoma and paraganglioma resection. Anesth Analg. 2000;91(5):1118–23. PubMed PMID: 11049893. Epub 2000/10/26. eng
8. Kramer CK, Leitao CB, Azevedo MJ, Canani LH, Maia AL, Czepielewski M, et al. Degree of catecholamine hypersecretion is the most important determinant of intra-operative hemodynamic outcomes in pheochromocytoma. J Endocrinol Investig. 2009;32(3):234–7. PubMed PMID: 19542740. Epub 2009/06/23. eng
9. Chang RY, Lang BH, Wong KP, Lo CY. High pre-operative urinary norepinephrine is an independent determinant of peri-operative hemodynamic instability in unilateral pheochromocytoma/paraganglioma removal. World J Surg. 2014;38(9):2317–23. PubMed PMID: 24782037. Epub 2014/05/02. eng
10. Namekawa T, Utsumi T, Kawamura K, Kamiya N, Imamoto T, Takiguchi T, et al. Clinical predictors of prolonged postresection hypotension after laparoscopic adrenalectomy for pheochromocytoma. Surgery. 2016;159(3):763–70. PubMed PMID: 26477475. Epub 2015/10/20. eng
11. Phitayakorn R, McHenry CR. Perioperative considerations in patients with adrenal tumors. J Surg Oncol. 2012;106(5):604–10. PubMed PMID: 22513507. Epub 2012/04/20. Eng
12. Challis BG, Casey RT, Simpson HL, Gurnell M. Is there an optimal preoperative management strategy for phaeochromocytoma/paraganglioma? Clin Endocrinol. 2017;86(2):163–7. PubMed PMID: 27696513. Epub 2016/10/25. eng
13. Brunaud L, Boutami M, Nguyen-Thi PL, Finnerty B, Germain A, Weryha G, et al. Both preoperative alpha and calcium channel blockade impact intraoperative hemodynamic stability similarly in the management of pheochromocytoma. Surgery. 2014;156(6):1410–7. discussion7-8. PubMed PMID: 25456922. Epub 2014/12/03. eng
14. Wachtel H, Kennedy EH, Zaheer S, Bartlett EK, Fishbein L, Roses RE, et al. Preoperative Metyrosine improves cardiovascular outcomes for patients undergoing surgery for Pheochromocytoma and Paraganglioma. Ann Surg Oncol. 2015;22(Suppl 3):S646–54. PubMed PMID: 26374407. Epub 2015/09/17. eng
15. Roizen A. Prospective randomized trial of four anesthetic techniques for resection of pheochromocytoma. Anesthesiology. 1982;57: A43.
16. Practice guidelines for preoperative fasting and the use of pharmacologic agents to reduce the risk of pulmonary aspiration: application to healthy patients undergoing elective procedures: an updated report by the American Society of Anesthesiologists Task Force on preop-

erative fasting and the use of pharmacologic agents to reduce the risk of pulmonary aspiration. Anesthesiology. 2017 PubMed PMID: 28045707. Epub 2017/01/04. eng.

17. STANDARDS FOR BASIC ANESTHETIC MONITORING [Web Document]. http://www.asahq.org/quality-and-practice-management/standards-and-guidelines: American Society of Anesthesiologists; 2015 [updated October 28, 2015; cited 2017 2/6/2017].
18. Khan FA, Ullah H. Pharmacological agents for preventing morbidity associated with the haemodynamic response to tracheal intubation. Cochrane Database Syst Rev, 2013; July 03 (7):Cd004087. PubMed PMID: 23824697. Epub 2013/07/05. eng
19. Usubiaga JE, Wikinski JA, Usubiaga LE. Use of lidocaine and procaine in patients with pheochromocytoma. Anesth Analg. 1969;48(3):443–53. PubMed PMID: 5815109. Epub 1969/05/01. eng
20. Ebert TJ, Muzi M, Berens R, Goff D, Kampine JP. Sympathetic responses to induction of anesthesia in humans with propofol or etomidate. Anesthesiology. 1992;76(5):725–33. PubMed PMID: 1575340. Epub 1992/05/01. eng
21. Stoner TR Jr, Urbach KF. Cardiac arrhythmias associated with succinylcholine in a patient with pheochromocytoma. Anesthesiology. 1968;29(6):1228–9. PubMed PMID: 5726757. Epub 1968/11/01. eng
22. Joffe D, Robbins R, Benjamin A. Caesarean section and phaeochromocytoma resection in a patient with von Hippel Lindau disease. Can J Anaesth J Can d'anesthesie. 1993;40(9):870–4. PubMed PMID: 8403182. Epub 1993/09/01. eng
23. Tomulic K, Saric JP, Kocman B, Skrtic A, Filipcic NV, Acan I. Successful management of unsuspected retroperitoneal paraganglioma via the use of combined epidural and general anesthesia: a case report. J Med Case Rep. 2013;7:58. PubMed PMID: 23448279. Pubmed Central PMCID: PMC3599738. Epub 2013/03/02. eng
24. Nizamoglu A, Salihoglu Z, Bolayrl M. Effects of epidural-and-general anesthesia combined versus general anesthesia during laparoscopic adrenalectomy. Surg Laparosc Endosc Percutan Tech. 2011;21(5):372–9. PubMed PMID: 22002277. Epub 2011/10/18. eng
25. Luo A, Guo X, Yi J, Ren H, Huang Y, Ye T. Clinical features of pheochromocytoma and perioperative anesthetic management. Chin Med J. 2003;116(10):1527–31. PubMed PMID: 14570616. Epub 2003/10/23. eng
26. O'Riordan JA. Pheochromocytomas and anesthesia. Int Anesthesiol Clin. 1997;35(4):99–127. PubMed PMID: 9444533. Epub 1998/01/28. eng
27. Ebert TJ, Muzi M. Sympathetic hyperactivity during desflurane anesthesia in healthy volunteers. A comparison with isoflurane. Anesthesiology. 1993;79(3):444–53. PubMed PMID: 8363068. Epub 1993/09/01. eng
28. El-Galley R, Hammontree L, Urban D, Pierce A, Sakawi Y. Anesthesia for laparoscopic donor nephrectomy: is nitrous oxide contraindicated? J Urol. 2007;178(1):225–7. discussion 7. PubMed PMID: 17512015. Epub 2007/05/22. eng
29. Sun R, Jia WQ, Zhang P, Yang K, Tian JH, Ma B, et al. Nitrous oxide-based techniques versus nitrous oxide-free techniques for general anaesthesia. Cochrane Database Syst Rev. 2015; Nov 6 (11):Cd008984. PubMed PMID: 26545294. Epub 2015/11/07. eng
30. Breslin DS, Farling PA, Mirakhur RK. The use of remifentanil in the anaesthetic management of patients undergoing adrenalectomy: a report of three cases. Anaesthesia. 2003;58(4):358–62. PubMed PMID: 12648118. Epub 2003/03/22. Eng
31. Ali Erdogan M, Selim Ozkan A, Ozgul U, Colak Y, Ucar M. Dexmedetomidine, Remifentanil, and Sevoflurane in the perioperative Management of a Patient during a laparoscopic Pheochromocytoma resection. J Cardiothorac Vasc Anesth. 2015;29(6):e79–80. PubMed PMID: 26411814. Epub 2015/09/29. Eng
32. Hughes RE, Magovern GJ. The relationship between right atrial pressure and blood volume. AMA Arch Surg. 1959;79(2):238–43. PubMed PMID: 13669851. Epub 1959/08/01. eng
33. Wilson JN, Grow JB, Demong CV, Prevedel AE, Owens JC. Central venous pressure in optimal blood volume maintenance. Arch Surg (Chicago, Ill: 1960). 1962;85:563–78. PubMed PMID: 14001047. Epub 1962/10/01. eng

34. Marik PE, Baram M, Vahid B. Does central venous pressure predict fluid responsiveness? A systematic review of the literature and the tale of seven mares. Chest. 2008;134(1):172–8. PubMed PMID: 18628220. Epub 2008/07/17. eng
35. Marik PE, Cavallazzi R. Does the central venous pressure predict fluid responsiveness? An updated meta-analysis and a plea for some common sense. Crit Care Med. 2013;41(7):1774–81. PubMed PMID: 23774337. Epub 2013/06/19. eng
36. Legrand G, Ruscio L, Benhamou D, Pelletier-Fleury N. Goal-directed fluid therapy guided by cardiac monitoring during high-risk abdominal surgery in adult patients: cost-effectiveness analysis of esophageal Doppler and arterial pulse pressure waveform analysis. Value Health J Int Soc Pharmacoeconomics Outcomes Res. 2015;18(5):605–13. PubMed PMID: 26297088. Epub 2015/08/25. eng
37. Hack H. Use of the esophageal Doppler machine to help guide the intraoperative management of two children with pheochromocytoma. Paediatr Anaesth. 2006;16(8):867–76. PubMed PMID: 16884470. Epub 2006/08/04. eng
38. Kinney MA, Narr BJ, Warner MA. Perioperative management of pheochromocytoma. J Cardiothorac Vasc Anesth. 2002;16(3):359–69. PubMed PMID: 12073213. Epub 2002/06/20. eng
39. Subramaniam R. Pheochromocytoma – current concepts in diagnosis and management. Trends Anaesth Crit Care. 2011;1(2):104–10.
40. Friederich JA, Butterworth JF. Sodium nitroprusside: twenty years and counting. Anesth Analg. 1995;81(1):152–62. PubMed PMID: 7598246. Epub 1995/07/01. eng
41. Boden WE, Padala SK, Cabral KP, Buschmann IR, Sidhu MS. Role of short-acting nitroglycerin in the management of ischemic heart disease. Drug Des Devel Ther. 2015;9:4793–805. PubMed PMID: 26316714. Pubmed Central PMCID: PMC4548722. Epub 2015/09/01. eng
42. Lord MS, Augoustides JG. Perioperative management of pheochromocytoma: focus on magnesium, clevidipine, and vasopressin. J Cardiothorac Vasc Anesth. 2012;26(3):526–31. PubMed PMID: 22361482. Epub 2012/03/01. Eng
43. Kwon SY, Lee KS, Lee JN, Ha YS, Choi SH, Kim HT, et al. Risk factors for hypertensive attack during pheochromocytoma resection. Investig Clin Urol. 2016;57(3):184–90. PubMed PMID: 27194549. Pubmed Central PMCID: PMC4869566. Epub 2016/05/20. Eng
44. Kiernan CM, Du L, Chen X, Broome JT, Shi C, Peters MF, et al. Predictors of hemodynamic instability during surgery for pheochromocytoma. Ann Surg Oncol. 2014;21(12):3865–71. PubMed PMID: 24939623. Pubmed Central PMCID: PMC4192065. Epub 2014/06/19. Eng
45. Treschan TA, Peters J. The vasopressin system: physiology and clinical strategies. Anesthesiology. 2006;105(3):599–612. quiz 39-40. PubMed PMID: 16931995. Epub 2006/08/26. eng
46. Roth JV. Use of vasopressin bolus and infusion to treat catecholamine-resistant hypotension during pheochromocytoma resection. Anesthesiology. 2007;106(4):883–4. PubMed PMID: 17413940. Epub 2007/04/07. eng
47. Tan SG, Koay CK, Chan ST. The use of vasopressin to treat catecholamine-resistant hypotension after phaeochromocytoma removal. Anaesth Intensive Care. 2002;30(4):477–80. PubMed PMID: 12180588. Epub 2002/08/16. eng
48. Brunaud L, Nguyen-Thi PL, Mirallie E, Raffaelli M, Vriens M, Theveniaud PE, et al. Predictive factors for postoperative morbidity after laparoscopic adrenalectomy for pheochromocytoma: a multicenter retrospective analysis in 225 patients. Surg Endosc. 2016;30(3):1051–9. PubMed PMID: 26092019. Epub 2015/06/21. Eng
49. Srougi V, Chambo JL, Tanno FY, Soares IS, Almeida MQ, Pereira MA, et al. Presentation and surgery outcomes in elderly with pheocromocytoma: a comparative analysis with young patients. Int Braz J Urol Off J Braz Soc Urol. 2016;42(4):671–7. PubMed PMID: 27564276. Pubmed Central PMCID: PMC5006761. Epub 2016/08/27. eng
50. Dugas G, Fuller J, Singh S, Watson J. Pheochromocytoma and pregnancy: a case report and review of anesthetic management. Can J Anaesth J Can d'anesthesie. 2004;51(2):134–8. PubMed PMID: 14766689. Epub 2004/02/10. Eng
51. Jayatilaka G, Abayadeera A, Wijayaratna C, Senanayake H, Wijayaratna M. Phaeochromocytoma during pregnancy: anaesthetic management for a caesarean section combined with bilateral adrenalectomy. Ceylon Med J. 2013;58(4):173–4. PubMed PMID: 24385061. Epub 2014/01/05. Eng

Chapter 10
Surgery for Pheochromocytoma

Benjamin Deschner and Dina Elaraj

Introduction

Pheochromocytomas and paragangliomas are tumors that arise in chromaffin tissue and produce catecholamines. Rarely, these tumors can be biochemically silent and only produce symptoms due to mass effect [1]. Pheochromocytomas arise in the adrenal medulla, and paragangliomas (also referred to as extra-adrenal pheochromocytomas) arise in the sympathetic and, rarely, parasympathetic ganglia. The treatment of these tumors is usually surgical after appropriate preoperative preparation. The preoperative preparation of a patient with a catecholamine-producing tumor is described in a prior chapter and includes alpha-blockade, beta-blockade, and volume expansion. In addition, since 25–75% of patients with catecholamine-producing tumors will have hyperglycemia, glucose control is also important [2]. Furthermore, since almost 40% of patients with pheochromocytomas and paragangliomas will harbor a germline mutation [3], patients should be referred for genetic testing and genetic counseling prior to surgery, if possible, as knowledge of the specific gene mutation will allow for optimal surgical planning.

Given that the majority of patients with catecholamine-producing tumors have adrenal pheochromocytomas, this chapter will focus on the techniques of adrenalectomy. Adrenalectomy may be performed via an open incision or via a minimally

B. Deschner
Department of Surgery, Northwestern University Feinberg School of Medicine, Chicago, IL, USA

D. Elaraj (✉)
Department of Surgery, Northwestern University Feinberg School of Medicine, Chicago, IL, USA

Section of Endocrine Surgery, Northwestern University Feinberg School of Medicine, Chicago, IL, USA
e-mail: delaraj@nm.org

L. Landsberg (ed.), *Pheochromocytomas, Paragangliomas and Disorders of the Sympathoadrenal System*, Contemporary Endocrinology,
https://doi.org/10.1007/978-3-319-77048-2_10

invasive approach and may involve removing the entire adrenal gland or partially resecting the adrenal gland. Open adrenalectomy may be performed via the transabdominal (anterior), thoracoabdominal, or retroperitoneal (posterior or flank) approaches. Minimally invasive adrenalectomy may be performed via the laparoscopic transperitoneal (transabdominal) or retroperitoneoscopic approaches. Decisions regarding operative approach and extent of adrenalectomy will depend on tumor size, suspicion for malignancy, the patient's body mass index and past surgical history, genetic testing results, and surgeon experience.

Surgical Anatomy

The adrenal glands are paired, slightly asymmetric structures overlying the superior pole of each kidney. Each gland normally weighs between 4 and 6 grams and consists of an outer cortex and an inner catecholamine-secreting medulla. The cortex has a golden yellow-orange color, which visually distinguishes the adrenal gland from the surrounding pale-yellow perinephric fat. The adrenal glands are located in the perinephric fat within Gerota's fascia.

Exposure and dissection of the adrenal glands requires knowledge of the many adjacent structures. The right adrenal gland sits slightly more superiorly than the left, lying posterolateral to the inferior vena cava (IVC) and right lobe of the liver. The left adrenal gland lies lateral to the aorta and posterior to the tail of the pancreas, splenic artery, and stomach, with the peritoneum of the lesser sac overlying the gland's anterior aspect.

One of the most important surgical anatomic considerations is the blood supply to the adrenal glands. The arterial blood supply is similar in both adrenal glands, with fine arterial branches (as opposed to a solitary discrete vessel) perfusing the glands from the superior, middle, and inferior adrenal arteries (which are branches off the inferior phrenic artery, aorta, and renal artery, respectively). In contrast, the venous supply is quite different and typically consists of a dominant adrenal vein with varying numbers of smaller accessory veins. The right adrenal vein typically exits the gland inferiorly and anteromedially, taking a short course into the posterolateral aspect of the IVC. The left adrenal vein is longer, exiting the hilum of the gland to join with the left inferior phrenic vein, with the confluence of these veins draining into the left renal vein.

Perioperative Management and Technical Considerations

Regardless of the operative approach, several considerations are necessary to optimize outcomes in patients with pheochromocytomas. These include appropriate deep vein thrombosis prophylaxis, intraoperative hemodynamic monitoring via arterial line, placement of a large-bore central venous catheter for the rapid administration of crystalloid and rarely blood products, placement of a Foley catheter, and close communication between the surgical and anesthesia teams. Close communication between the surgical and anesthesia teams is critical, as tumor manipulation by the surgeon may cause release of catecholamines with resultant tachycardia and hypertension. Furthermore, it is essential for the surgeon to communicate when the main adrenal vein will be ligated, as the patient may develop hypotension at this point in the operation due to unopposed alpha-blockade from the preoperative preparation and may require treatment with vasopressors. Gentle manipulation and dissection is critical, as intraoperative fracture of the pheochromocytoma can result in seeding and recurrence, either in the adrenalectomy bed or throughout the peritoneal cavity [4]. Postoperatively, patients should be closely monitored in the recovery room, a step-down unit, or the surgical intensive care unit, depending on resources available.

Minimally Invasive Adrenalectomy

Minimally invasive adrenalectomy may be performed via the laparoscopic transperitoneal or retroperitoneoscopic approaches. Minimally invasive approaches have been shown to be associated with significantly less pain and morbidity than open adrenalectomy, as well as shorter hospital length of stay and improved patient satisfaction [5, 6].

Laparoscopic transperitoneal adrenalectomy was first reported in 1992 by Gagner and colleagues [7] and since then has become the most widespread minimally invasive approach to the resection of adrenal tumors. The operation is most commonly performed with the patient in the lateral decubitus position and is indicated for the treatment of pheochromocytomas <6 cm without evidence of local invasion or metastasis [8]. Technical factors largely limit laparoscopy for the resection of larger tumors, but laparoscopic resection of benign pheochromocytomas >6 cm is possible, particularly on the left side, and an individualized approach should be undertaken. Retroperitoneoscopic adrenalectomy was first reported in 1995 by Mercan and colleagues [9] and has further advanced the field of minimally invasive adrenalectomy. Since the initial report, other authors have reported their modifications of the technique [10, 11]. It is performed with the patient in the prone jackknife position.

Outcomes of laparoscopic transperitoneal adrenalectomy and retroperitoneoscopic adrenalectomy are similar with respect to operative time, blood loss, complication rates, and length of stay [12–14]. There are, however, advantages and disadvantages to each. Advantages of laparoscopic transperitoneal adrenalectomy include the ability perform an intra-abdominal evaluation, the ability to dissect larger tumors, and the ease of converting to an open procedure, if necessary. Disadvantages include the need to reposition the patient in cases of bilateral pheochromocytomas. Advantages of the retroperitoneoscopic approach include the avoidance of scar tissue in patients who have undergone previous abdominal surgery and the ability to perform bilateral adrenalectomy without repositioning the patient. Disadvantages of the retroperitoneoscopic approach include limitations in the size of the tumor amenable to this approach [5].

Laparoscopic Transperitoneal Adrenalectomy

Laparoscopic transperitoneal adrenalectomy is most commonly performed with the patient in the lateral decubitus position, which allows for passive retraction of adjacent abdominal viscera by gravity (Fig. 10.1). The patient is cradled by a vacuum bean-bag immobilizer with an axillary roll and all pressure points generously padded. The patient is positioned, so the break in the table is between the costal margin and the iliac crest, and the table is then flexed.

The first step in the procedure involves gaining peritoneal access and port placement. The abdominal cavity is entered with either a Veress needle or an open technique, and a pneumoperitoneum with carbon dioxide is established. Standard port placement involves four 11 mm ports placed equally spaced along the costal margin (Fig. 10.2); left adrenalectomy can potentially be done with three ports if the spleen and tail of the pancreas can be adequately retracted with gravity.

The next step in the procedure involves gaining exposure to the adrenal gland. On the right side, this involves mobilizing the liver anteromedially by incising the lateral attachments and right triangular ligament. Once the liver is mobilized and retracted, the peritoneum along the posterior aspect of the liver is incised, thus exposing the adrenal gland and IVC. On the left side, exposure to the adrenal gland involves mobilizing the splenic flexure of the colon inferiorly and incising the splenorenal ligament, allowing the spleen and tail of the pancreas to be mobilized anteromedially. Once the spleen and tail of the pancreas are retracted, Gerota's fascia medial to the adrenal gland is incised, thus exposing the adrenal gland.

The next step in the procedure is mobilization of the adrenal gland itself. This is initially done in a cephalad-to-caudad direction along the medial aspect of the adrenal gland while retracting the gland laterally. This allows for devascularization of the small adrenal arteries along the medial aspect of the gland. Next, the inferior aspect of the gland is dissected after incising the peritoneum along the inferior aspect of the gland. At this point, the adrenal vein is identified and either sealed and

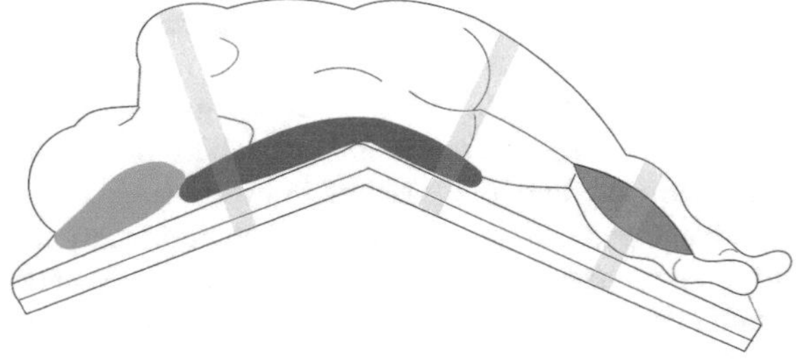

Fig. 10.1 Lateral decubitus position for laparoscopic transperitoneal right adrenalectomy

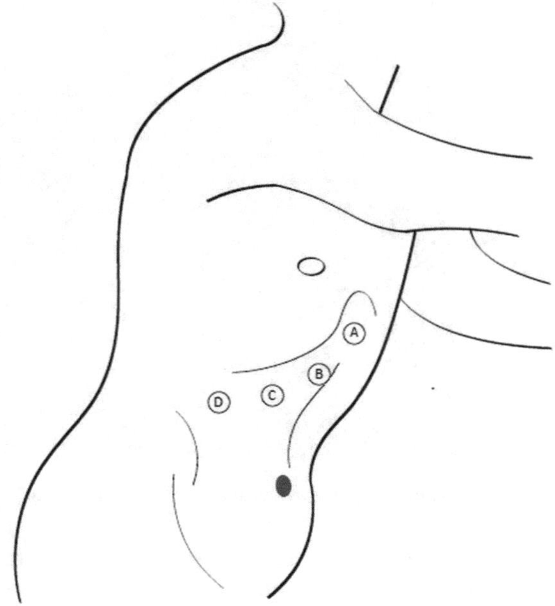

Fig. 10.2 Port site placement for laparoscopic transperitoneal right adrenalectomy. *A*: liver retractor, *B*: laparoscope, *C* and *D*: dissecting instruments

divided with an energy device or clipped and divided with scissors. It is important to note that if the adrenal vein is divided before sufficiently devascularizing the arterial blood supply, the pheochromocytoma may become engorged and bleed, potentially precluding completion of the procedure laparoscopically. The hypertensive episodes characteristic to the dissection of pheochromocytomas may also lead to increased blood loss and obscure the visualization of important structures. As previously mentioned, it is also important to communicate the timing of division of the main adrenal vein to the anesthesia team.

The last step of the procedure is dissection of the adrenal gland away from the renal hilum and off the anterior-superior aspect of the kidney. This is done by retracting the adrenal gland superolaterally away from the superior pole of the kidney and taking the remaining posterior and lateral attachments with an energy device. Retraction is crucial at this point, since if this space is not opened adequately, a superior pole renal artery branch may be mistaken for an inferior adrenal artery; injury to a superior pole renal artery branch can result in renovascular hypertension.

Retroperitoneoscopic Adrenalectomy

Retroperitoneoscopic adrenalectomy is performed with the patient in the prone jackknife position with the chest and abdomen supported by parallel bolsters. The extremities are cradled with generous padding.

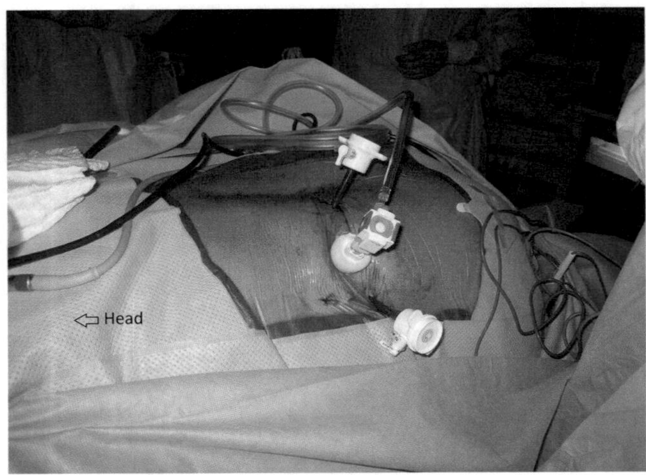

Fig. 10.3 Port site placement for retroperitoneoscopic left adrenalectomy

The first step in the procedure involves gaining retroperitoneal access and port placement. Standard port placement involves three ports spaced 4–5 cm apart, placed below the tips of the 12th and 11th ribs: a 12 mm trocar containing a spherical dissecting balloon and two 5 mm trocars placed on either side (Fig. 10.3). The spherical dissecting balloon is used to develop the retroperitoneal space posterior and superior to the kidney, and the retroperitoneal space is insufflated with carbon dioxide.

The next step in the procedure involves identification of the adrenal gland. Since the adrenal gland is a retroperitoneal structure, no adjacent organs have to be mobilized in order to expose the gland. The superior pole of the kidney is identified and retracted caudad. The inferior aspect of the adrenal gland is then dissected away from the superior pole of the kidney. The dissection then continues along the medial aspect of the gland. The small adrenal arteries along the medial aspect of the gland are devascularized. On the right side, it is important to note that these vessels cross the IVC posteriorly. The adrenal vein is next identified and controlled. Lastly, the superolateral attachments are taken. It is important to leave these attachments for last, as they help hold the adrenal gland in place during other aspects of the dissection.

Open Adrenalectomy

Open adrenalectomy may be performed via the transabdominal (anterior), thoracoabdominal, or retroperitoneal (posterior or flank) approaches. In the current minimally invasive era, the transabdominal and thoracoabdominal approaches are reserved for large tumors or those with invasion into surrounding structures

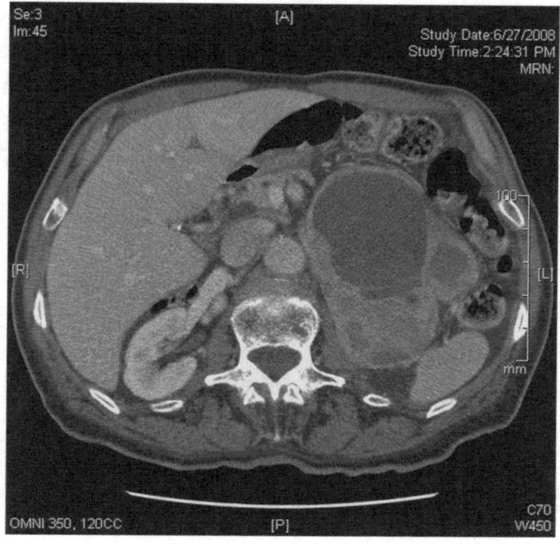

Fig. 10.4 Axial computed tomography image from an 83-year-old male patient with a 16 cm left adrenal pheochromocytoma which required resection via an open transperitoneal approach

requiring en bloc resection or may be necessary for resection of a recurrent pheochromocytoma in a previously dissected area. Figure 10.4 shows a computed tomography scan of an 83-year-old patient with a 16 cm left adrenal pheochromocytoma that required resection via an open transabdominal approach. The open retroperitoneal approach is not commonly performed and is almost of historical interest only, since large or invasive tumors should be resected via a transabdominal or thoracoabdominal approach, and smaller tumors that may be considered for a retroperitoneal approach due to a history of prior abdominal surgery, for example, should be resected retroperitoneoscopically.

Open transperitoneal and thoracoabdominal adrenalectomy are performed with the patient in the supine position. If a thoracoabdominal approach is to be undertaken, a bolster should be placed under the flank of the side of the adrenal tumor. Open transperitoneal adrenalectomy may be done via multiple incisions including subcostal, extended subcostal (extending cephalad through the xiphoid), bilateral subcostal, or vertical midline, depending on tumor size and invasiveness/relationship to surrounding structures. The thoracoabdominal incision begins as an upper midline incision and then curves to follow the course of the 8th or 9th rib to the posterior axillary line. It is deepened through the latissimus dorsi, serratus anterior, and intercostal muscles, and the pleura is entered. A segment of the rib is removed to improve exposure, and the diaphragm is divided along its periphery.

The next step in the procedure involves exposure of the adrenal gland. On the right side, this involves mobilizing the liver anteromedially by not only incising the lateral attachments and right triangular and coronary ligaments, but by also dividing the falciform ligament and incising the left triangular and coronary ligaments, as well. Sometimes it is necessary to mobilize the hepatic flexure of the colon inferiorly. A Kocher maneuver of the duodenum is useful to expose the infrahepatic IVC. If tumor invasion of the IVC is suspected, vascular control of both the suprahepatic and infrahepatic IVC is critical before beginning the tumor dissection. On the left side, exposure to the adrenal gland involves mobilizing the splenic flexure of the colon inferiorly and mobilizing the spleen and tail of the pancreas anteromedially. An alternative approach involves dividing the gastrocolic ligament and entering the lesser sac. The peritoneum inferior to the pancreas is next incised. Sometimes both techniques are necessary in order to obtain adequate exposure. Once the adrenal gland has been exposed, it is dissected from its surrounding structures. If there is invasion into adjacent organs, en bloc resection should be performed. Even in the case of malignant pheochromocytomas that are not completely resectable, surgical debulking has been advocated for palliation, both to reduce the levels of circulating catecholamines and to facilitate uptake of postoperative 131-I-meta-iodobenzylguanidine radiotherapy [15].

Partial Adrenalectomy

As previously discussed, up to 40% of patients with pheochromocytomas or paragangliomas will have a germline mutation [3]. Because germline mutations can lead to the development of bilateral pheochromocytomas, necessitating potential treatment with bilateral adrenalectomy and subsequent lifelong steroid hormone dependence, the technique of partial adrenalectomy (sometimes referred to as subtotal, cortical-sparing, or adrenal-sparing adrenalectomy) has been advocated. This technique was first reported for the treatment of bilateral pheochromocytomas by multiple authors in the 1980s [16–18]. The potential to avoid lifelong steroid hormone dependence and risk of Addisonian crisis is of particular importance in patients with bilateral pheochromocytomas associated with genetic syndromes, since the requirement for steroid hormone replacement can complicate the treatment (both surgical and systemic) of other manifestations of the syndrome.

The technique of partial adrenalectomy for bilateral pheochromocytomas usually involves a subtotal adrenalectomy on the side with the larger tumor with careful evaluation of the adrenal gland remnant. It has been determined that a remnant size of about 1/3 of the entire gland should provide adequate cortical function [19]. If the remnant appears sufficiently vascularized, a total adrenalectomy is then performed on the contralateral side. If the initial adrenal gland remnant does not appear sufficiently vascularized, then it is resected and a subtotal resection is attempted on the contralateral side. This strategy limits the potential for reoperation for recurrence to one side, as opposed to bilateral partial adrenalectomy, which has also been described.

It is important to note that it may not be technically feasible to perform partial adrenalectomy, and this is an intraoperative decision made by the surgeon. Tumors amenable to this technique are tumors located at the periphery of the gland, where a rim of normal-appearing adrenal cortex can be distinguished and separated from the pheochromocytoma. Adrenal glands with large or multiple pheochromocytomas will probably not be amenable to this technique. It is also important to note that pheochromocytomas arise from the adrenal medulla and that when an adrenal gland is partially resected, some adrenal medullary tissue may be left behind and is at risk for the development of recurrent pheochromocytoma.

After resection of bilateral pheochromocytomas via the described technique, the remnant cortical tissue should be assessed for function by measuring the serum or plasma cortisol the morning after surgery. The diagnosis of adrenal insufficiency is highly likely if the morning cortisol is <5 mcg/dL (140 nmol/L) [20]. If the morning cortisol is low or equivocal, a cosyntropin stimulation test should be performed, which involves administration of 250 mcg cosyntropin intravenously and measurement of cortisol 30–60 min later. A peak-stimulated cortisol level <18 mcg/dL (500 nmol/L) indicates inadequate adrenal reserve, and glucocorticoid therapy should be initiated [20].

Outcomes of partial adrenalectomy are evaluated by the rate of steroid hormone independence and the rate of recurrent pheochromocytoma. The rate of steroid hormone independence has been reported to range from 57% to 100% in a review of ten studies containing at least ten patients each with hereditary pheochromocytoma undergoing adrenal-sparing adrenalectomy [21]. In the two largest series, the rate of steroid hormone independence was 57% for 114 patients with multiple endocrine neoplasia type 2 (MEN2) [22] and 91% for 57 patients with both MEN2 and von Hippel-Lindau (VHL) syndrome [23].

The estimation of risk of recurrent pheochromocytoma after partial adrenalectomy is limited by small numbers of patients in published series, short follow-up times, and how recurrence is defined by different authors. Some authors define this as contralateral recurrence after total unilateral adrenalectomy, while other authors define this as local recurrence on the ipsilateral side of a partial adrenalectomy. The former definition provides information regarding the time interval between an initial adrenalectomy and the development of a pheochromocytoma on the contralateral side, while the latter definition provides the true recurrence rate of the technique of partial adrenalectomy. In a review of ten studies containing at least ten patients each with hereditary pheochromocytoma undergoing adrenal-sparing adrenalectomy, the risk of recurrence ranged from 0% to 21% at a mean follow-up ranging from 36 to 138 months [21]. In the two largest series, the rate of recurrence was 3% at a mean follow-up of 120 months for 114 patients with MEN2 [22] and 0% at 48 months for 57 patients with both MEN2 and VHL [23].

Summary

In summary, optimal outcomes for patients with pheochromocytomas require appropriate preoperative genetic testing, adequate preoperative alpha- and beta-blockade, intraoperative hemodynamic monitoring, meticulous surgical technique, and close communication between the surgical and anesthesia teams. The choice of operative approach (open vs minimally invasive) and decisions regarding extent of adrenalectomy will depend on tumor size, suspicion for malignancy, patient factors, genetic testing results, and surgeon experience.

References

1. Timmers HJ, Pacak K, Huynh TT, et al. Biochemically silent abdominal paragangliomas in patients with mutations in the succinate dehydrogenase subunit B gene. J Clin Endocrinol Metab. 2008;93:4826–32.
2. Wiesner TD, Bluher M, Windgassen M, Paschke R. Improvement of insulin sensitivity after adrenalectomy in patients with pheochromocytoma. J Clin Endocrinol Metab. 2003;88:3632–6.
3. Gupta G, Pacak K, Committee AAS. Precision Medicine: an update on genotype-biochemical phenotype relationships in Pheochromocytoma/Paraganglioma patients. Endocr Pract Off J Am Coll Endocrinol Am Assoc Clin Endocrinol. 2017;23:690.
4. Li ML, Fitzgerald PA, Price DC, Norton JA. Iatrogenic pheochromocytomatosis: a previously unreported result of laparoscopic adrenalectomy. Surgery. 2001;130:1072–7.
5. Gumbs AA, Gagner M. Laparoscopic adrenalectomy. Best Pract Res Clin Endocrinol Metab. 2006;20:483–99.
6. Agarwal G, Sadacharan D, Aggarwal V, et al. Surgical management of organ-contained unilateral pheochromocytoma: comparative outcomes of laparoscopic and conventional open surgical procedures in a large single-institution series. Langenbeck's Arch Surg. 2012;397:1109–16.
7. Gagner M, Lacroix A, Bolte E. Laparoscopic adrenalectomy in Cushing's syndrome and pheochromocytoma. N Engl J Med. 1992;327:1033.
8. Lenders JW, Duh QY, Eisenhofer G, et al. Pheochromocytoma and paraganglioma: an endocrine society clinical practice guideline. J Clin Endocrinol Metab. 2014;99:1915–42.
9. Mercan S, Seven R, Ozarmagan S, Tezelman S. Endoscopic retroperitoneal adrenalectomy. Surgery. 1995;118:1071–5. discussion 5-6
10. Siperstein AE, Berber E, Engle KL, Duh QY, Clark OH. Laparoscopic posterior adrenalectomy: technical considerations. Arch Surg. 2000;135:967–71.
11. Walz MK, Alesina PF, Wenger FA, et al. Posterior retroperitoneoscopic adrenalectomy--results of 560 procedures in 520 patients. Surgery. 2006;140:943–8. discussion 8-50
12. Berber E, Tellioglu G, Harvey A, Mitchell J, Milas M, Siperstein A. Comparison of laparoscopic transabdominal lateral versus posterior retroperitoneal adrenalectomy. Surgery. 2009;146:621–5. discussion 5-6
13. Lezoche E, Guerrieri M, Feliciotti F, et al. Anterior, lateral, and posterior retroperitoneal approaches in endoscopic adrenalectomy. Surg Endosc. 2002;16:96–9.
14. Rubinstein M, Gill IS, Aron M, et al. Prospective, randomized comparison of transperitoneal versus retroperitoneal laparoscopic adrenalectomy. J Urol. 2005;174:442–5. discussion 5
15. Scholz T, Eisenhofer G, Pacak K, Dralle H, Lehnert H. Clinical review: current treatment of malignant pheochromocytoma. J Clin Endocrinol Metab. 2007;92:1217–25.
16. Irvin GL 3rd, Fishman LM, Sher JA. Familial pheochromocytoma. Surgery. 1983;94:938–40.
17. van Heerden JA, Sizemore GW, Carney JA, Brennan MD, Sheps SG. Bilateral subtotal adrenal resection for bilateral pheochromocytomas in multiple endocrine neoplasia, type IIa: a case report. Surgery. 1985;98:363–6.
18. Giordano WC. Preservation of adrenocortical function during surgery for bilateral pheochromocytoma. J Urol. 1982;127:100–2.
19. Brauckhoff M, Thanh PN, Gimm O, Bar A, Brauckhoff K, Dralle H. Functional results after endoscopic subtotal cortical-sparing adrenalectomy. Surg Today. 2003;33:342–8.
20. Bornstein SR, Allolio B, Arlt W, et al. Diagnosis and treatment of primary adrenal insufficiency: an Endocrine Society clinical practice guideline. J Clin Endocrinol Metab. 2016;101:364–89.
21. Castinetti F, Taieb D, Henry JF, et al. MANAGEMENT OF ENDOCRINE DISEASE: outcome of adrenal sparing surgery in heritable pheochromocytoma. Eur J Endocrinol. 2016;174:R9–18.
22. Castinetti F, Qi XP, Walz MK, et al. Outcomes of adrenal-sparing surgery or total adrenalectomy in phaeochromocytoma associated with multiple endocrine neoplasia type 2: an international retrospective population-based study. Lancet Oncol. 2014;15:648–55.
23. Alesina PF, Hinrichs J, Meier B, Schmid KW, Neumann HP, Walz MK. Minimally invasive cortical-sparing surgery for bilateral pheochromocytomas. Langenbeck's Arch Surg. 2012;397:233–8.

Chapter 11
Pheochromocytoma in Pregnancy

Kenneth K. Chen

The prevalence of pheochromocytoma in pregnancy has been estimated to be 1 in 54,000 pregnancies [1, 2]. Despite it being an uncommon condition, it is important to diagnose it promptly, and the most common reason for overlooking this is the much higher prevalence of pregnancy-related hypertensive conditions such as gestational hypertension and preeclampsia. Other presenting symptoms such as headaches, dyspnea, palpitations, nausea, flushing, and anxiety are nonspecific and can easily be overlooked, especially in a pregnant woman who may experience these symptoms as part of normal pregnancy.

Maternal pheochromocytoma can have profound effects on both mother and fetus, and so it is important that it be considered as part of the differential diagnosis for severe or paroxysmal hypertension in the pregnant woman particularly in the first half of pregnancy. There is minimal placental transfer of catecholamines due to the placental expression of catecholamine-metabolizing enzymes such as monoamine oxidase and catechol-O-methyltransferase [3]; this serves as a protective barrier for the fetus against excessive maternal catecholamine exposure. Adverse fetal effects are usually a result of catecholamine-induced uteroplacental vasoconstriction which in turn can cause intrauterine hypoxia and/or placental abruption [4]. Unrecognized pheochromocytoma is associated with a maternal and fetal mortality rate of up to 50% at induction of anesthesia or during labor [5]. In contrast, after early diagnosis and proper treatment, maternal mortality has declined substantially to <5% and fetal mortality to <15% [6, 7]. A review in 1999 estimated that antenatal diagnosis of pheochromocytoma was made in 83% of cases [8], and a more recent review published in 2013 estimated that the current rate has declined slightly to 73% [9].

K. K. Chen (✉)
Division & Fellowship Director, Obstetric & Consultative Medicine Staff Endocrinologist, Women & Infants' Hospital of Rhode Island, Alpert Medical School of Brown University, Providence, RI, USA
e-mail: kenneth_k_chen@brown.edu

L. Landsberg (ed.), *Pheochromocytomas, Paragangliomas and Disorders of the Sympathoadrenal System*, Contemporary Endocrinology,
https://doi.org/10.1007/978-3-319-77048-2_11

There are certain signs and symptoms which may be of some help in differentiating pheochromocytoma from pregnancy-related hypertension. With the latter, the hypertension is very unlikely to be paroxysmal and develops after 20 weeks. Excessive ankle edema, proteinuria, or clinical features of the HELLP syndrome are not compatible with pheochromocytoma. The presence of clinical signs such as cafe au lait spots, skin freckling, or cutaneous fibromas would make the possibility of pheochromocytoma very compelling given its association with neurofibromatosis type 1. It should be noted that both conditions can give rise to an elevated hemoglobin level and hematocrit – the former due to tumor-associated erythropoietin production and the latter due to hemoconcentration from intravascular fluid shifts.

Catecholamine production generally remains unchanged throughout pregnancy, and the levels are not increased in preeclampsia [10]. Fasting plasma metanephrine levels are the most sensitive and specific diagnostic test though it should be noted that falsely elevated levels can be caused by pharmacologic agents such as tricyclic antidepressants, labetalol, methyldopa, prochlorperazine, and decongestants. It is not recommended that pregnant women be subjected to pharmacodynamic tests such as the glucagon stimulation test or the clonidine suppression test given the risk of serious side-effects. There is currently no established data which necessitates the use of different reference values for plasma or urinary metanephrines in pregnant women.

Anatomical localization is required for definitive treatment once a biochemical diagnosis has been made. In pregnancy, the modality of choice to achieve this is T2-weighted magnetic resonance imaging (MRI) with gadolinium contrast given that computed tomography (CT) scanning involves significant radiation exposure to the fetus. Nuclear scanning with metaiodobenzylguanidine (MIBG) is contraindicated in pregnancy as it has been shown that there is evidence that this molecule crosses the placenta [11]. Anatomical localization is also important as a growing, gravid uterus can impact particularly extra-adrenal lesions as they tend to be more influenced by changes in position or by uterine contractions. Physical compression of these lesions can cause hemorrhage into the tumor and/or precipitate a hypertensive crisis.

Medical therapy in the form of alpha-blockade should be initiated once a biochemical diagnosis is made; phenoxybenzamine is considered the agent of choice as it provides long-acting, stable, and noncompetitive blockade. It should be noted that the target blood pressure should not be too low as this may compromise the uteroplacental circulation. Placental transfer of phenoxybenzamine does occur, but it is generally considered to be safe [12], though neonatal hypotension has been reported in newborns of mothers treated with it prior to delivery [13]. Beta-blockade is then instituted after alpha-blockade is achieved to avoid tachyarrhythmias; the dose should be titrated to achieve a maternal heart rate of 80–100 beats per minute. Metoprolol is the preferred agent as others such as atenolol have been associated with fetal bradycardia and/or intrauterine fetal growth restriction [14]. Hypertensive crises should be treated with intravenous phentolamine or nitroprusside, although the latter should be limited due to the risk of fetal cyanide toxicity. It is important to avoid commonly used medications which can precipitate a crisis, such as metoclopramide or contrast media. It is also important for the obstetrician to minimize abdominal palpation as this can invoke a sudden and strong tumoral release of catecholamines.

Surgery in the form of laparoscopic adrenalectomy can be considered once adequate medical therapy and localization of the lesion have been achieved. No reliable data exist comparing outcomes regarding timing of surgery (prior to 24 weeks where diagnosed, at term, postpartum) or mode of delivery (vaginal or C-section). Most institutions advocate that if the lesion is diagnosed during the first two trimesters, the best time to operate is during the second trimester; and if the lesion is diagnosed during the third trimester, surgery should be delayed until at least the time of delivery though the timing of this will need to be brought forward if the mother remains symptomatic despite the medical blockade. It is well documented that the best time for elective surgeries to occur for a pregnant woman is during the second trimester as there is an increased risk of spontaneous abortion and preterm labor if they occurred during the first and third trimesters, respectively. Curiously, a systematic review published in 2013 found that there was no definite advantage in proceeding with tumor removal during the second trimester even if it had been diagnosed early in pregnancy [9].

In the instance where the pheochromocytoma is not removed before 24 weeks gestation, there is considerable debate as to whether it should be removed at the time of delivery via an elective C-section or whether it should be removed laparoscopically a few weeks postpartum. Proponents of the latter approach give the advantages of a faster operative recovery as well as the ability to utilize MIBG and/or positron emission tomography (PET) to exclude multiple or metastatic disease [15] prior to surgery. An elective C-section is the delivery method of choice as the process of labor may result in uncontrolled release of catecholamines secondary to pain and uterine contractions. That being said, there are many instances where a planned induction of labor with assisted vaginal delivery is equally as safe (see clinical case #2 below). In those patients in whom the tumor has been removed successfully by surgery during the second trimester, they are at significant risk of postoperative hypotension due to the prolonged action of phenoxybenzamine as well as increased plasma volume during this time. Hence, they are advised to increase their salt and fluid intake for the preceding 2 weeks prior to surgery. These patients can have their delivery done by either method.

It has been known for some years that magnesium reduces catecholamine release from both the adrenal medulla and peripheral adrenergic nerve terminals [16]. It is also a highly effective direct alpha-adrenergic antagonist as well as anti-arrhythmic in the setting of high-dose epinephrine infusions [17]. Magnesium sulfate infusions are efficacious in the management of hypertension and arrhythmias during operative removal of pheochromocytoma, and case reports describe its successful use in patients with pheochromocytoma crisis including those with catecholamine-induced cardiomyopathy [18, 19]. Obstetricians and maternity units are very experienced with the use of magnesium sulfate infusions for the prevention of seizures in patients with preeclampsia; hence it is this author's recommendation that they be routinely considered during labor and delivery and/or operative removal of the tumor in pregnant patients with pheochromocytoma.

This author also recommends that genetic screening should be considered in all pregnant women with pheochromocytoma given that patients with germline mutations tend to be younger. This is especially so in those patients with paragangliomas, bilateral adrenal pheochromocytomas, a positive family history, and those with clinical findings suggestive of associated syndromic disorders such as multiple endocrine neoplasia type 2, neurofibromatosis type 1, von Hippel-Lindau syndrome, or the familial paraganglioma syndromes (SDHB, SDHD). A hereditary basis may be found in up to 24% of patients, and detection of pheochromocytoma in the proband may result in early diagnosis and intervention of other affected family members [20, 21].

Clinical Case #1

A 29-year-old primigravida presented for her routine prenatal visit at 16+ weeks gestation. She has no documented medical or significant family history, and her pregnancy had been uneventful to date, but it was noted at this visit that her blood pressure was elevated at 150/95 mmHg. Her ob-gyn sent off preeclampsia labs which were all normal. The decision was made to observe the patient given that she was completely asymptomatic at this time. She denied any symptoms suggestive of obstructive sleep apnea.

She presented for her level 2 ultrasound at 19 weeks gestation, and it was noted at this time that her blood pressure was still elevated at 160/100 mmHg and she had an elevated heart rate of 125–130 beats per minute. She was still asymptomatic at this time, but she was admitted to hospital under the maternal-fetal medicine service for further management.

A urinary drug screen was negative. Preeclampsia labs were again found to be completely normal. In any case, preeclampsia did not explain the patient's sinus tachycardia, and it is extremely rare for preeclampsia to present before 20 weeks gestation unless the patient had a molar pregnancy or had severe preexisting maternal medical disease such as chronic renal insufficiency. A secondary cause of hypertension was suspected, and given her concurrent tachycardia, thyroid function tests and fasting plasma metanephrines were ordered first up with a view that further testing for other endocrinopathies or primary renal disease would occur should they be negative. Fasting plasma normetanephrine level was found to be significantly elevated at 2.5 nmol/L (upper limit of normal = 0.90 nmol/L), and a subsequent 24 h urinary norepinephrine level of 1024 nmol/day (upper limit of normal = 505 nmol/day) is consistent with a diagnosis of pheochromocytoma.

This case illustrates the importance of considering a secondary cause of hypertension for patients who present in early pregnancy with such and that pheochromocytoma should always be considered in these instances. Preeclampsia is and should always be considered as a possibility though it is important to recognize that it usually presents after 20 weeks gestation and that there are usually maternal and/or fetal features which reflect the placental insufficiency associated with this condition (e.g., maternal proteinuria, maternal HELLP syndrome, fetal growth restriction).

Clinical Case #2

A 26-year-old G3P2 presented to her regional hospital at 12 weeks gestation with a hypertensive emergency. A secondary work-up was ordered, and her fasting plasma normetanephrine was significantly elevated. A diagnosis of pheochromocytoma was made, but she was not transferred to our maternal-fetal medicine service for further management of her pregnancy until 24 weeks gestation due to geographical barriers.

She was commenced on phenoxybenzamine which was increased gradually, and she was maintained on a dose of 20 mg po QID between 28 weeks gestation to the time of her delivery. She was added on labetalol therapy at 34 weeks gestation to help control her sinus tachycardia. A MRI scan of her abdomen was performed at 25 weeks gestation which revealed a solitary lesion measuring 35 mm in diameter just inferior to the medial limb of her left adrenal gland.

A maternal cardiac echocardiography was performed at the beginning of the third trimester to exclude left ventricular dysfunction due to catecholamine cardiomyopathy. Serial growth ultrasounds were performed which showed that her baby was measuring at 10th percentile throughout the third trimester. The decision was made to induce her at 36 weeks gestation given that both of her previous deliveries were uncomplicated vaginal deliveries with relatively short duration of labor; it was decided that she should have an assisted second stage of labor to avoid prolonged pushing. Regional anesthesia was administered early on to minimize pain, and she was commenced on a magnesium sulfate infusion at this time. Her blood pressure was well-maintained throughout her labor which lasted only 4 h in total.

Her postpartum course was uneventful. The infant was monitored in the NICU for the first 72 h and fortunately did not experience any hypotension or respiratory depression. She elected not to breastfeed given that there is a paucity of data on the transfer of phenoxybenzamine to the infant via lactation. A MIBG scintiscan was performed at 1 month postpartum which confirmed that there was no avid disease other than the left adrenal gland. She had an elective laparoscopic left adrenalectomy at 5 weeks postpartum which was uncomplicated. She was successfully titrated off all her antihypertensive medications afterward and has remained well since then with normal documented levels of plasma and urine metanephrines. Histopathology confirmed a 33 mm pheochromocytoma which stained positive for succinate dehydrogenase complex subunit B (SDHB).

A few multidisciplinary meetings were convened throughout the course of this lady's pregnancy between her maternal-fetal medicine specialist, endocrinologist, endocrine surgeon, obstetric anesthesiologist, and neonatologist. The individualized management plan (especially the mode of delivery and the timing of surgery) which was based upon repeated multidisciplinary discussion brought about the good outcomes experienced by both mother and baby.

References

1. Harrington JL, Farley DR, van Heerden JA, Ramin KD. Adrenal tumors and pregnancy. World J Surg. 1999;23:182–6.
2. Lindsay JR, Nieman LK. Adrenal disorders in pregnancy. Endocrinol Metab Clin N Am. 2006;35:1–20.
3. Dahia PLM, Hayashida CY, Strunz C, et al. Low cord blood levels of catecholamine from a newborn of a pheochromocytoma patient. Eur J Endocrinol. 1994;130:217–9.
4. Combs CA, Easterling TR, Schmucker BC. Hemodynamic observations during paroxysmal hypertension in a pregnancy with pheochromocytoma. Obstet Gynecol. 1989;74:439–41.
5. Lau P, Permezel M, Dawson P, et al. Pheochromocytoma in pregnancy. Aust N Z J Obstet Gynecol. 1996;36:472–6.
6. Sarathi V, Lila AR, Bandgar TR, et al. Phaeochromocytoma and pregnancy: a rare but dangerous combination. Endocr Pract. 2010;16:300–9.
7. Lenders JWM. Pheochromocytoma and pregnancy: a deceptive connection. Eur J Endocrinol. 2012;166:143–50.
8. Ahlawart SK, Jain S, Kumari S, et al. Phaeochromocytoma associated with pregnancy: case report & review of the literature. Obstet Gynecol Surv. 1999;54:728–37.
9. Biggar MA, Lennard TWJ. Systematic review of phaeochromocytoma in pregnancy. Br J Surg. 2013;100:182–90.
10. Pedersen EB, Christensen NJ, Christensen P, et al. Preeclampsia - a state of prostaglandin deficiency? Urinary prostaglandin secretion, the renin-aldosterone system, and circulating catecholamines in preeclampsia. Hypertension. 1983;5:105–11.
11. Ilias I, Sahdev A, Reznek RH, et al. The optimal imaging of adrenal tumours: a comparison of different methods. Endocr Relat Cancer. 2007;14:587–99.
12. Santeiro ML, Stromquist C, Wyble L. Phenoxybenzamine placental transfer during the third trimester. Ann Pharmacother. 1996;30:1249–51.
13. Aplin SC, Yee KF, Cole MJ. Neonatal effects of long-term phenoxybenzamine therapy. Anesthesiology. 2004;100:1608–10.
14. Lydakis C, Lip GY, Beevers M, Beevers DG. Atenolol and fetal growth in pregnancies complicated by hypertension. Am J Hypertens. 1999;12:541–7.
15. Junglee N, Harries SE, Davies N, et al. Pheochromocytoma in pregnancy: when is operative intervention indicated? J Women's Health. 2007;16:1362–5.
16. Douglas WW, Rubin RP. The mechanism of catecholamine release from the adrenal medulla and the role of calcium in stimulus-secretion coupling. J Physiol. 1963;167:288–310.
17. Mayer DB, Miletich DJ, Feld JM, Albrecht RF. The effects of magnesium salts on the duration of epinephrine-induced ventricular tachyarrhythmias in anesthetized rats. Anesthesiology. 1989;71:923–8.
18. James MF, Cronje L. Pheochromocytoma crisis: the use of magnesium sulfate. Anesth Analg. 2004;99:680–6.
19. Strachan AN, Claydon P, Caunt JA. Phaeochromocytoma diagnosed during labour. Br J Anaesth. 2000;85:635–7.
20. Neumann HP, Bausch B, McWhinney SR, et al. Germ-line mutations in non-syndromic pheochromocytoma. N Engl J Med. 2002;346:1459–66.
21. Bryant J, Farmer J, Kessler LJ, et al. Pheochromocytoma: the expanding genetic differential diagnosis. J Natl Cancer Inst. 2003;95:1196–204.

Chapter 12
Pure Autonomic Failure: Diagnosis, Differential Diagnosis, and Natural History

Pearl K. Jones and Roy Freeman

Introduction

Pure autonomic failure (PAF), previously called idiopathic orthostatic hypotension, is an uncommon, idiopathic neurodegenerative disorder with primarily peripheral autonomic manifestations. The disorder is characterized by the abnormal accumulation of the protein alpha-synuclein within autonomic nerves. Sometimes called the Bradbury-Eggleston syndrome, the disorder was first described in 1925 by Bradbury and Eggleston in a report of three patients with peripheral autonomic dysfunction. These patients demonstrated a slow, fixed heart rate, with orthostatic hypotension, and evidence of diffuse peripheral autonomic impairment including thermoregulatory, gastrointestinal, erectile, and sudomotor dysfunction [1]. The authors speculated that this presentation represented a disorder affecting the autonomic nervous system. Subsequent studies demonstrated neuropathological degeneration of sympathetic postganglionic neurons [2, 3] and, importantly, key evidence of the pathogenesis, in an autopsy report of a patient with typical Lewy bodies identical to those found in Parkinson's disease [4]. Further studies of PAF patients have confirmed the presence of Lewy bodies as a pathologic hallmark of the disorder.

While Bradbury and Eggleston's initial description continues to provide the defining characteristics of this disorder – namely, an isolated peripheral autonomic disorder restricted to the peripheral autonomic nervous system – studies over the past two decades have suggested that the disorder has greater heterogeneity. Since their initial report more than 90 years ago, a vast literature of neuropathologic

P. K. Jones
Lotus Spine and Pain, San Antonio, TX, USA

R. Freeman (✉)
Autonomic and Peripheral Nerve Laboratory, Department of Neurology, Beth Israel Deaconess Medical Center, Boston, MA, USA
e-mail: rfreeman@bidmc.harvard.edu

L. Landsberg (ed.), *Pheochromocytomas, Paragangliomas and Disorders of the Sympathoadrenal System*, Contemporary Endocrinology,
https://doi.org/10.1007/978-3-319-77048-2_12

Table 12.1 The α-synucleinopathies

Disease	Pathological hallmark
Multiple system atrophy	Glial cytoplasmic inclusions
Pure autonomic failure	Lewy bodies and Lewy neurites
Parkinson's disease	Lewy bodies and Lewy neurites
Dementia with Lewy bodies	Lewy bodies and Lewy neurites

studies and clinical reports has emerged to further characterize PAF. Although the initial presentation may be one of isolated peripheral autonomic impairment, over a period of time, some patients may develop extensive motor and cognitive deficits that indicate central neuronal degeneration and a phenotype consistent with Parkinson's disease, dementia with Lewy bodies, or multiple system atrophy [5, 6].

Pathophysiology

The alpha-synucleinopathies, PAF, Parkinson's disease, Lewy body dementia, and multiple system atrophy, are a heterogenous group of disorders characterized by abnormal accumulation of the presynaptic protein alpha-synuclein, in the central and/or peripheral nervous system. The disorders PAF, Parkinson's disease, and dementia with Lewy bodies all share common neuropathologic features, i.e., alpha-synuclein deposition in Lewy bodies and Lewy neurites, whereas in multiple system atrophy, alpha-synuclein is deposited in the glia, forming glial cytoplasmic inclusion bodies (see Table 12.1). The anatomic location of the abnormal deposition, and consequent neuronal degeneration, in large part defines the clinical phenotype.

In PAF, alpha-synuclein deposition and neuronal degeneration occur primarily in peripheral autonomic neurons and are documented in the sympathetic ganglia, thoracolumbar and sacral spinal cord, autonomic axons in the epicardial fat, autonomic nerve fascicles in periadrenal adipose tissue, and the autonomic nerves in the muscularis of the urinary bladder [7–10]. Despite the finding in PAF autopsy reports of typical and atypical Lewy bodies in central locations such as the substantia nigra, locus coeruleus, and substantia innominata [7], in these autopy studies, there is no neuronal loss evident in these locations, which may underlie the minimal central features in PAF.

Clinical Features

Patients with PAF are typically middle-aged [5, 6], although rarely, late-onset cases may occur [11]. The onset of symptoms is gradual, and the presenting feature is characteristically orthostatic hypotension. Other commonly reported features of autonomic failure include constipation, bladder dysfunction, erectile dysfunction, and sweating abnormalities.

Patients report a constellation of symptoms associated with OH including dizziness, light-headedness, and pre-syncope with standing. Less common symptoms include shortness of breath due to ventilation-perfusion mismatch in the lung apices

[12], chest pain due to myocardial hypoperfusion, headache, fatigue, confusion, or difficulty concentrating [13]. Some patients describe neck pain or neck discomfort on standing, a symptom called the "coat-hanger headache," which is due to hypoperfusion of the trapezius and shoulder girdle muscles [14]. Visual blurring or dimming may also occur, likely due to retinal or occipital lobe ischemia.

Supine hypertension frequently coexists with orthostatic hypotension in patients with autonomic failure and may be present in up to 50% of PAF patients [15]. The mechanisms underlying supine hypertension are incompletely understood. Possible mechanisms include the absence of the baroreflex buffering in the setting of residual sympathetic activity, elevation of angiotensin II, and inappropriate mineralocorticoid receptor activation [16–18]. In addition, most of the pharmacotherapies for orthostatic hypotension result in or exacerbate supine hypertension.

Orthostatic hypotension and symptoms of orthostatic intolerance tend to be worse in the early morning hours, especially in those individuals who have supine hypertension, due to a pressure-induced nocturnal diuresis and diurnal fluid shifts that lead to early morning hypotension. The early morning hypotension is a reversal of the normal circadian variation in blood pressure [19]. Supine hypertension in PAF may be associated with end-organ damage including left ventricular hypertrophy and impaired renal function [15].

Some PAF patients report symptoms of rapid eye movement (REM) behavioral sleep disorder. This disorder is characterized by abnormal vocalization, motor behavior, and dream mentation and manifests by patients acting out their dreams. Features may include shouting, screaming, and limb movements resembling kicking, swinging, and punching. These manifestations are a consequence of attenuation of the descending central inhibition of the anterior horn cells, which innervate the bulbar, trunk, and limb muscles, that occurs during REM sleep [20, 21]. The proposed pathoanatomy of REM sleep behavioral disorder, which includes central structures such as the subdorsolateral nucleus and procoeruleus complex and the magnocellular complex [20, 21], supports the involvement of the central nervous system in some patients. The prevalence of REM behavioral disorder in PAF is not known; estimates range from 40% to 60% [22, 23].

Hyposmia, which may be subclinical or clinically evident, is a frequent concomitant finding in PAF patients. Hyposmia is a well-established finding in patients with Parkinson's disease and is independent of the severity or duration of the movement disorder; indeed deposition of alpha-synuclein in the olfactory bulb is an early pathologic finding in Parkinson's disease [24] and may be associated with loss of peripheral cardiac noradrenergic innervation [25]. The prevalence of hyposmia in PAF is not known [26, 27].

Phenotype Conversion

Patients with PAF are at risk for conversion to one of the central alpha-synucleinopathies, Parkinson's disease, dementia with Lewy bodies, and multiple system atrophy. Two recent studies examined the conversion rate and the predictors of conversion.

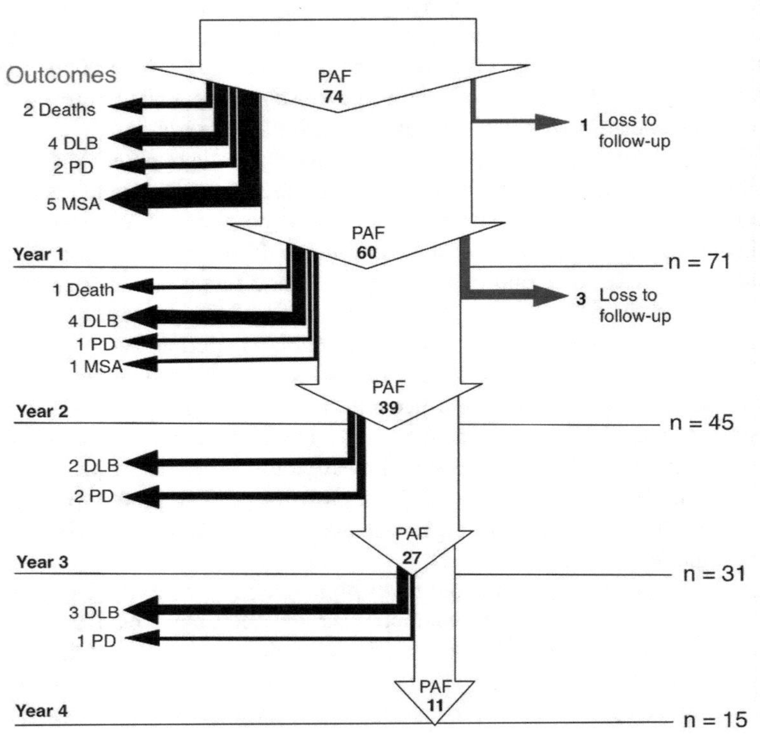

Fig. 12.1 Outcome of the natural history of pure autonomic failure. Arrows denote subject flow through the natural history study. Endpoint outcomes are listed on the left. This 4-year prospective study suggests a >10% cumulative risk of conversion to a central synucleinopathy per year. *DLB* dementia with Lewy bodies, *PD* Parkinson's disease, *PAF* pure autonomic failure. [From Kaufmann et al. [5], with permission]

One multicenter study prospectively followed 74 patients [5]. Of these, 34% (25/74) developed a central alpha-synucleinopathy [Parkinson's disease (n = 6), dementia with Lewy bodies (n = 13), and multiple system atrophy (n = 6)] (see Fig. 12.1). Those patients who phenoconverted to multiple system atrophy had younger age at onset of autonomic failure, severe bladder/bowel dysfunction, preserved olfaction, and a cardiac chronotropic response upon head-up tilt test >10 beats per minute, whereas those who phenoconverted to Parkinson's disease or dementia with Lewy bodies had decreased olfaction, a lesser chronotropic response to head-up tilt test, and a longer duration of illness.

Of the 42 patients who still had a diagnosis of PAF at their last evaluation, 30 had additional nonspecific features suggesting CNS involvement (i.e., probable RBD, impaired olfaction, and/or subtle motor signs). Only 12 subjects with PAF remained completely free of signs suggesting CNS involvement. Those patients who retained the PAF phenotype (i.e., without evidence of REM sleep behavioral disorder, hyposmia, or subtle neurological findings) had very low plasma norepinephrine levels, slow resting heart rate, no REM sleep behavior disorder, and a preserved sense of smell.

Although none of the PAF patients in this cohort met the clinical diagnostic criteria for Parkinson's disease, multiple system atrophy, or dementia with Lewy bodies, subtle nonspecific deficits were present in many patients on initial clinical examination. These deficits included mild generalized slowness/bradykinesia (12%), minimal hypomimia or reduced blinking frequency (26%), reduced unilateral arm swing when walking (12%), and mild slowing/reduction in amplitude in rapid alternating movements (22%). Resting tremor or rigidity was not present in any patient on initial evaluation [5].

In a retrospective single-center study [6], investigators reviewed the medical records of 318 patients that fulfilled the criteria for possible PAF. Only 79 of these had sufficient follow-up data. Forty-one patients (41/79, 53%, vs. 41/318, 13%) retained the PAF phenotype, whereas 37 patients (37/79, 47%, vs. 37/318, 12%) converted to a central alpha-synucleinopathy. Of those who converted, 22 (59%) developed multiple system atrophy, 11 (30%) developed Parkinson's disease or dementia with Lewy bodies, and 4 (11%) remained indeterminate [6].

Predictors of conversion to MSA in this study included a mild degree of cardiovagal impairment on cardiovascular autonomic reflex testing, a preganglionic pattern of sweat loss assessed by the quantitative sudomotor axon reflex test, severe bladder dysfunction, a supine norepinephrine level >100 pg/mL, and subtle motor signs at first presentation.

Those patients who converted to the Lewy body disorders, Parkinson's disease, and dementia with Lewy bodies, in comparison with PAF patients, had subtle motor signs at first presentation, worse autonomic function, and higher increases in venous plasma norepinephrine on standing.

Diagnostic and Research Investigations

The diagnosis of pure autonomic failure is based on the characteristic clinical phenotype of peripheral autonomic dysfunction with no further evidence of central neuronal degeneration. The differentiation from an early presentation of the central alpha-synucleinopathies may be challenging, particularly when subtle motor findings are present. The autonomic peripheral neuropathies are also part of the differential diagnosis. Laboratory chemistry tests (see Table 12.2) should be carried out on all patients with the pure autonomic failure phenotype to exclude a treatable autonomic peripheral neuropathy.

Cardiovascular and sudomotor autonomic testing may help in the differentiation among the alpha-synucleinopathies (see differences above), although there is some overlap in autonomic test results among the different disorders. Autonomic testing also helps in differentiating PAF from the non-autonomic causes of orthostatic hypotension.

Neurochemical tests may provide additional insight into the disorder. Norepinephrine is a key neurotransmitter in the sympathetic vascular nervous sys-

Table 12.2 Laboratory testing for pure autonomic failure patients

Fasting or random plasma glucose, oral glucose tolerance test, or HbA1c to assess for diabetes. If normal, assess for prediabetic state
Vitamin B12 levels. Measure metabolites (methylmalonic acid and homocysteine) if borderline value
Serum protein immunofixation electrophoresis
Nicotinic acetylcholine receptor antibodies to assess for autoimmune autonomic ganglionopathy
Additional tests based on concomitant clinical features
Supine and standing venous plasma catecholamines

tem and can be used as a surrogate for sympathoneural activity. In all four alpha-synucleinopathies, the increment in plasma norepinephrine associated with orthostatic change is attenuated. But in PAF, in contrast to MSA and Parkinson's disease, supine plasma norepinephrine levels tend to be low [28, 29].

Plasma levels of dihydroxyphenylglycol (DHPG) may also contribute to the diagnosis. Plasma DHPG is derived almost entirely from the actions of monoamine oxidase on norepinephrine in the sympathetic axoplasm. Because, most axoplasmic norepinephrine under resting conditions comes from net leakage of norepinephrine from storage vesicles, as opposed to reuptake of released norepinephrine, plasma DHPG may provide a better measure of noradrenergic innervation [30, 31]. Plasma levels of DHPG are low in patients with PAF but also in those patients with Parkinson's disease who have orthostatic hypotension [32].

Cardiac sympathetic neuroimaging may contribute to assessment of the diagnosis of the central and peripheral alpha-synucleinopathies. In imaging studies using radioactive agents, such as [^{123}I]metaiodobenzylguanidine ([^{123}I]MIBG) single-photon emission computed tomographic scanning and 6-[^{18}F]fluorodopamine positron emission tomographic scanning, cardiac noradrenergic denervation – the hallmark of the peripheral alpha-synucleinopathies – is present in PAF but also in patients with PD (particularly those with neurogenic orthostatic hypotension).

Several studies have also evaluated skin biopsies in patients with pure autonomic failure [33–35]. In the first of these [33], a case study, phosphorylated alpha-synuclein, was present as dot-like or linear immunoreactivity in a thin (5 μ) cross section of a nerve fascicle and in the wall of a blood vessel. Subsequent controlled studies, using thicker (50 μ) sections, demonstrated decreased cutaneous somatic and autonomic innervation and alpha-synuclein deposition in cutaneous postganglionic sympathetic and cholinergic nerve fibers [34, 35].

Treatment of Orthostatic Hypotension

Non-pharmacologic

Patient education is the first step in the treatment of orthostatic hypotension [36, 37]. Non-pharmacological interventions should be initiated prior to any pharmacotherapy. Patients should be made aware of situations that exacerbate symptoms including warmer temperatures and hot baths and showers, which may promote peripheral vasodilation. Symptoms may be worse in early mornings due to nocturnal diuresis, particularly those patients with supine hypertension. Raising the head of the bed may attenuate this diuresis [38]. Discussion of prodromal symptoms of syncope is also important, and instruction on maneuvers to reduce venous pooling can be helpful. Patients are advised to increase fluid and salt intake with salt tablets or increased dietary intake. Patients may also use abdominal binders and/or compression stockings. Abdominal binders may be more effective and have been shown to increase systolic blood pressure by around 11 mm Hg [39].

Pharmacologic

There are several medications that can be used in conjunction with non-pharmacologic strategies for the symptomatic treatment of orthostatic hypotension. The goal of treatment is for improvement, rather than reversal of the orthostatic blood pressure fall. The primary therapies are fludrocortisone, midodrine, droxidopa, and pyridostigmine. Fludrocortisone, a synthetic mineralocorticoid that increases renal sodium resorption, improves orthostatic tolerance and standing blood pressures by increasing intravascular compartment volume. Common side effects include peripheral edema, hypokalemia, and headache. Midodrine is a selective α-1 adrenergic agonist with a 3–4-h duration of action. Midodrine significantly increases standing blood pressures while decreasing symptoms of orthostatic intolerance [40, 41]. The side effects include supine hypertension, piloerection, urinary retention, and scalp tingling. Droxidopa is a synthetic precursor of norepinephrine that is converted to norepinephrine by aromatic L-amino acid decarboxylase. It is FDA approved for the treatment of neurogenic orthostatic hypotension. Studies with droxidopa have demonstrated a significant increase in standing systolic blood pressures and improvement in patient symptoms [42, 43]. Additional medications include pyridostigmine, an acetylcholinesterase inhibitor which was initially used for the treatment of myasthenia gravis. Pyridostigmine may increase standing blood pressure by enhancing sympathetic ganglionic transmission [44]. Additional treatments are listed in Table 12.3.

Table 12.3 Medications used for symptomatic treatment of orthostatic hypotension

Medication	Dose	Adverse effects
Midodrine	2.5–10 mg PO q4H, as needed	Supine hypertension, piloerection, urinary retention, scalp tingling
Fludrocortisone	0.05–0.2 mg PO daily	Supine hypertension, headache, hypokalemia, edema
Droxidopa	100 mg TID up to total daily dose 1800 mg as needed	Supine hypertension
Pyridostigmine	30–60 mg PO TID	Excessive salivation, abdominal cramping, nausea, and vomiting

Abbreviations: oral (PO); every four hours (q4H); three times a day (TID); hypertension (HTN)

Clinical Case

A 65-year-old male with no past medical history presented to the outpatient neurology clinic with complaints of dizziness and light-headedness with standing that had a gradual onset. He reported one episode of syncope. He noted that dizziness occurred primarily when standing, no symptoms when laying down or sitting. He also reported light-headedness after having large meals. On further review, he also reported constipation and erectile dysfunction. There was no report of weakness or sensory symptoms.Vital signs were notable for a supine blood pressure of 150/85 mm Hg and a heart rate of 80 beats per minute. After standing for 3 min, blood pressure was 90/70 mm Hg and heart rate 82 beats per minute. Neurologic exam was notable for normal mental status, normal cranial nerve exam, and normal strength and reflexes. MRI of the brain and MRA of the head and neck were normal. Laboratory chemistries were normal. Autonomic testing revealed severe orthostatic hypotension, together with abnormal measures of sympathetic adrenergic, sudomotor, and parasympathetic function.Over 4 years of follow-up, his orthostatic hypotension responded well to treatment. He developed symptoms consistent with rapid eye movement (REM) behavioral disorder. His neurological examination was unchanged.

Conclusion

Pure autonomic failure is an alpha-synucleinopathy, characterized clinically by significant orthostatic hypotension in the absence of significant extrapyramidal, cerebellar, or pyramidal features. It is regarded as a slowly progressive disorder, with a good prognosis if the clinical features remain restricted to the peripheral autonomic nervous system. However, phenotype conversion to one of the central alpha-synucleinopathies occurs in a significant number of patients. Careful follow-up of PAF patients is necessary, monitoring for the predictors of phenotype conversion, such as REM behavioral disorder and hyposmia, and for changes in the features of the clinical examination.

References

1. Bradbury S, Eggleston C. Postural hypotension: report of 3 cases. Am Heart J. 1925;1:73–86.
2. Goodall MC, Harlan WR Jr, Alton H. Decreased noradrenaline (norepinephrine) synthesis in neurogenic orthostatic hypotension. Circulation. 1968;38:592–603.
3. Bannister R, Crowe R, Eames R, Burnstock G. Adrenergic innervation in autonomic failure. Neurology. 1981;31:1501–6.
4. Johnson RH, Lee Gde J, Oppenheimer DR, Spalding JM. Autonomic failure with orthostatic hypotension due to intermediolateral column degeneration. A report of two cases with autopsies. Q J Med. 1966;35(138):276–92.

5. Kaufmann H, Norcliffe-Kaufmann L, Palma JA, Biaggioni I, Low PA, Singer W, et al. Natural history of pure autonomic failure: a United States prospective cohort. Ann Neurol. 2017;81(2):287–97.
6. Singer W, Berini SE, Sandroni P, Fealey RD, Coon EA, Suarez MD, et al. Pure autonomic failure: predictors of conversion to clinical CNS involvement. Neurology. 2017;88(12):1129–36.
7. Hague K, Lento P, Morgello S, Caro S, Kaufmann H. The distribution of Lewy bodies in pure autonomic failure: autopsy findings and review of the literature. Acta Neuropathol(Berl). 1997;94(2):192–6.
8. Arai K, Kato N, Kashiwado K, Hattori T. Pure autonomic failure in association with human alpha-synucleinopathy. Neurosci Lett. 2000;296(2–3):171–3.
9. Kaufmann H, Hague K, Perl D. Accumulation of alpha-synuclein in autonomic nerves in pure autonomic failure. Neurology. 2001;56(7):980–1.
10. Hague K, Lento P, Morgello S, Caro S, Kaufmann H. The distribution of Lewy bodies in pure autonomic failure: autopsy findings and review of the literature. [review] [16 refs]. Acta Neuropathol(Berl). 1997;94(2):192–6.
11. Fanciulli A, Stefanova N, Scherfler C, Moser P, Seppi K, Gizewski ER, et al. Very late-onset pure autonomic failure. Mov Disord Off J Mov Disord Soc. 2017;32(7):1106–8.
12. Gibbons CH, Freeman R. Orthostatic dyspnea: a neglected symptom of orthostatic hypotension. Clin Auton Res. 2005;15(1):40–4.
13. Centi J, Freeman R, Gibbons CH, Neargarder S, Canova AO, Cronin-Golomb A. Effects of orthostatic hypotension on cognition in Parkinson disease. Neurology. 2017;88(1):17–24.
14. Robertson D, Kincaid DW, Haile V, Robertson RM. The head and neck discomfort of autonomic failure: an unrecognized aetiology of headache. Clin Auton Res. 1994;4(3):99–103.
15. Garland EM, Gamboa A, Okamoto L, Raj SR, Black BK, Davis TL, et al. Renal impairment of pure autonomic failure. Hypertension. 2009;54(5):1057–61.
16. Arnold AC, Okamoto LE, Gamboa A, Black BK, Raj SR, Elijovich F, et al. Mineralocorticoid receptor activation contributes to the supine hypertension of autonomic failure. Hypertension. 2016;67(2):424–9.
17. Arnold AC, Okamoto LE, Gamboa A, Shibao C, Raj SR, Robertson D, et al. Angiotensin II, independent of plasma renin activity, contributes to the hypertension of autonomic failure. Hypertension. 2013;61(3):701–6.
18. Shannon JR, Jordan J, Diedrich A, Pohar B, Black BK, Robertson D, et al. Sympathetically mediated hypertension in autonomic failure. Circulation. 2000;101(23):2710–5.
19. Mann S, Altman DG, Raftery EB, Bannister R. Circadian variation of blood pressure in autonomic failure. Circulation. 1983;68:477–83.
20. Boeve BF. Idiopathic REM sleep behaviour disorder in the development of Parkinson's disease. Lancet Neurol. 2013;12(5):469–82.
21. Boeve BF, Silber MH, Saper CB, Ferman TJ, Dickson DW, Parisi JE, et al. Pathophysiology of REM sleep behaviour disorder and relevance to neurodegenerative disease. Brain. 2007;130(Pt 11):2770–88.
22. Miglis MG, Muppidi S, During E, Jaradeh S. A case series of REM sleep behavior disorder in pure autonomic failure. Clin Auton Res Off J Clin Auton Res Soc. 2017;27(1):41–4.
23. Plazzi G, Cortelli P, Montagna P, De Monte A, Corsini R, Contin M, et al. REM sleep behaviour disorder differentiates pure autonomic failure from multiple system atrophy with autonomic failure. J Neurol Neurosurg Psychiatry. 1998;64(5):683–5.
24. Braak H, Ghebremedhin E, Rub U, Bratzke H, Del Tredici K. Stages in the development of Parkinson's disease-related pathology. Cell Tissue Res. 2004;318(1):121–34.
25. Lee PH, Yeo SH, Kim HJ, Youm HY. Correlation between cardiac 123I-MIBG and odor identification in patients with Parkinson's disease and multiple system atrophy. Mov Disord Off J Mov Disord Soc. 2006;21(11):1975–7.
26. Silveira-Moriyama L, Mathias C, Mason L. Best C, Quinn NP, Lees AJ. Hyposmia in pure autonomic failure. Neurology. 2009;72(19):1677–81.
27. Goldstein DS, Sewell L. Olfactory dysfunction in pure autonomic failure: implications for the pathogenesis of Lewy body diseases. Parkinsonism Relat Disord. 2009;15(7):516–20.

28. Goldstein DS, Polinsky RJ, Garty M, Robertson D, Brown RT, Biaggioni I, et al. Patterns of plasma levels of catechols in neurogenic orthostatic hypotension. Ann Neurol. 1989;26:558–63.
29. Goldstein DS, Sharabi Y. Neurogenic orthostatic hypotension: a pathophysiological approach. Circulation. 2009;119(1):139–46.
30. Goldstein DS, Holmes C, Kopin IJ, Sharabi Y. Intra-neuronal vesicular uptake of catecholamines is decreased in patients with Lewy body diseases. J Clin Invest. 2011;121(8):3320–30.
31. Goldstein DS, Eisenhofer G, Kopin IJ. Sources and significance of plasma levels of catechols and their metabolites in humans. J Pharmacol Exp Ther. 2003;305(3):800–11.
32. Goldstein DS, Holmes C, Sharabi Y, Brentzel S, Eisenhofer G. Plasma levels of catechols and metanephrines in neurogenic orthostatic hypotension. Neurology. 2003;60(8):1327–32.
33. Shishido T, Ikemura M, Obi T, Yamazaki K, Terada T, Sugiura A, et al. Alpha-synuclein accumulation in skin nerve fibers revealed by skin biopsy in pure autonomic failure. Neurology. 2010;74(7):608–10.
34. Donadio V, Incensi A, Piccinini C, Cortelli P, Giannoccaro MP, Baruzzi A, et al. Skin nerve misfolded alpha-synuclein in pure autonomic failure and Parkinson disease. Ann Neurol. 2016;79(2):306–16.
35. Donadio V, Incensi A, Cortelli P, Giannoccaro MP, Jaber MA, Baruzzi A, et al. Skin sympathetic fiber alpha-synuclein deposits: a potential biomarker for pure autonomic failure. Neurology. 2013;80(8):725–32.
36. Freeman R. Clinical practice. Neurogenic orthostatic hypotension. N Engl J Med. 2008;358(6):615–24.
37. Gibbons CH, Schmidt P, Biaggioni I, Frazier-Mills C, Freeman R, Isaacson S, et al. The recommendations of a consensus panel for the screening, diagnosis and treatment of neurogenic orthostatic hypotension and associated supine hypertension. J Neurol. 2017;264:1567.
38. Omboni S, Smit AA, van Lieshout JJ, Settels JJ, Langewouters GJ, Wieling W. Mechanisms underlying the impairment in orthostatic tolerance after nocturnal recumbency in patients with autonomic failure. Clin Sci(Lond). 2001;101(6):609–18.
39. Smit AA, Wieling W, Fujimura J, Denz JC, Opfer-Gehrking TL, Akarriou M, et al. Use of lower abdominal compression to combat orthostatic hypotension in patients with autonomic dysfunction. Clin Auton Res. 2004;14(3):167–75.
40. Wright RA, Kaufmann HC, Perera R, Opfer-Gehrking TL, McElligott MA, Sheng KN, et al. A double-blind, dose response study of midodrine in neurogenic orthostatic hypotension. Neurology. 1998;51(1):120–4.
41. Low PA, Gilden JL, Freeman R, Sheng KN, McElligott MA. Efficacy of midodrine vs placebo in neurogenic orthostatic hypotension. A randomized, doubleblind multicenter study. Midodrine study group. JAMA. 1997;277(13):1046–51.
42. Biaggioni I, Freeman R, Mathias CJ, Low P, Hewitt LA, Kaufmann H, et al. Randomized withdrawal study of patients with symptomatic neurogenic orthostatic hypotension responsive to Droxidopa. Hypertension. 2015;65(1):101–7.
43. Kaufmann H, Freeman R, Biaggioni I, Low P, Pedder S, Hewitt LA, et al. Droxidopa for neurogenic orthostatic hypotension: a randomized, placebo-controlled, phase 3 trial. Neurology. 2014;83(4):328–35.
44. Singer W, Sandroni P, Opfer-Gehrking TL, Suarez GA, Klein CM, Hines S, et al. Pyridostigmine treatment trial in neurogenic orthostatic hypotension. Arch Neurol. 2006;63(4):513–8.

Chapter 13
Hypoglycemia-Associated Autonomic Failure in Diabetes

Philip E. Cryer and Ana Maria Arbelaez

The Problem of Hypoglycemia in Diabetes

Iatrogenic hypoglycemia is the limiting factor in the glycemic management of absolute endogenous insulin-deficient diabetes mellitus [1]. Hypoglycemia causes recurrent morbidity in most people with type 1 diabetes (T1D) and many with advanced type 2 diabetes (T2D) and is sometimes fatal. It generally precludes maintenance of euglycemia over a lifetime in such patients and, thus, full realization of the benefits of glycemic control. As discussed in this chapter, hypoglycemia impairs defenses against subsequent hypoglycemia and, thus, causes a vicious cycle of recurrent hypoglycemia.

An estimated 415 million people worldwide had diabetes in 2015 that is projected to increase to 642 million people by 2040 [2]. Approximately 5% have T1D, and many of the remainder have long-standing, advanced T2D with absolute endogenous insulin deficiency. Thirty to forty percent of those with T1D suffer one to three episodes of severe iatrogenic hypoglycemia (that requiring the assistance of another person) each year [3]. The vast majority suffer one to two episodes of symptomatic hypoglycemia each week. Virtually all have frequent continuous glucose monitoring levels <70 mg/dL (3.9 mmol/L) [4]. The incidence of hypoglycemia in insulin-treated T2D is about one-third of that in T1D [3, 5] although it is similar in T2D and T1D matched for duration of insulin therapy [6]. Because T2D is approximately 20-fold more prevalent than T1D and most people with T2D ultimately require treatment with insulin, most episodes of iatrogenic hypoglycemia, including severe hypoglycemia, occur in T2D.

P. E. Cryer (✉) · A. M. Arbelaez
Washington University School of Medicine, St. Louis, MO, USA
e-mail: pcryer@wustl.edu

L. Landsberg (ed.), *Pheochromocytomas, Paragangliomas and Disorders of the Sympathoadrenal System*, Contemporary Endocrinology,
https://doi.org/10.1007/978-3-319-77048-2_13

Episodes of hypoglycemia can cause anxiety, embarrassment, aberrant behavior, an array of unpleasant symptoms, impairment of physical performance, confusion, seizure, coma, injuries, or transient neurological deficits [1]. An estimated 4–10% of deaths of people with T1D are attributed to hypoglycemia and thought to be the result of cardiac arrhythmias [1, 7, 8].

Iatrogenic hypoglycemia in diabetes is typically the result of the interplay of therapeutic insulin excess and compromised physiologic and behavioral defenses against the resulting falling plasma glucose concentrations [1]. Insight into those compromised defenses developed over the past four decades by the senior author and his colleagues and incorporated into his concept of hypoglycemia-associated autonomic failure in diabetes [1, 9] is the focus of this chapter. Our development of a sensitive and specific single isotope derivative (radioenzymatic) method for the measurement of epinephrine and norepinephrine [10, 11] in the early 1970s was key. That then unique analytical method enabled us to study the human sympathoadrenal system [12–14] and made our comprehensive studies of the physiology and pathophysiology of glucose counterregulation in humans [1] possible.

The Physiology of Glucose Counterregulation

The senior author and his colleagues defined the physiology of glucose counterregulation—the mechanisms that normally prevent or rapidly correct hypoglycemia—in humans [15–19] (Fig. 13.1). In our early study of glucose kinetics during hypoglycemia induced by intravenous insulin injection, the finding that plasma insulin concentrations were still greater than tenfold higher than baseline at the time of reversal of insulin-suppressed glucose production and of insulin-stimulated glucose utilization [15] made it clear that the correction of hypoglycemia is not due solely to waning of the glucose-lowering hormone insulin. Additional glucose-raising (glucose counterregulatory) factors must be involved. Among the latter, our findings [16–18] that glucose counterregulation during hypoglycemia (1) is not impaired by pharmacologic adrenergic blockade (or epinephrine deficiency) and (2) is only partially impaired by infusion of somatostatin (an effect reversed by glucagon replacement) but (3) fails completely during adrenergic blockade combined with somatostatin-induced glucagon deficiency established that there are multiple glucose counterregulatory factors, a key fail-safe system, and that there is a hierarchy among those factors. As plasma glucose concentrations fall, the physiologic defenses against hypoglycemia are a decrease in the secretion of the glucose-lowering pancreatic beta-cell hormone insulin, an increase in the secretion of the glucose-raising pancreatic alpha-cell hormone glucagon, and an increase in the secretion of the glucose-raising adrenomedullary hormone epinephrine [19]. Of these, two points warrant emphasis. First, a decrease in insulin secretion as plasma glucose concentrations fall within the physiological range is a key glucose counterregulatory event. Second, when glucagon secretion is intact, epinephrine is not required for restoration of plasma glucose. Epinephrine does, however, provide an

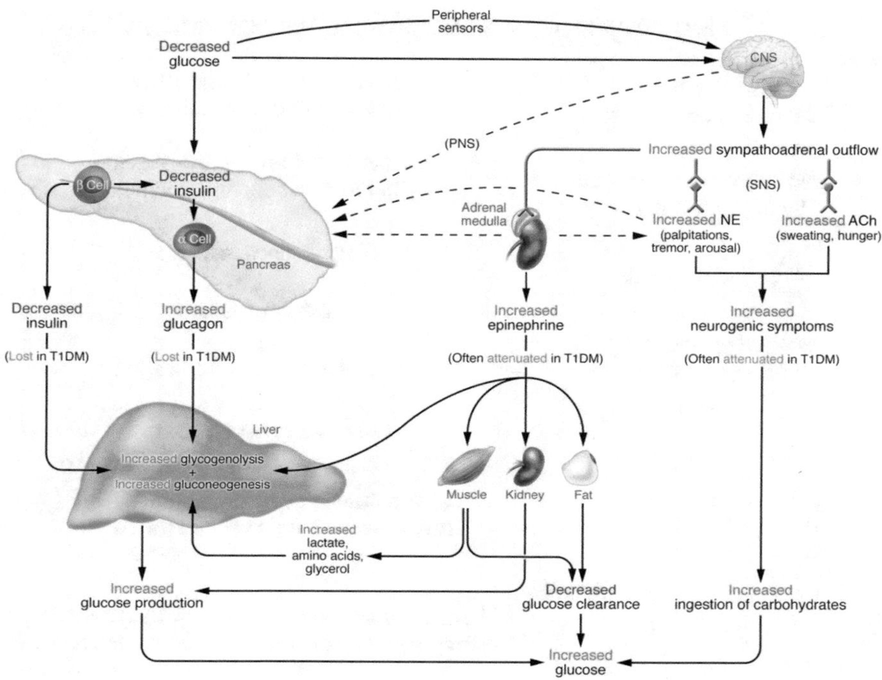

Fig. 13.1 Physiologic and behavioral defenses against hypoglycemia in humans. Decrements in insulin and increments in glucagon are lost, and increments in epinephrine and neurogenic symptoms are typically attenuated in absolute endogenous insulin-deficient diabetes, T1D and advanced T2D. *SNS* sympathetic nervous system, *PNS* parasympathetic nervous system. (From Cryer [77], with permission)

early warning signal in the form of tremor, anxiety, and palpitations. Epinephrine becomes critical to glucose counterregulation when glucagon secretion is deficient. The behavioral defense against hypoglycemia is carbohydrate ingestion [1, 19] prompted by recognition of neurogenic (autonomic) symptoms [20] that largely originate from the adrenal medullary response [21]. The effectiveness of these defenses ensures a continuous supply of glucose and thus survival.

The Pathophysiology of Glucose Counterregulation

The concept of hypoglycemia-associated autonomic failure in diabetes Hypoglycemia is uncommon in patients with diabetes caused by relative pancreatic beta-cell failure, early T2D. But hypoglycemia is common in those with absolute pancreatic beta-cell failure, advanced T2D and T1D, in whom defenses against hypoglycemia are compromised [1]. The concept of hypoglycemia-associated autonomic failure (HAAF) in diabetes [1, 9] (Fig. 13.2) posits that in

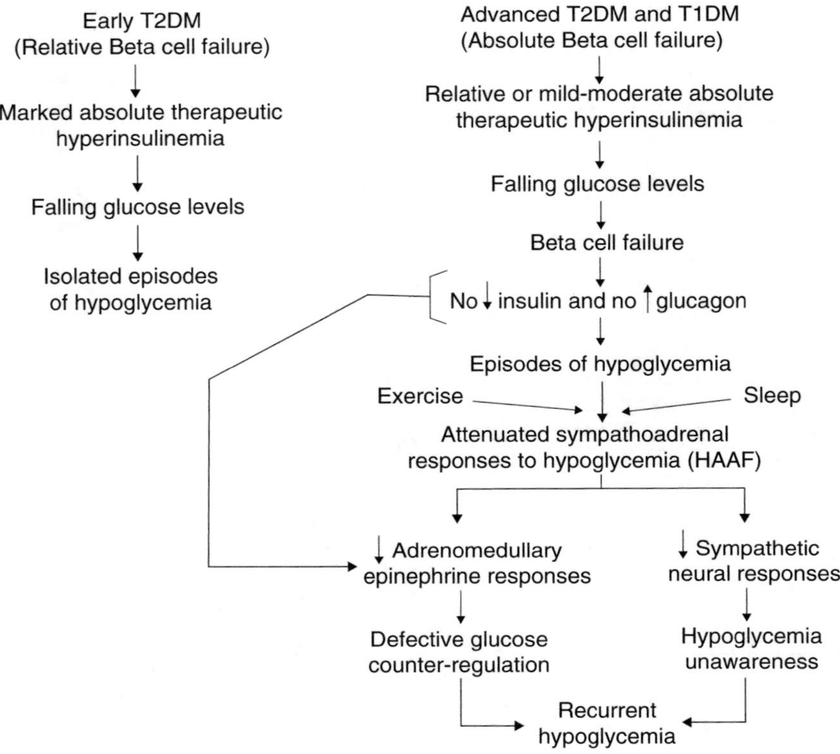

Fig. 13.2 The concept of hypoglycemia-associated autonomic failure (HAAF) in diabetes. (From Cryer [1], with permission)

the latter, patients' necessarily imperfect insulin replacement (or sulfonylurea- or glinide-stimulated insulin secretion) results in falling plasma glucose concentrations, but no decrease in insulin secretion and no increase in glucagon secretion, and, thus, leads to episodes of hypoglycemia. Those episodes (like sleep or prior exercise) attenuate adrenomedullary epinephrine secretion during subsequent hypoglycemia. In the setting of absent insulin and glucagon responses, the attenuated epinephrine responses cause the clinical syndrome of defective glucose counterregulation [22] which is associated with a 25-fold [22] or greater [23] increased risk of severe iatrogenic hypoglycemia during intensive glycemic therapy. The attenuated adrenal medullary responses cause the clinical syndrome of hypoglycemia unawareness (impaired awareness of hypoglycemia) which is associated with at least a sixfold increased risk of severe iatrogenic hypoglycemia during intensive glycemic therapy [24]. The resulting recurrent hypoglycemia further attenuates the adrenal medullary response to falling plasma glucose concentrations.

HAAF in diabetes is a functional disorder distinct from classical diabetic autonomic neuropathy [1, 25]. Unlike the latter, HAAF can be induced by prior hypoglycemia, sleep, or exercise and at least partially reversed by short-term scrupulous avoidance of hypoglycemia and is manifested clinically by recurrent iatrogenic hypoglycemia.

There are at least three forms of HAAF [1, 26]: (1) hypoglycemia-related HAAF, (2) sleep-related HAAF [27–29], and [3] exercise-related HAAF [30]. With respect to the latter, recent evidence indicates that a decrease in the plasma glucose concentration during exercise can cause HAAF [31].

Critical findings leading to the concept of HAAF Made possible by the availability of assays for the precise and accurate measurement of epinephrine and norepinephrine [10–14], the concept of HAAF in diabetes evolved from a series of findings, all in humans. Those included our insight into the physiology of glucose counterregulation [15–19] just summarized; our discovery of the clinical syndrome of defective glucose counterregulation in diabetes [22]; our pivotal finding that hypoglycemia today reduces neuroendocrine (including glucagon and epinephrine) and symptomatic defenses against hypoglycemia tomorrow [32]; our finding, with others, that hypoglycemia unawareness in diabetes is reversible by short-term scrupulous avoidance of iatrogenic hypoglycemia [33]; and our finding that the glucagon response to hypoglycemia is lost late in advanced T2D [34] as it is lost early in T1D [22, 35].

We found that an intravenous insulin infusion identifies some patients with T1D whose plasma glucose concentrations decline progressively and others in whom it declines but then stabilizes normally [22]. Compared with nondiabetic individuals, plasma glucagon responses to hypoglycemia are absent in both patient groups, but plasma epinephrine responses to hypoglycemia are reduced only in the patients with defective glucose counterregulation (Fig. 13.3). The latter patients have a 25-fold higher incidence of severe iatrogenic hypoglycemia during subsequent intensive glycemic therapy [22], a finding confirmed by others [23]. Those studies documented that glucose counterregulation is compromised, and the frequency of iatrogenic hypoglycemia is increased, by the combination of absent glucagon and attenuated epinephrine secretory responses to falling plasma glucose concentrations, the clinical syndrome of defective glucose counterregulation in diabetes.

Our pivotal finding was that 2 h of interval of afternoon hyperinsulinemic hypoglycemia, compared with interval of afternoon hyperinsulinemic euglycemia, reduces the neuroendocrine (including plasma glucagon and epinephrine) and symptomatic responses to hypoglycemia the following morning in nondiabetic individuals [32] (Fig. 13.4) and in patients with T1D [36]. Obviously, that now well-established phenomenon is central to the concept of HAAF in diabetes.

The dynamic nature of HAAF in diabetes was further underscored by our finding that hypoglycemia unawareness is reversible in most affected patients with T1D by 3–4 weeks of scrupulous avoidance of iatrogenic hypoglycemia [33] (Fig. 13.5). That finding was also reported by others [37–39] at the same time.

Our finding that the glucagon response to hypoglycemia is also lost in advanced T2D [34] (Fig. 13.6) extended the concept of HAAF in diabetes from T1D to advanced T2D.

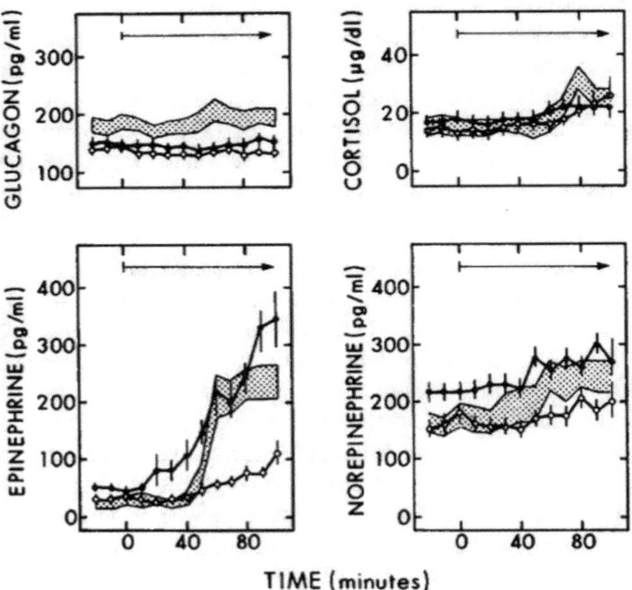

Fig. 13.3 Plasma glucagon, epinephrine, norepinephrine, and cortisol concentrations during insulin infusions (40 mU/kg/hour, horizontal arrows) in nondiabetic humans (shaded areas) and in patients with T1D who had adequate glucose counterregulation (closed symbols) or patients with T1D who had inadequate (defective) glucose counterregulation (open symbols). The latter patients had a 25-fold higher incidence of severe iatrogenic hypoglycemia during subsequent intensive glycemic therapy. (From White et al. [22], with permission)

Findings relevant to the mechanisms of HAAF Our findings relevant to the mechanism of HAAF in diabetes, which are discussed shortly, again all in humans, included evidence that a decrease in pancreatic beta-cell insulin secretion normally signals an increase in pancreatic alpha-cell glucagon secretion during hypoglycemia [40, 41]; there is no increase in blood-to-brain glucose transport in a model of HAAF [42]; the glycemic threshold for a decrease in brain glucose metabolism is less than 50 mg/dL (2.8 mmol/L) [43]; there are regional increments in brain synaptic activity during hypoglycemia and increased thalamic activation in a model of HAAF [44–46]; and experimental HAAF is prevented by nonselective adrenergic blockade [47].

Mechanisms of the Absent Insulin and Glucagon Secretory Responses in HAAF

Insulin In the absence of endogenous insulin secretion, circulating insulin levels are simply a function of the absorption and clearance of injected exogenous insulin. Intraislet endogenous insulin secretion, as measured by circulating C-peptide concentrations, cannot decrease as plasma glucose concentrations fall.

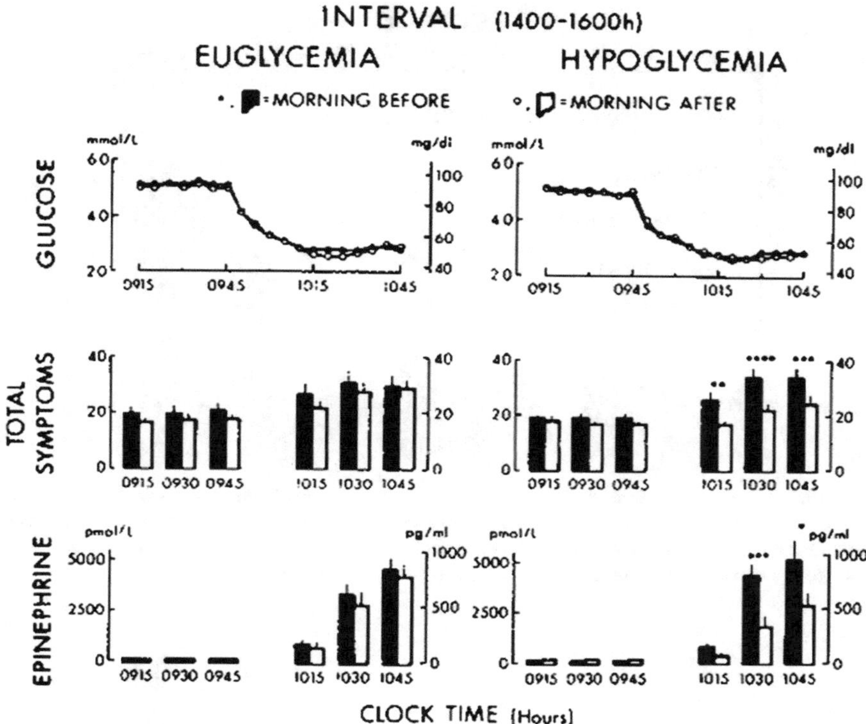

Fig. 13.4 Mean plasma glucose concentrations, total symptom scores, and plasma epinephrine concentrations during hyperinsulinemic euglycemia then hypoglycemic clamps on consecutive mornings before and after interval of afternoon hyperinsulinemic euglycemia (left) and before and after interval of afternoon hyperinsulinemic hypoglycemia (right) in nondiabetic humans. (From Heller and Cryer [32], with permission)

Glucagon The absence of an increase in glucagon secretion during hypoglycemia in HAAF in diabetes is also best attributed to pancreatic beta-cell failure, specifically the lack of a decrease in the intraislet pancreatic alpha-cell inhibitory signal of beta-cell insulin during hypoglycemia [1, 9]. The evidence for that conclusion is substantial. First, loss of the insulin and glucagon responses to falling plasma glucose concentrations are correlated, developing early in T1D and late in T2D, and precede attenuation of the sympathoadrenal response [35]. Second, loss of the glucagon response cannot be attributed to islet denervation. Normal glucagon secretion in response to hypoglycemia occurs in humans with a transplanted (denervated) pancreas [48] and in those with spinal cord transections and, thus, no sympathoadrenal outflow from the brain to the islets [49]. It also occurs in dogs with a denervated pancreas [50]. Furthermore, glucagon release occurs in response to low glucose from the perfused rodent pancreas and from perifused rodent and human islets. Thus, the defect in HAAF must be within the islets. Third, since there is a glucagon secretory response to administered amino acids

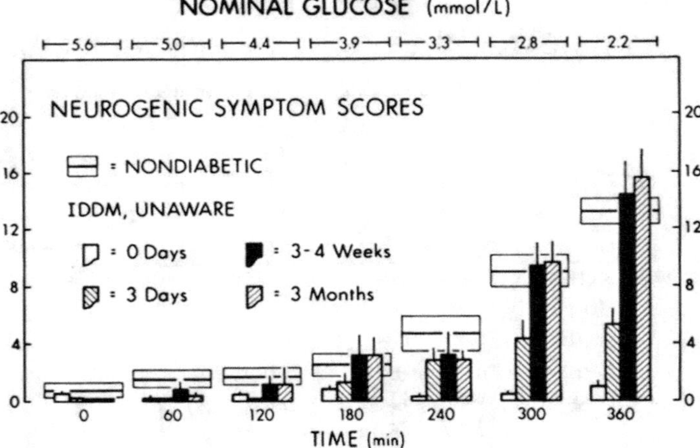

Fig. 13.5 Mean neurogenic symptom scores during hyperinsulinemic stepped hypoglycemic clamps in nondiabetic humans (rectangles) and patients with T1D with hypoglycemia unawareness studied at baseline (0 days) and again at 3 days, 3–4 weeks, and 3 months of scrupulous avoidance of hypoglycemia. [From Dagogo-Jack et al. [33], with permission]

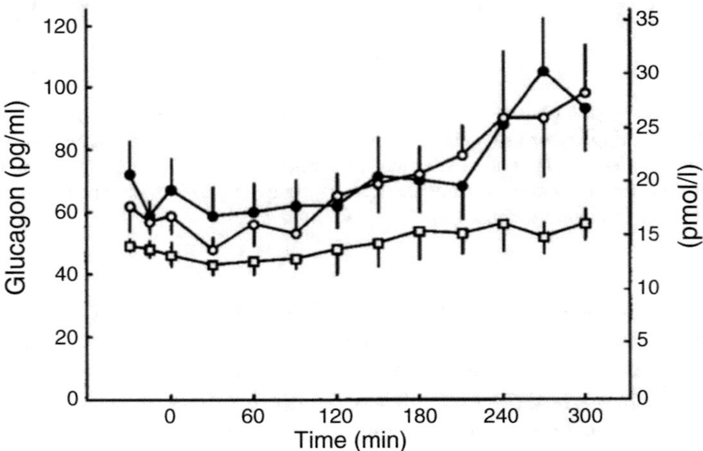

Fig. 13.6 Mean plasma glucagon concentrations during hyperinsulinemic stepped hypoglycemic clamps in nondiabetic humans (closed circles), patients with T2D treated with oral antidiabetic agents (open circles), and patients with T2D treated long term with insulin (open squares). (From Segel et al. [34], with permission)

in patients with HAAF (e.g., 41), loss of the glucagon response to hypoglycemia must be the result of reduced signaling to functioning alpha-cells. Fourth, because insulin normally regulates glucagon secretion in a reciprocal fashion in humans [40, 41], it follows that loss of beta-cell insulin secretion would result in loss of the signal of a decrease in intraislet insulin to increase glucagon secretion during hypoglycemia.

The lack of a decrease in insulin and the lack of an increase in glucagon as glucose concentrations fall are prerequisites for defective glucose counterregulation but do not cause defective glucose counterregulation or hypoglycemia unawareness. The latter two components of HAAF in diabetes develop only when the sympathoadrenal and resulting symptomatic responses to hypoglycemia become attenuated.

Mechanism of the Attenuated Sympathoadrenal Responses in HAAF

Unlike the loss of the insulin and glucagon responses at the islet level, the alteration resulting in attenuated adrenal medullary responses must reside within the central nervous system or its afferent or efferent connections. Despite an array of hypotheses, summarized in the paragraphs that follow, the mechanism of the attenuated adrenal medullary response to hypoglycemia in HAAF in diabetes is not known.

The systemic mediator hypothesis The systemic mediator hypothesis postulates that an increase in a circulating factor during recent antecedent hypoglycemia (or prior exercise) acts on the brain to attenuate the adrenal and related symptomatic responses to subsequent hypoglycemia [51, 52]. It was originally suggested that cortisol might be that factor [51, 52], but neither prior cortisol elevations similar to those that occur during hypoglycemia [53, 53] nor inhibition of the cortisol response to prior hypoglycemia with metyrapone [54] prevents the attenuated epinephrine and symptomatic responses to subsequent hypoglycemia in humans. Recent data in humans [55] suggest that endorphins or epinephrine might be that factor. Prior morphine injection reduced plasma epinephrine and symptomatic responses to subsequent hypoglycemia. In data presented but not reported in the abstract, prior epinephrine injection reduced symptomatic responses and tended to reduce plasma epinephrine responses to subsequent hypoglycemia. Nonetheless, earlier data [56] indicated that prior epinephrine administration did not reduce the plasma epinephrine response to subsequent hypoglycemia. The extent to which the recent findings [55] are physiologic or pharmacologic is unknown.

The brain fuel transport hypothesis The brain fuel transport hypothesis postulates that recent antecedent hypoglycemia causes increased blood-to-brain transport of glucose (or of an alternative metabolic fuel) and that attenuates sympathoadrenal and symptomatic responses to subsequent hypoglycemia. Despite some seemingly consistent early data (reviewed 1,9), global blood-to-brain glucose transport, measured with [1-^{11}C]glucose positron emission tomography, is not reduced in patients with poorly controlled T1D [57] and is not increased after nearly 24 h of interprandial hypoglycemia [42] which produces a model of HAAF (including attenuated plasma epinephrine and neurogenic symptom responses to hypoglycemia) in nondiabetic humans.

A premise of the brain glucose transport hypothesis is that hypoglycemia causes a decrease in the rate of cerebral glucose metabolism which in turn causes an increase in sympathoadrenal activity and a decrease in cognitive function and that an increase in blood-to-brain glucose transport during subsequent hypoglycemia would preserve brain glucose metabolism and, thus, attenuate sympathoadrenal and symptomatic responses. However, there is evidence that the sympathoadrenal response to hypoglycemia is a signaling event, and not a response to a decrease in brain glucose metabolism, in that the neuroendocrine response occurs at a higher plasma glucose concentration than that required to cause a decrease in brain glucose metabolism and that the glycemic threshold for a decrease in brain glucose metabolism is less than 50 mg/dL (2.8 mmol/L) [43]. If so, an increase in blood-to-brain glucose transport at a plasma glucose concentration greater than 50 mg/dL would not be expected to reduce the sympathoadrenal or symptomatic responses to hypoglycemia.

If the normally small astrocytic brain glycogen pool [1] increases substantially above baseline after hypoglycemia, that expanded source of glucose within the brain might fulfill this hypothesis. However, the notion of brain glycogen supercompensation has not been supported in patients with T1D and hypoglycemia unawareness [58] or in a model of HAAF in nondiabetic individuals [59].

Neurons also oxidize lactate, but that lactate is largely derived from glucose within the brain [1]. An increase in blood-to-brain lactate transport could fulfill the brain fuel transport hypothesis, albeit also with the assumption that mild to moderate hypoglycemia causes a decrease in brain oxidative metabolism that causes an increase in adrenal medullary activity and a decrease in cognitive function discussed above. As reviewed previously [9], lactate infusions reduce adrenal and symptomatic responses to hypoglycemia, but brain lactate uptake does not increase [60] or increases only to a small extent [61] during hypoglycemia in humans. Nonetheless, increased brain lactate uptake without increased oxidation of lactate during hypoglycemia in patients with T1D has been reported [62], and lactate infusions that caused only a small increase in brain lactate metabolism were found to result in maintenance of brain glucose metabolism during subsequent hypoglycemia in rats subjected to recurrent hypoglycemia [63].

The brain metabolism hypothesis The brain metabolism hypothesis postulates that recent antecedent hypoglycemia somehow alters central nervous system metabolic regulation resulting in attenuated adrenal medullary responses to declining plasma glucose concentrations and, thus, HAAF in diabetes. The molecular and cellular studies of the phenomenon in rodents have largely focused on the ventromedial hypothalamus [64–66]. A recent construct is that recurrent hypoglycemia increases brain lactate uptake [63] that stimulates gamma-aminobutyric acid (GABA) producing hypothalamic neurons and that the failure of hypothalamic GABA levels to decrease normally causes an attenuated adrenal response to hypoglycemia [64, 65]. Interestingly, partial blockade of nicotinic acetylcholine receptors was found to improve the adrenomedullary epinephrine response to hypoglycemia in a rodent model of HAAF [66] suggesting that increased preganglionic adrenal nerve stimulation (i.e., a central nervous system effect) contributes to the development of HAAF.

In apparent contrast, however, a decrease in brain lactate concentrations, measured with proton magnetic resonance spectroscopy, during hypoglycemia has been reported in patients with T1D and impaired awareness of hypoglycemia [67].

Potential pharmacologic manipulations that might ameliorate HAAF in diabetes were reviewed previously [9].

The cerebral network hypothesis The cerebral network hypothesis is distinguished from the brain metabolism hypothesis in that it postulates that recent antecedent hypoglycemia acts through a network of interconnected brain regions to inhibit hypothalamic activation and, thus, attenuates the adrenal and symptomatic responses to subsequent hypoglycemia [1, 9]. In contrast to the brain metabolism hypothesis, the cerebral network hypothesis has been developed largely in humans [44–46].

As reviewed previously [9], the cerebral network hypothesis is largely based on findings from functional neuroimaging in humans during hypoglycemia, particularly [^{15}O]water positron emission tomography measurements of regional cerebral blood flow as an index of regional brain synaptic activity [44–46], and the psychophysiological concept of habituation of the response to a given stress and its proposed mechanism [68, 69]. The posterior paraventricular nucleus of the thalamus is the brain site at which previous stress acts to attenuate responses to subsequent episodes of that specific stress in rats. The effect of recent antecedent hypoglycemia to attenuate the adrenal response to subsequent hypoglycemia, the core feature of HAAF in diabetes, is an example of habituation of the adrenal medullary response to hypoglycemia in humans.

Hypoglycemia increases synaptic activity in the human dorsal midline thalamus among other sites [44–46] and increases synaptic activity to a greater extent after recent antecedent hypoglycemia (i.e., in a model of HAAF in diabetes in nondiabetic humans) only in the dorsal midline thalamus [45] (Fig. 13.7). That is the site of the posterior paraventricular nucleus of the thalamus [69]. Thus, thalamic inhibition of the adrenal response to hypoglycemia could be a component of the mechanism of HAAF in diabetes [45]. Additional potential links in the cerebral network, including the medial prefrontal cortex, have been reviewed [9].

Using arterial spin labeling magnetic resonance imaging to measure cerebral blood flow (CBF), others [70] reported increments in global CBF during hypoglycemia in patients with T1D and impaired awareness of hypoglycemia but not in patients with T1D and normal awareness of hypoglycemia or in nondiabetic individuals. They suggested that an increase in global CBF may enhance nutrient supply to the brain, hence suppressing symptomatic awareness of hypoglycemia. However, their finding rests on a very small difference in global CBF during hypoglycemia between patients with impaired awareness of hypoglycemia ($+8 \pm 3\%$, $P < 0.05$) and patients with normal awareness of hypoglycemia ($+5 \pm 2\%$, $P < 0.08$)

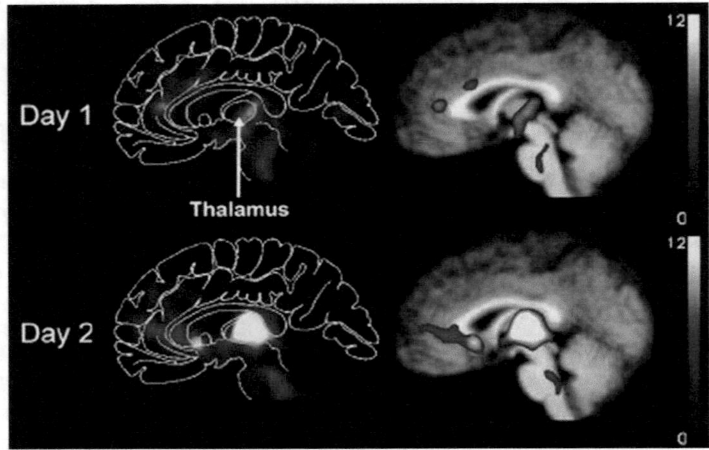

Fig. 13.7 Increased thalamic response to hypoglycemia in a model of HAAF. Synaptic activation during hypoglycemia, measured with [^{15}O]water positron emission tomography in nondiabetic humans, at baseline (Day 1) with interval hypoglycemia resulting in attenuated plasma epinephrine and symptomatic responses to hypoglycemia associated with a greater increase in synaptic activation in the dorsal midline thalamus (yellow) on Day 2. (From Arbelaez et al. [45], with permission)

[compared with −2 ± 2% in nondiabetic individuals] in seven subjects in each of the three groups. The authors' interpretation also rests on the validity of the brain glucose transport hypothesis discussed earlier. Those authors [70] also noted no redistribution of regional CBF to the thalamus during hypoglycemia in patients with T1D and impaired awareness of hypoglycemia, a finding seemingly at variance with our earlier finding in a model of HAAF [45] but consistent with another report [71].

Eliminating Hypoglycemia in Diabetes

It is possible to minimize the risk of hypoglycemia in insulin-, sulfonylurea-, and glinide-treated diabetes. A pragmatic approach to that has been published [72]. A major step forward would be to eliminate the use of sulfonylureas and glinides and to limit the use of insulin in T2D. These are feasible given the recent availability of glucose-lowering drugs for the treatment of T2D that do not in themselves cause hypoglycemia such as DPP-IV inhibitors, GLP-1 receptor agonists, SGLT2 inhibitors, and thiazolidinediones. But it is not possible to consistently eliminate hypoglycemia from the lives of persons with insulin-treated diabetes. That may become possible if automated insulin delivery systems become totally closed-loop and consistently reliable. Successful islet transplantation eliminates hypoglycemia but only as long as the graft remains functional.

Although prolonged, profound hypoglycemia can cause brain death directly, most fatal hypoglycemic episodes are the result of cardiac arrhythmias [1]. Recent antecedent hypoglycemia causes cardiovascular HAAF including reduced baroreflex sensitivity [73] and the resulting increased vulnerability to a ventricular arrhythmia. In that setting, the adrenal medullary response to an episode of hypoglycemia could trigger a fatal arrhythmia by activating beta-adrenergic receptors [74] in the heart, specifically beta-1 adrenergic receptors [75]. Nonselective adrenergic blockade prevents the effect of recent antecedent hypoglycemia to produce the HAAF phenomenon in humans [47]. There is evidence that treatment with a β-adrenergic antagonist reduces cardiovascular mortality during intensive glycemic therapy of diabetes [76]. Given these findings, it is conceivable that treatment with a relatively selective β_1-adrenergic receptor antagonist might prevent HAAF in diabetes without compromising the glycemic and symptom-generating actions of the catecholamines which are mediated through β_2-adrenergic receptors [1]. If so, that treatment would reduce the frequency of iatrogenic hypoglycemia in diabetes substantially.

Illustrative Case

A 53-year-old man with a 15-year history of type 2 diabetes and a 5-year history of treatment with insulin reports he feels well. He is using a basal (insulin glargine at bedtime)-bolus (insulin lispro before meals) regimen. His SMPG values generally range from 140 mg/dL (7.8 mmol/L) to 220 mg/dL (12.2 mmol/L). His hemoglobin A1c is 6.9% (52 mmol/mol). Review of his SMPG log reveals two morning glucose levels less than 50 mg/dL (2.8 mmol/L) in the past month, but he does not recall any symptoms at those times.

This patient almost assuredly has hypoglycemia unawareness caused by recurrent iatrogenic hypoglycemia, probably mostly at night. Therefore, he is at risk for an episode of dangerous, potentially fatal hypoglycemia in the future. The fact that his hemoglobin A1c is low relative to the vast majority of his recorded SMPG values is a clue that he has recurrent hypoglycemia somewhere in the 24-h period, probably at night when SMPG is rarely performed. His morning SMPG values of less than 50 mg/dL (2.8 mmol/L), distinctly hypoglycemic values, apparently without symptoms make the diagnosis of hypoglycemia unawareness likely. Continuous glucose monitoring would almost assuredly document recurrent nocturnal hypoglycemia without symptoms. The probable culprit is his bedtime insulin glargine.

Acknowledgments This chapter was prepared by the authors without external support. Dr. Cryer has served as a consultant to Novo Nordisk A/S in recent years. Dr. Arbelaez has nothing to declare.

Many of the early studies cited were supported by grants to Dr. Cryer from the National Institutes of Health (e.g., R01 DK27085) and from the American Diabetes Association and by a general clinical research center grant (M01 RR00036) from NIH.

References

1. Cryer PE. Hypoglycemia in diabetes, pathophysiology, prevalence and prevention. 3rd ed. Alexandria: American Diabetes Association; 2016.
2. International Diabetes Federation. IDF Diabetes Atlas. 7th ed. Brussels: International Diabetes Federation; 2015. (http://www.diabetesatlas.org).
3. U. K. Hypoglycemia Study Group. Risk of hypoglycaemia in types 1 and 2 diabetes: effects of treatment modalities and their duration. Diabetologia. 2007;50:1140–7.
4. Juvenile Diabetes Research Foundation (JDRF) Continuous Glucose Monitoring Study Group. Prolonged nocturnal hypoglycemia is common during 12 months of continuous glucose monitor-ing in children and adults with type 1 diabetes. Diabetes Care. 2010;33:1004–8.
5. Donnelly LA, Morris AD, Frier BM, Ellis JD, Donnan PT, Durant R, Band MM, Reekie G, Leese GP for the DARTS/MEMO Collaboration. Frequency and predictors of hypoglycaemia in type 1 and insulin-treated type 2 diabetes: a population-based study. Diabet Med. 2005;22:749–55.
6. Hepburn DA, MacLeod KM, Pell AC, Scougal IJ, Frier BM. Frequency and symptoms of hypoglycaemia experienced by patients with type 2 diabetes treated with insulin. Diabet Med. 1993;10:231–7.
7. Cryer PE. Glycemic goals in diabetes: trade-off between glycemic control and iatrogenic hypoglycemia. Diabetes. 2014;63:2188–95.
8. Writing Group for the DCCT/EDIC Research Group. Association between 7 years of intensive treatment of type 1 diabetes and long-term mortality. JAMA. 2015;313:45–53.
9. Cryer PE. Mechanisms of hypoglycemia-associated autonomic failure in diabetes. N Engl J Med. 2013;369:362–272.
10. Cryer PE, Santiago JV, Shah SD. Measurement of norepinephrine and epinephrine in small volumes of human plasma by a single isotope derivative method: response to the upright posture. J Clin Endocrinol Metab. 1974;39:1025–9.
11. Shah SD, Clutter WE, Cryer PE. External and internal standards in the single isotope derivative (radioenzymatic) measurement of norepinephrine and epinephrine. J Lab Clin Med. 1985;106:624–9.
12. Clutter WE, Bier DM, Shah SD, Cryer PE. Epinephrine plasma metabolic clearance rate and physiologic thresholds for metabolic and hemodynamic actions in man. J Clin Invest. 1980;66:94–101.
13. Berk MA, Clutter WE, Skor DA, Shah SD, Gingerich RP, Parvin CA, Cryer PE. Ehanced glycemic responsiveness to epinephrine in insulin dependent diabetes is the result of the inability to secrete insulin. J Clin Invest. 1985;75:1842–51.
14. Cryer PE. Physiology and pathophysiology of the human sympathoadrenal neuroendocrine system. N Engl J Med. 1980;303:436–44.
15. Garber AJ, Cryer PE, Santiago JV, Haymond MW, Pagliara AS, Kipnis DM. The role of adrenergic mechanisms in the substrate and hormonal response to insulin-induced hypoglycemia in man. J Clin Invest. 1976;58:7–15.
16. Clarke WL, Santiago JV, Thomas L, Haymond MW, Ben-Galim E, Cryer PE. Adrenergic mechanisms in recovery from hypoglycemia in man: adrenergic blockade. Am J Physiol Endocrinol Metab. 1979;236:E147–52.
17. Gerich J, Davis L, Lorenzi M, Rizza R, Bohannon N, Karam J, Lewis S, Kaplan R, Schultz T, Cryer P. Hormonal mechanisms of recovery from hypoglycemia. Am J Physiol Endocrinol Metab. 1979;236:E380–5.
18. Rizza RA, Cryer PE, Gerich JE. Role of glucagon, catecholamines and growth hormone in human glucose counterregulation. J Clin Invest. 1979;64:62–71.
19. Cryer PE, Gerich JE. Glucose counterregulation, hypoglycemia and intensive therapy of diabetes mellitus. N Engl J Med. 1985;313:232–41.
20. Towler DA, Havlin CE, Craft S, Cryer PE. Mechanisms of awareness of hypoglycemia: perception of neurogenic (predominantly cholinergic) rather than neuroglycopenic symptoms. Diabetes. 1993;42:1791–8.

21. DeRosa MA, Cryer PE. Hypoglycemia and the sympathoadrenal system: neurogenic symptoms are largely the result of sympathetic neural rather adrenomedullary activation. Am J Physiol Endocrinol Metab. 2004;287:E32–41.
22. White NH, Skor DA, Cryer PE, Levandoski LA Bier DM, Santiago JV. Identification of type 1 diabetic patients at increased risk for hypoglycemia during intensive therapy. N Engl J Med. 1983;308:485–91.
23. Bolli GB, De Feo P, De Cosmo S, Perriello G, Ventura MM, Massi-Benedetti M, Santeusanio F, Gerich JE, Brunetti P. A reliable and reproducible test for adequate glucose counterregulation in type 1 diabetes mellitus. Diabetes. 1994;33:732–7.
24. Geddes J, Schopman JE, Zammitt NN, Frier BM. Prevalence of impaired awareness of hypoglycaemia in adults with type 1 diabetes. Diabet Med. 2008;25:501–4.
25. Ryder REJ, Owens DR, Hayes TM, Ghatei MA, Bloom SR. Unawareness of hypoglycemia and inadequate hypoglycemic counterregulation: no causal relation with diabetic autonomic neuropathy. BMJ. 1990;301:783–7.
26. Cryer PE. Diverse causes of hypoglycemia-associated autonomic failure in diabetes. N Engl J Med. 2004;350:2272–9.
27. Jones TW, Porter P, Sherwin RS, Davis EA, O'Leary P, Frazer F, Byrne G, Stick S, Tamborlane WV. Decreased epinephrine responses to hypoglycemia during sleep. N Engl J Med. 1998;338:1657–62.
28. Banarer S, Cryer PE. Sleep-related hypoglycemia-associated autonomic failure in type 1 diabetes. Diabetes. 2003;52:1195–203.
29. Schultes B, Jauch-Chara K, Gais S, Hallschmid M, Reiprich E, Kern W, Oltmanns KM, Peters A, Fehm HL, Born J. Defective awakening response to nocturnal hypoglycemia in patients with type 1 diabetes mellitus. PLoS Med. 2007;4:e69.
30. Sandoval DA, Aftab Guy DL, Richardson MA, Ertl AC, Davis SN. Effects of low and moderate antecedent exercise on counterregulatory responses to subsequent hypoglycemia in type 1 diabetes. Diabetes. 2004;52:1798–806.
31. Cade WT, Khoury N, Nelson S, Shackleford A, Semenkovich K, Krauss MJ, Arbelaez AM. Hypoglycemia during moderate intensity exercise reduces counterregulatory responses to subsequent hypoglycemia. Physiol Rep. 2016;4:e12848.
32. Heller SR, Cryer PE. Reduced neuroendocrine and symptomatic responses to subsequent hypoglycemia after 1 episode of hypoglycemia in nondiabetic humans. Diabetes. 1991;40:223–6.
33. Dagogo-Jack S, Rattarasarn C, Cryer PE. Reversal of hypoglycemia unawareness, but not defective glucose counterregulation, in IDDM. Diabetes. 1994;43:1426–34.
34. Segel SA, Paramore DS, Cryer PE. Hypoglycemia-associated autonomic failure in type 2 diabetes. Diabetes. 2002;51:724–33.
35. Arbelaez AM, Xing D, Cryer PE, Kollman C, Beck RW, Sherr J, kRuedy KJ, Tamborlane WV, Mauras N, Tsalikian E, Wilson DM, White NH for the DirecNet Study Group. Blunted glucagon but not epinephrine responses to hypoglycemia occur in youth with less than one year duration of type 1 diabetes mellitus. Pediatr Diabetes. 2014;15:127–34.
36. Dagogo-Jack SE, Craft S, Cryer PE. Hypoglycemia-associated autonomic failure in insulin-dependent diabetes mellitus. J Clin Invest. 1993;91:819–28.
37. Fanelli CG, Epifano L, Rambotti AM, Pampanelli S, Di Vincenzo A, Modarelli F, Lepore M, Annibale B, Ciofetta M, Bottini P, Porcelati F, Scionti L, Santeusanio F, Brunetti P, Bolli GB. Meticulous prevention of hypoglycemia normalizes the glycemic thresholds and magnitude of most neuroendocrine responses to , symptoms of, and cognitive function during hypoglycemia in intensively treated patients with short-term IDDM. Diabetes. 1993;42:1683–9.
38. Fanelli C, Pampanelli S, Epifano L, Rambotti AM, Di Vincenzo A, Modarelli F, Ciofetta M, Lepore M, Annibale B, Torlone E, Perriello G, De Feo P, Santeusanio F, Brunetti P, Bolli GB. Long-term recovery from unawareness, deficient counterregulation and lack of cognitive dysfunction during hypoglycaemia following institution of rational intensive therapy in IDDM. Diabetologia. 1994;37:1265–76.
39. Cranston I, Lomas J, Maran A, Macdonald I, Amiel SA. Restoration of hypoglycaemia awareness in patients with long-duration insulin-dependent diabetes. Lancet. 1994;344:283–7.

40. Raju B, Cryer PE. Loss of the decrement in intraislet insulin plausibly explains loss of the glucagon response to hypoglycemia in insulin-deficient diabetes. Diabetes. 2005;54:757–64.
41. Cooperberg BA, Cryer PE. Insulin reciprocally regulates glucagon secretion in humans. Diabetes. 2010;59:2936–40.
42. Segel SA, Fanelli CG, Dence CS, Markham J, Videen TO, Paramore DS, Powers WJ, Cryer PE. Blood-to-brain glucose transport, cerebral glucose metabolism and cerebral blood flow are not increased after hypoglycemia. Diabetes. 2001;50:1911–7.
43. Lee JJ, Khoury N, Shackleford AM, Nelson S, Herrera H, Antenor-Dorsey JA, Semenkovich K, Shimony JS, Powers WJ, Cryer PE, Arbelaez AM. Dissociation between hormonal counter-regulatory responses and cerebral glucose metabolism during hypoglycemia. In Preparation.
44. Teves D, Videen TO, Cryer PE, Powers WJ. Activation of human medial prefrontal cortex during autonomic responses to hypoglycemia. Proc Natl Acad Sci U S A. 2004;101:6217–21. A
45. Arbelaez AM, Powers WJ, Videen TO, Price JL, Cryer PE. Attenuation of counterregulatory responses to recurrent hypoglycemia by active thalamic inhibition. A mechanism for hypoglycemia-associated autonomic failure. Diabetes. 2008;57:270–475.
46. Arbelaez AM, Rutlin JR, Hershey T, Powers WJ, Videen TO, Cryer PE. Thalamic activation during slightly subphysiological glycemia in humans. Diabetes Care. 2012;35:2570–4.
47. Ramanathan RP, Cryer PE. Adrenergic mediation of hypoglycemia-associated autonomic failure. Diabetes. 2011;60:602–6.
48. Diem P, Redmon JB, kAbid M, Moran A, Sutherland DE, Halter JB, Robertson RP. Glucagon, catecholamine and pancreatic polypeptide secretion in type 1 diabetic recipients of pancreatic allografts. J Clin Invest. 1990;86:2008–13.
49. Palmer JP, Henry DP, Benson JW, Johnson DG, Ensinck JW. Glucagon response to hypoglycemia in sympathectomized man. J Clin Invest. 1976;57:522–5.
50. Sherck SM, Shiota M, Saccomando J, Cardin S, Allen EJ, Hastings JR, Neal DW, Williams PE, Cherrington AD. Pancreatic response to mild non-insulin-induced hypoglycemia does not involve extrinsic neural input. Diabetes. 2001;50:2487–96.
51. Davis SN, Shavers C, Costa F, Mosqueda-Garcia R. Role of cortisol in the pathogenesis of deficient counterregulation after antecedent hypoglycemia in normal humans. J Clin Invest. 1996;98:680–91.
52. Davis SN, Shavers C, Davis B, Costa F. Prevention of an increase in plasma cortisol during hypoglycemia preserves subsequent counterregulatory responses. J Clin Invest. 1997;100:429–38.
53. Raju B, McGregor VP, Cryer PE. Cortisol elevations comparable to those that occur during hypoglycemia do not cause hypoglycemia-associated autonomic failure. Diabetes. 2003;52:2083–9.
54. Goldberg PA, Weiss R, McCrimmon RJ, Hintz EV, Dziura JD, Sherwin RS. Antecedent hypercortisolemia is not primarily responsible for generating hypoglycemia-associated autonomic failure. Diabetes. 2006;55:1121–6.
55. Gospin R, Tiwari A, Carey M, Tomuta N, Shamoon H, Bariely I, Hawkins M, Mbanya A. Hypoglycemia-associated autonomic failure (HAAF) is induced by opioid but not adrenergic receptor activation (abstract). Diabetes. 2016;65:A39.
56. de Galan BE, Rietjens SJ, Tack CJ, van der Werf SP, Sweep CGJ, Lenders JWM, Smits P. Antecedent adrenaline attenuates the responsiveness to, but not the release of, counter-regulatory hormones during subsequent hypoglycemia. J Clin Endocrinol Metab. 2003;88:5462–7.
57. Fanelli CG, Dence CS, Markham J, Videen TO, Paramore DS, Cryer PE, Powers WJ. Blood-to-brain glucose transport and cerebral glucose metabolism are not reduced in poorly controlled type 1 diabetes. Diabetes. 1998;47:1444–50.
58. Oz G, Tesfaye N, Kumar A, Declchand DK, Eberly LE, Seaquist ER. Brain glycogen content and metabolism in subjects with type 1 diabetes and hypoglycemia unawareness. J Cereb Blood Flow Metab. 2012;32:256–63.
59. Oz G, Moheet A, Dinuzzo M, Kumar A, Khowaja AA, Kubisizak K, Eberly LE, Seaquist ER. Cerebral glycogen in humans following acute and recurrent hypoglycemia:53. Implications for a role in hypoglycemia-associated autonomic failure (HAAF) (abstract). Diabetes. 2016;65:A105.

60. Wahren J, Ekberg K, Fernqvist-Forbes E, Nair S. Brain substrate utilization during acute hypoglycemia. Diabetes. 1999;42:812–7.
61. Lubow JM, Pinon IG, Avogaro A, Cobelli C, Treeson DM, Mandeville KA, Tofolo G, Boyle PJ. Brain oxygen utilization is unchanged by hypoglycemia in normal humans: lactate, alanine and leucine uptake are not sufficient to offset energy deficit. Am J Physiol Endocrinol Metab. 2006;290:E149–53.
62. De Feyter HM, Mason GF, Shulman GI, Rothman DL, Petersen KF. Increased brain lactate concentrations without increased lactate oxidation during hypoglycemia in type 1 diabetic individuals. Diabetes. 2013;62:3075–80.
63. Herzog RJ, Jiang L, Herman P, Zhao C, Sanganahalli BG, Mason GF, Hyder F, Rothman DL, Sherwin RS, Behar KL. Lactate preserves neuronal metabolism and functions following antecedent recurrent hypoglycemia. J Clin Invest. 2013;123:1988–98.
64. Chan O, Sherwin RS. Influence of VMH fuel sensing on hypoglycemic responses. Trends Endocrinol Metab. 2013;24:616–24.
65. Chan O, Paranjape SA, Horblitt A, Zhu W, Sherwin RS. Lactate-induced release of GABA in the ventromedial hypothalamus contributes to counterregulatory failure in recurrent hypoglycemia and diabetes. Diabetes. 2013;62:4239–46.
66. LaGamma EF, Kirtok N, Chan O, Nankova BB. Partial blockade of nicotinic acetylcholine receptors improves the counterregulatory response to hypoglycemia in recurrently hypoglycemic rats. Am J Physiol Endocrinol Metab. 2014;307:E580–8.
67. Wiegers EC, Rooijackers HM, Tack CJ, Heerschap A, de Galan BE, van der Graaf M. Brain lactate concentration falls in response to hypoglycemia in patients with type 1 diabetes and impaired awareness of hypoglycemia. Diabetes. 2016;65:1601–5.
68. Grissom N, Bhatnagar S. Habituation to repeated stress: get used to it. Neurobiol Learn Mem. 2009;92:215–24.
69. Bhatnagar S, Huber R, Nowak N, Trotter P. Lesions of the posterior paraventricular thalamus block habituation of hypothalamic-pituitary-adrenal response to repeated restraint. J Neuroendocrinol. 2002;14:403–10.
70. Wiegers EC, Becker KM, Rooijackers HM, von Samson-Himmelstjerma FC, Tack CJ, Heerschap A, de Galan BE, van der Graaf M. Cerebral blood flow response to hypoglycemia is altered in patients with type 1 diabetes and impaired awareness of hypoglycemia. J Cereb Blood Flow Metab 2016; 37:1994–2001.
71. Mangia S, Tesfaye N, De Martino F, Kumar AF, Kollasch P, Moheet AA, Eberly LE, Seaquist ER. Hypoglycemia-induced increases in thalamic cerebral blood flow are blunted in subjects with type 1 diabetes and hypoglycemia unawareness. J Cereb Blood Flow Metab. 2012;32:2084–90.
72. International Hypoglycemia Study Group. Minimizing hypoglycemia in diabetes. Diabetes Care. 2015;38:1583–91.
73. Rao AD, Bonyhay I, Dankwa J, Baimas-George M, Kneen L, Ballatori S, Freeman R, Adler GK. Baroreflex sensitivity impairment during hypoglycemia: implications for cardiovascular control. Diabetes. 2016;65:209–15.
74. Reno CM, Daphna-Iken D, Chen YS, VanderWeele J, Jethi K, Fisher SJ. Severe hypoglycemia-induced lethal cardiac arrhythmias are mediated by sympathoadrenal activation. Diabetes. 2013;62:3570–81.
75. Reno CM, Skinner A, Malik N, Viera de Abreu A, Chen YS, Daphna-Iken D, Fisher SJ. Beta1-adrenergic receptor blockade reduces severe hypoglycemia-induced cardiac arrhythmias in nondiabetic and diabetic rats (abstract). Diabetes. 2016;65:A102.
76. Tsujimoto T, Sugiyama T, Noda M, Kajio H. Intensive glycemic therapy in patients with type 2 diabetes on beta-blockers. Diabetes Care. 2016;39:1818–26.
77. Cryer PE. Mechanisms of sympathoadrenal failure and hypoglycemia in diabetes. J Clin Invest. 2006;116:1470–3.

Chapter 14
The Sympathetic Nervous System in Hypertension

Gino Seravalle, Giuseppe Mancia, and Guido Grassi

Introduction

Cumulative evidence collected in the last few decades have investigated the behavior of sympathetic cardiovascular drive in essential hypertension. These observations have shown that several excitatory influences of the adrenergic nervous system on the heart and on peripheral circulation are already detectable in the early stages and contribute to sustain this pathophysiological condition and also to the disease progression and the development of target organ damage. This chapter will provide an overview of the noradrenergic abnormalities characterizing the hypertensive states and the possible pathophysiological mechanisms.

Mechanisms Regulating Adrenergic Tone

The sympathetic nervous system is a major regulator of cardiac output and systemic vascular resistance, the major components of neural blood pressure regulation. Tonic sympathetic activity is mainly generated by neurons located in the

G. Seravalle
Cardiologia, Ospedale San Luca, IRCCS Istituto Auxologico Italiano, Milan, Italy

G. Mancia
Università Milano Bicocca, Monza, Italy

G. Grassi (✉)
Clinica Medica, Università Milano-Bicocca, Monza, and IRCCS Multimedica, Sesto San Giovanni/Milan, Italy

Clinica Medica, Ospedale S. Gerardo dei Tintori, Monza, Italy
e-mail: guido.grassi@unimib.it

L. Landsberg (ed.), *Pheochromocytomas, Paragangliomas and Disorders of the Sympathoadrenal System*, Contemporary Endocrinology,
https://doi.org/10.1007/978-3-319-77048-2_14

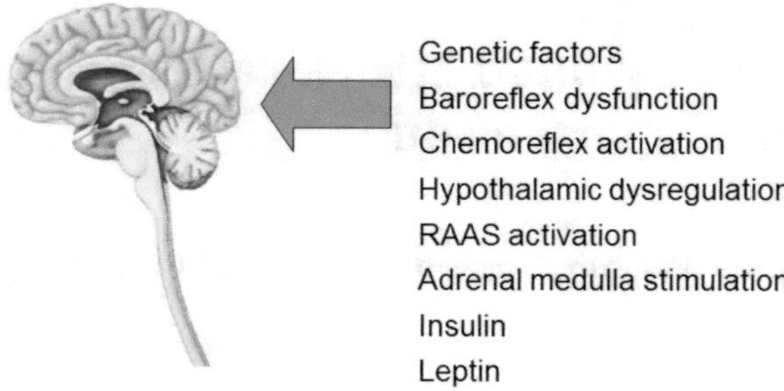

Fig. 14.1 Schematic illustration of the possible mechanisms responsible for the potentiation of the sympathetic activation in essential hypertension

rostral ventrolateral medulla (RVLM) and regulated by arterial baroreceptors, cardiopulmonary mechanoreceptors, and chemoreceptors (Fig. 14.1). Sympathetic activity is also modulated by neurons in the limbic system, the hypothalamus, and the cortex [1–4].

A large body of evidence has also shown that blood pressure and blood volume regulation closely depend on the interactions between sympathetic nervous system, the renin-angiotensin system, and renal sodium excretion [5–7].

Physiologically, elevated blood pressure caused by increased sympathetic activity leads to baroreflex activation, in turn resulting in inhibition of the sympathetic activity and the return of blood pressure toward baseline values. It appears well established now that baroreceptors contribute not only to short- but also long-term regulation of blood pressure levels [2, 7, 8]. In addition it is likely that the anteroventral region of the third ventricle plays an important role in the long-term regulation of blood pressure, sympathetic activity, and fluid/volume homeostasis. This region of the brain is sensitive to circulating hormones, blood pressure, and fluid/volume changes. Input from these pathways is integrated and routed to the paraventricular nucleus of the hypothalamus which is the transmitter of excitatory and inhibitory signals for long-term blood pressure control.

It is also suggested that the metabolic alterations frequently detectable in hypertension, such as the hyperinsulinemic state and the related insulin resistance, may be the triggering factors. This hypothesis is based on the evidence that insulin may have central sympathoexcitatory effects which may thus be enhanced in hypertensive patients' adrenergic drive [9].

Gene Polymorphisms

The hypothesis of a neurogenic cause at the basis of the hypertensive state is supported by studies showing that the genetic background of a given patient may interfere with the sympathetic neural function. This has been observed in a study showing that normotensive subjects with a family history of hypertension have already an increased sympathetic neural drive [10] (Fig. 14.2). This has been more recently supported by the evidence that mutations of single genes directly or indirectly involved in cardiovascular regulation may affect blood pressure,

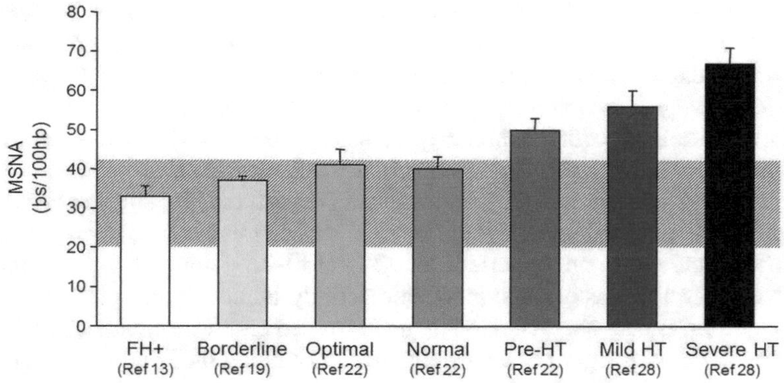

Fig. 14.2 Mean values of muscle sympathetic nerve activity (MSNA) expressed as burst incidence corrected for heart rate values in different group of subjects. Data obtained from Ref in the brackets. The gray zone refers to the area of sympathetic activity recorded in healthy normal subjects. These levels of normalcy may be different in different studies and depend on several factors (age, gender, etc.). *FH+* positive familiarity for hypertension, *HT* hypertension

sympathetic function, and cardiovascular responses to stress. This is the case for the gene encoding melanocortin-4 receptor, which participates not only at energy balance control but also at blood pressure regulation. A melanocortin-4 receptor deficiency is accompanied by a reduced adrenergic function and low blood pressure values [11]. This is also the case for the gene encoding phosducin, which participates at cardiovascular homeostasis control by regulating G proteins. Phosducin plays a role in modulating the adrenergic and blood pressure responses to stress and thus in determining stress-induced hypertension [12, 13]. Another observation derives from the presence of specific polymorphisms of α-1A-adrenoceptor gene associated with hyperadrenergic tone in hypertensive patients with the metabolic syndrome [14]. These findings strongly support the concept that genetic factors may participate at the phenotypic expression of an adrenergic overdrive.

Prehypertension and "Borderline" Hypertension

Evidence from several sources have clearly documented that sympathetic neural factors and an abnormality in sympathetic control of the cardiovascular system participate in the early blood pressure increase occurring in the initial clinical phase of the hypertensive disease.

It has been shown that a resting tachycardia, associated with a hyperkinetic state, is frequently present in a consistent fraction of young hypertensives [15]. These hemodynamic abnormalities are accompanied by a significant increase in circulating plasma levels of noradrenaline. This evidence suggests that the inhibitory influences exerted by vagal tone on the sinus node are already lost and that the excitatory ones exerted by sympathetic drive are already potentiated.

Data obtained in the 1990s have also shown that in subjects with borderline or very mild hypertension, sympathetic nerve traffic is increased, indicating that central sympathetic outflow is already activated [16, 17]. The use of a different technique to investigate the adrenergic system, the norepinephrine spillover techniques, has shown in subject with essential hypertension that the cardiac and renal districts were those more involved by this sympathetic activation [18].

Recent evidences provided by Seravalle and coworkers [19] suggest that even in subjects in which blood pressure values are in the high/normal range on the basis of ESH/ESC guidelines on hypertension [20] (130–139 mm Hg or systolic and 85–89 mm Hg for diastolic), sympathetic activity is already elevated (Fig. 14.2). This condition is also characterized by an increased cardiovascular risk and higher mortality [21]. With regard to the mechanisms sustaining the hyperadrenergic tone, an impairment of baroreflex heart rate control appears very early in the clinical course of the hypertensive disease; a few mm Hg increase in blood pressure may be responsible for a functional baroreceptor impairment of heart rate control. These subjects were also characterized by an increase in HOMA index and in plasma insulin levels. As a hyperinsulinemic state may exert central sympathoexcitatory effects [22, 23], the possibility that the high-normal blood pressure-related sympathetic activation depends on this metabolic alteration is confirmed by the strong direct relation observed between HOMA index and sympathetic nerve traffic.

Mild and Severe Hypertension

A meta-analysis of the studies performed by employing plasma norepinephrine as a marker of sympathetic drive has shown that in a consistent number of hypertensive patients, the circulating levels of this adrenergic neurotransmitter are increased [24]. This increase is likely to depend on an enhanced central neuroadrenergic drive, given the evidence that direct recording of sympathetic nerve traffic has been shown to be considerably potentiated in essential hypertensive patients.

The magnitude of the sympathetic neural activation appears to parallel the clinical severity of the blood pressure elevation, from moderate hypertension to severe hypertensive state [25] (Fig. 14.2). This potentiation has been demonstrated to involve the sympathetic outflow to different cardiovascular districts, as documented by the increased norepinephrine spillover in cerebral, coronary, and renal circulation as well [18].

Isolated Systolic Hypertension

Only limited evidence is available in isolated systolic hypertension, a condition in which an important determinant of baroreflex control of sympathetic drive, such as diastolic blood pressure [26], is not increased or even reduced. Patients with systo-diastolic and isolated systolic hypertension have shown an increase in sympathetic nerve traffic [27], and this is not limited to young and middle-aged but is evident also in elderly patients. In both the systo-diastolic and isolated systolic hypertension, the ability of baroreflex stimulation and deactivation to modify heart rate is impaired, while the baroreflex control of sympathetic activity is not affected. This extends to old age the differential impairment between baroreceptor heart rate and baroreceptor sympathetic reflex that has been reported in younger subjects with essential hypertension [17, 25]. Also in this case, factors responsible for the adrenergic activation include an increased activity of the renin-angiotensin system, a hyperinsulinemia induced by insulin resistance, and an impairment of the cardiopulmonary reflex, because all these factors are known to lead to a stimulation of central sympathetic drive [28–30]. In elderly subjects, however, the last two factors are more likely to be involved than the first, because aging is accompanied by a reduction of plasma renin and angiotensin II levels [31]. In the elderly, the absence of tachycardia suggests that the sympathetic activation involves the peripheral circulation but not the heart, despite the impairment of both the peripheral and the cardiac modulation by baroreflex. This would be compatible with previous observations that (a) there is a lesser increase in norepinephrine spillover from cardiac sympathetic nerve terminals into the venous reservoir in elderly than in young hypertensive subjects [18] and (b) plasma norepinephrine and sympathetic nerve activity have only a very limited correlation with heart rate values [32].

Adrenergic Tone and Dipping Alterations

The use of ambulatory blood pressure monitoring allows identification of four different patterns of nocturnal blood pressure profile, i.e., the dipping, nondipping (defined as a < 10% fall in nocturnal BP relative to diurnal BP (i.e., [daytime BP – nighttime BP]/daytime BP × 100%), arithmetically equivalent to a night-to-day BP ratio > 0.9), extreme dipping (≥20% fall), and reverse dipping (<0% fall), associated with different rates of target organ damage and clinical outcome [33–35]. Reverse-dipping blood pressure pattern (i.e., the condition characterized by no reduction or an increase in nighttime blood pressure from the daytime values) is characterized by a sympathetic activation that is greater than that observed in the other forms of nighttime blood pressure fall [36] (Fig. 14.3). A close inverse relationship between the degree of sympathetic activation and the magnitude of the nighttime fall in systolic or diastolic blood pressure has been observed (Fig. 14.4). This means that in individuals with blood pressure elevation, a greater sympathetic activation is accompanied by reduced blood pressure at night due to the convergence of a variety of central and reflex influences. An inverse relationship has been observed in reverse dippers between HOMA index and plasma insulin levels and the magnitude of the nighttime BP fall confirming that the alterations in the dipping state are associated with insulin resistance [37, 38]. This reflects the multifold circulatory effects of insulin (vasomotor response, central action, alteration in neural sympathetic drive) [29]. Baroreflex mechanisms are unlikely to be involved in the determination of the magnitude of the blood pressure fall and increase in sympathetic activity at night, but this rather depends on other sympatho-modulating factors [36, 39]. There is a robust literature that speaks about the association between nocturnal hypertension and a multitude of

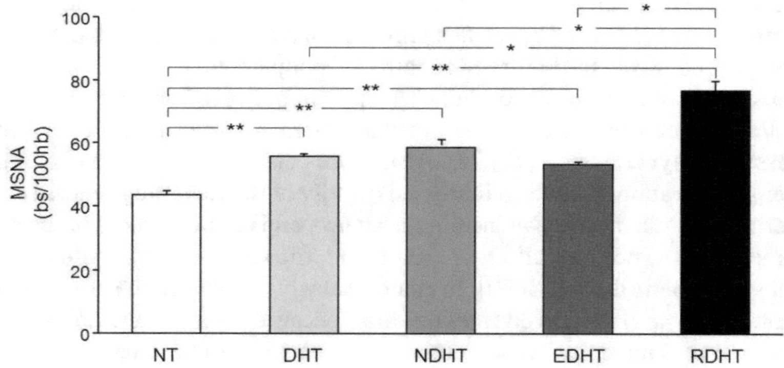

Fig. 14.3 Mean (±SEM) resting MSNA values expressed as burst incidence corrected for heart rate in normotensive dippers (NT) and hypertensive (HT) dippers (D), nondipper (ND), extreme dipper (ED), and reverse dipper (RD). * $p < 0.05$, ** $p < 0.01$. (Modified from Ref. [36], with permission)

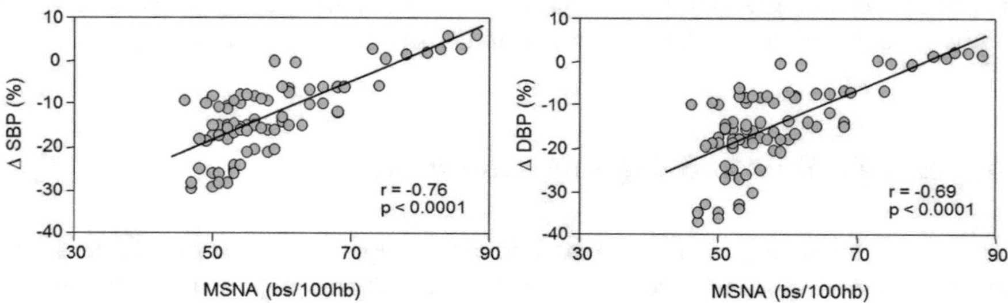

Fig. 14.4 Correlation between resting MSNA values corrected for heart rate and day-night changes in systolic BP (left) and diastolic BP (right) in the hypertensive patients of Fig. 14.3. Correlation coefficients (r) and levels of statistical significance (P) are shown. (Modified from Ref. [36], with permission)

unfavorable structural cardiovascular consequences (e.g., cardiac chamber dilatation, ventricular hypertrophy, carotid intima-media thickening, silent lacunae, leukoaraiosis, brain microbleeds) as well as functional alteration (e.g., diastolic dysfunction). The 24-h blood pressure overload, the altered or absent nocturnal hypotension, and the hyperadrenergic state are responsible for the increased incidence of cardiovascular and fatal events [34, 35, 40].

"White-Coat" and "Masked" Hypertension

The increasing use of 24-h blood pressure monitoring and the comparison with office and home blood pressure allow identification of two other different and opposite forms of hypertensive patients: the first, called white-coat hypertension, is characterized by an increase in blood pressure values during the visit of the doctor but not over the daytime [41, 42], while the second, called masked hypertension, is

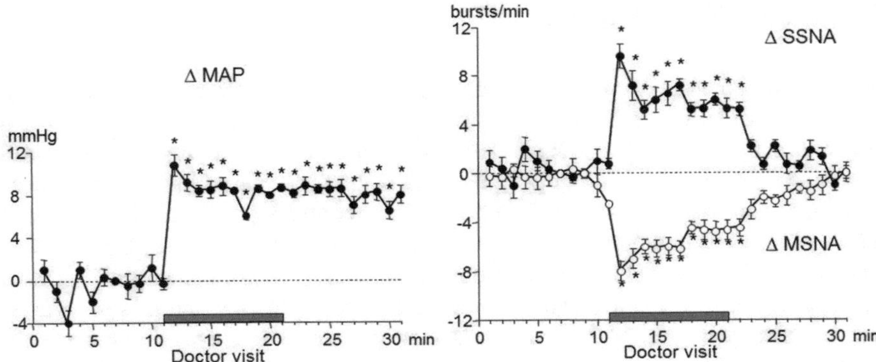

Fig. 14.5 Effects of sphygmomanometric blood pressure measurement by a doctor on mean arterial pressure (MAP) , muscle sympathetic nerve traffic (MSNA), and skin sympathetic nerve traffic (SSNA). Data are shown as mean (±SEM) changes as compared to the pre-visit values. * $p < 0.05$ refers to the statistical significance between single values obtained during doctor visit and pre-visit. (Unpublished figure drawn using data from Ref. [43], with permission)

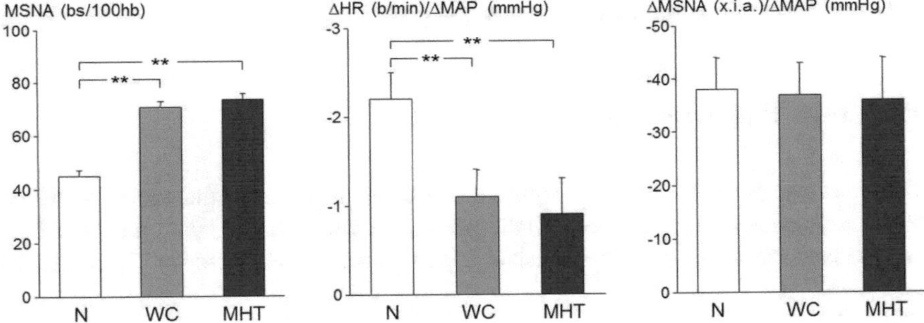

Fig. 14.6 Mean (±SEM) resting MSNA values (left) expressed as burst incidence corrected for heart rate in normotensive (N) subjects and in patients with white-coat (WC) and masked (M) hypertension (HT). Middle and right panels refer to baroreceptor HR and MSNA sensitivities, expressed as average ratios between changes in HR or MSNA over changes in mean arterial pressure (MAP) in the three groups. ** $p < 0.01$ vs N. (Modified from Ref. [44], with permission)

characterized by an increase in blood pressure values during the daily life but normal in the clinic environment. Both these two conditions are characterized by a marked sympathetic activation [43]. The emotional reaction is characterized by a behavior of the sympathetic nervous system that combines a skin sympathetic activation (and a resulting vasoconstriction) with a muscle sympathetic deactivation leading to muscle vasodilation [43–45] (Fig. 14.5). It has also been shown that sympathetic nerve traffic is about 30% greater in white-coat as compared to age-matched normotensives and that the magnitude of the adrenergic overdrive is almost superimposable to the one characterizing masked hypertension (Fig. 14.6). This hyperadrenergic state contributes to the adverse impact on organ damage and risk of cardiovascular events [46, 47].

Secondary Hypertension

Adrenergic tone in secondary hypertension varies in different disease states. Subjects with renovascular hypertension and pheochromocytoma show a sympathetic tone that is on average much lower than that of essential hypertensives with the same blood pressure levels [25], and this is the same for patients with primary aldosteronism [48]. Subjects with pheochromocytoma are characterized by high levels of catecholamines contributing to sympathoinhibitory effects on central sympathetic outflow. Surgical removal of the tumor results in a normalization of plasma catecholamine levels and blood pressure values and normalization of sympathetic nerve traffic [49] (Fig. 14.7). In renovascular hypertension, elevated plasma levels of angiotensin II may induce an increased release of norepinephrine from sympathetic nerve terminals [28]. In contrast, adrenergic tone is increased in chronic kidney disease. The marked sympathetic activation observed in renal failure [50] is already present in the early phase of this pathophysiological condition [51] and appears to be dependent on several mechanisms: (i) activation of renal chemoreceptors [52], (ii) activation of the renin-angiotensin-aldosterone system [53], (iii) increased circulating levels of endogenous inhibitors of the nitric oxide synthase [54], and (iv) the insulin resistance state [39].

Resistant Hypertension

True resistant hypertension is a diagnosis that depends upon (1) the exclusion of the secondary forms of hypertension, (2) the white-coat effect, and (3) poor patient adherence to prescribed therapy. True resistant hypertensives are characterized by a marked

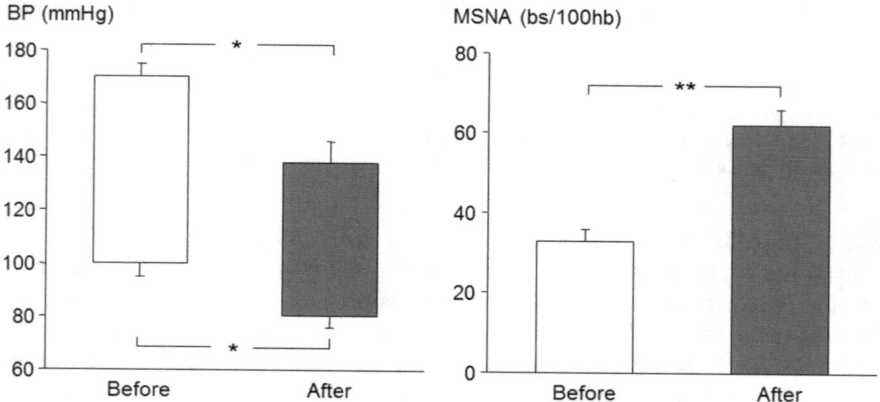

Fig. 14.7 Effects of surgical removal of pheochromocytoma on systolic and diastolic blood pressure (BP) (left) and muscle sympathetic nerve traffic (MSNA) (right). Data are expressed as mean (±SEM) before and after surgical procedure. $*p < 0.05$, $**p < 0.01$ vs presurgery. (Modified from Ref. [49], with permission)

sympathetic activation, greater than that observed in essential nonresistant hypertensive patients, as reported by studies with norepinephrine spillover and direct recording of muscle sympathetic nerve traffic [55, 56]. As regards the potential abnormalities associated with this condition, two deserve to be mentioned. The first refers to the finding that an aldosterone excess with its sympathoexcitatory effects has been repeatedly reported, representing another pathophysiological mechanism contributing to the adrenergic overdrive [57]. The second abnormality refers to the evidence that a consistent fraction of hypertensive patients resistant to antihypertensive drug treatment also displays sleep apnea syndrome [58], a condition that per se is characterized by a marked elevation in sympathetic nerve traffic as observed in lean normotensive subjects [59]. All these aspects represent the background for non-pharmacological and pharmacological interventions both in essential hypertensive and in true resistant hypertensive patients.

References

1. Guyenet PG. The sympathetic control of blood pressure. Nat Rev Neurosci. 2006;7:335–46.
2. Dampney RA, Coleman MJ, Fontes MA, Hirooka Y, Horluchi J, Li YW, McAllen RM. Central mechanisms underlying short- and long-term regulation of the cardiovascular system. Clin Exp Pharmacol Physiol. 2002;29:261–8.
3. Grassi G, Seravalle G. Sympatho-vagal imbalance in hypertension. In: Robertson D, Biaggioni I, Low PA, Paton JFR, editors. Primer on the autonomic nervous system. London: Academic Press; 2012. p. 345–8.
4. Grassi G, Seravalle G, Dell'Oro R, Turri C, Pasqualinotto L, Colombo M, Mancia G. Participation of the hypothalamus-hypophysis axis in the sympathetic activation of human obesity. Hypertension. 2001;38:1316–20.
5. Johns EJ, Kopp UC, DiBona GF. Neural control of renal function. Compr Physiol. 2011;1:731–67.
6. Iliescu R, Irwin ED, Georgakopoulos D, Lohmeier TE. Renal responses to chronic suppression of central sympathetic outflow. Hypertension. 2012;60:749–56.
7. Mancia G. The sympathetic nervous system in hypertension. J Hypertens. 1997;15:1553–65.
8. Lohmeier TE, Iliescu R. The baroreflex as a long-term controller of arterial pressure. Physiology. 2015;30:148–58.
9. Grassi G, Mancia G. Hyperadrenergic and labile hypertension. In: Lip GH, Hall J, editors. Comprehensive hypertension. Philadelphia: Mosby Elsevier; 2007. p. 719–26.
10. Yamada Y, Miyajima E, Tochikubo O, Matsukawa T, Shionoiri H, Ishii M, Kaneko Y. Impaired baroreflex changes in muscle sympathetic nerve activity in adolescents who have a family history of essential hypertension. J Hypertens. 1988;6:S525–8.
11. Greenfield JR, Miller JW, Keogh JM, Henning E, Satterwhite JH, Cameron GS, Atruc B, Mayer JP, Brage S, See TC, Lomas DJ, O'Rahilly S, Farooqi IS. Modulation of blood pressure by central melanocortinergic pathways. N Engl J Med. 2009;360:44–52.
12. Beets N, Harrison MD, Brede M, Zong X, Urbanski MJ, Sietmann A, Kaufling J, Barrot M, Seeliger MW, Vieira-Coelho MA, Hamet P, Gaudet D, Seda O, Tremblay J, Kotchen TA, Kaldunski M, Nusing R, Szabo B, Jacob HJ, Cowley AW Jr, Biel M, Stoll M, Lohse MJ, Broeckel U, Hein L. Phosducin influences sympathetic activity and prevents stress-induced hypertension in humans and mice. J Clin Invest. 2009;119:3597–612.
13. Grassi G. Phosducin – a candidate gene for stress-dependent hypertension. J Clin Invest. 2009;119:3515–8.

14. Grassi G, Padmanabhan S, Menna C, Seravalle G, Lee WK, Bombelli M, Brambilla G, Quarti Trevano F, Giannattasio C, Cesana G, Dominiczak A, Mancia G. Association between ADRA-1A gene and the metabolic syndrome: candidate genes and functional counterpart in the PAMELA population. J Hypertens. 2011;29:1121–7.
15. Julius S, Krause L, Schork NJ, Mejia AD, Jones KA, van de Ven C, Johnson EH, Sekkarie MA, Kjeldsen SE, Petrin J. Hyperkinetic borderline hypertension in Tecumseh, Michigan. J Hypertens. 1991;9:77–84.
16. Anderson EA, Sinkey CA, Lawton WJ, Mark AL. Elevated sympathetic nerve activity in borderline hypertensive humans. Evidences from direct intraneural recordings. Hypertension. 1989;14:177–83.
17. Floras JS, Hara K. Sympathoneural and haemodynamic characteristics of young subjects with mild essential hypertension. J Hypertens. 1993;11:647–55.
18. Esler M, Lambert G, Jennings G. Regional norepinephrine turnover in human hypertension. Clin Exp Hypertens. 1989;11(suppl 1):75–89.
19. Seravalle G, Lonati L, Buzzi S, Cairo M, Quarti Trevano F, Dell'Oro R, Facchetti R, Mancia G, Grassi G. Sympathetic nerve traffic and baroreflex function in optimal, normal, and high-normal blood pressure states. J Hypertens. 2015;33:1411–7.
20. Mancia G, Fagard R, Narkiewicz K, Redon J, Zanchetti A, Bohm M, et al. ESH/ESC guidelines for the management of hypertension. J Hypertens. 2013;31:1281–357.
21. Vasan RS, Larson MG, Leip EP, Evans JC, O'Donnell CJ, Kannel WB, Levy D. Impact of high-normal blood pressure on the risk of cardiovascular disease. N Engl J Med. 2001;345:1291–7.
22. Berne C, Fagius J, Pollare T, Hjemdahl P. The sympathetic response to euglycemic hyperinsulinemia. Evidence from microelectrode recordings in healthy subjects. Diabetologia. 1992;35:873–9.
23. Vollenweider P, Randin D, Tappy L, Jequier E, Nicod P, Scherrer U. Impaired insulin-induced sympathetic neural activation and vasodilation in skeletal muscle in obese humans. J Clin Invest. 1994;93:2365–71.
24. Goldstein DS. Plasma catecholamines and essential hypertension. An analytical review. Hypertension. 1983;5:86–99.
25. Grassi G, Cattaneo BM, Seravalle G, Lanfranchi A, Mancia G. Baroreflex control of sympathetic nerve activity in essential and secondary hypertension. Hypertension. 1998;31:68–72.
26. Sanders JS, Ferguson DW. Diastolic pressure determines autonomic responses to pressure perturbation in humans. J Appl Physiol. 1989;66:800–7.
27. Grassi G, Seravalle G, Bertinieri G, Turri C, Dell'Oro R, Stella ML, Mancia G. Sympathetic and reflex alterations in systo-diastolic and systolic hypertension of the elderly. J Hypertens. 2000;18:587–93.
28. Zimmerman BG. Evaluation of peripheral and central components of action of angiotensin on the sympathetic nervous system. J Pharmacol Exp Ther. 1967;158:1–10.
29. Reaven GM, Lithell H, Landsberg L. Hypertension and associated metabolic abnormalities – the role of insulin resistance and the sympathoadrenal system. N Engl J Med. 1996;334:374–81.
30. Mark AL, Mancia G. Cardiopulmonary baroreflexes in humans. In: Shepherd JT, Abboud FM, editors. Handbook of physiology, section 2: the cardiovascular system. Bethesda: American Physiological Society; 1983. p. 795–813.
31. Crane MG, Harris JJ. Effect of ageing on renin activity and aldosterone excretion. J Lab Clin Med. 1976;87:947–59.
32. Grassi G, Vailati S, Bertinieri G, Seravalle G, Stella ML, Dell'Oro R, Mancia G. Heart rate as a marker of sympathetic activity. J Hypertens. 1998;16:1635–9.
33. O'Brien E, Asmar R, Beilin L, Imai Y, Mallion JM, Mancia G, Mengden T, Myers M, Padfield P, Palatini P, Parati G, Pickering T, Redon J, Staessen J, Stergiou G, Verdecchia P, European Society of Hypertension Working Group on Blood Pressure Monitoring. European Society of Hypertension recommendations for conventional, ambulatory and home blood pressure measurement. J Hypertens. 2003;21:821–48.

34. Verdecchia P, Schillaci G, Borgioni C, Ciucci A, Gattobigio R, Guerrieri M, Comparato E, Benemio G, Porcellati C. Altered circadian blood pressure profile and prognosis. Blood Press Monit. 1997;2:347–52.
35. Ohkubo T, Imai Y, Tsuji I, Nagai K, Watanabe N, Minami N, Kato J, Kikuchi N, Nishiyama A, Aihara A, Sekino M, Satoh H, Hisamichi S. Relation between nocturnal decline in blood pressure and mortality. The Ohasama study. Am J Hypertens. 1997;10:1201–7.
36. Grassi G, Seravalle G, Quarti Trevano F, Dell'Oro R, Bombelli M, Cuspidi C, Facchetti R, Bolla GB, Mancia G. Adrenergic, metabolic, and reflex abnormalities in reverse and extreme dipper hypertensives. Hypertension. 2008;52:925–31.
37. Vyssoulis GP, Karpanou EA, Kyvelou SM, Adamopoulos DN, Deligeorgis AD, Spanos PG, Pietri PG, Cokkinos DF, Stefanadis CI. Nocturnal blood pressure fall and metabolic syndrome score in hypertensive patients. Blood Press Monit. 2007;12:351–6.
38. Brasil RR, Soares DV, Spina LD, Lobo PM, da Silva EM, Mansur VA, Pinheiro MF, Coceicao FL, Vaisman M. Association of insulin resistance and nocturnal fall of blood pressure in GH-deficient adults during GH replacement. J Endocrinol Investig. 2007;30:306–12.
39. Mancia G, Grassi G, Giannattasio C, Seravalle G. Sympathetic activation in the pathogenesis of hypertension and progression of organ damage. Hypertension. 1999;34:724–8.
40. Cuspidi C, Macca G, Sampieri L, Fusi V, Severgnini B, Michev I, Salerno M, Magrini F, Zanchetti A. Target organ damage and non-dipping pattern defined by two sessions of ambulatory blood pressure monitoring in recently diagnosed essential hypertensive patients. J Hypertens. 2001;19:1539–45.
41. Mancia G, Bertinieri G, Grassi G, Parati G, Pomidossi G, Ferrari A, Gregorini L, Zanchetti A. Effects of blood pressure measurements by the doctor on patient's blood pressure and heart rate. Lancet. 1983;II:695–8.
42. Pierdomenico SD, Bucci A, Costantini F, Lapenna D, Cuccurullo F, Mezzetti A. Twenty-four hour autonomic nervous function in sustained and "white-coat" hypertension. Am Heart J. 2000;140:672–7.
43. Grassi G, Turri C, Vailati S, Dell'Oro R, Mancia G. Muscle and skin sympathetic nerve traffic during "white-coat" effect. Circulation. 1999;100:222–5.
44. Grassi G, Seravalle G, Quarti Trevano F, Dell'Oro R, Bolla GB, Cuspidi C, Arenare F, Mancia G. Neurogenic abnormalities in masked hypertension. Hypertension. 2007;50:537–42.
45. Brod J, Fenci V, Hejl Z, Jirka J. Circulatory changes underlying blood pressure elevation during acute emotional stress in normotensive and hypertensive subjects. Clin Sci. 1959;18:269–79.
46. Mancia G, Facchetti R, Bombelli M, Grassi G, Sega R. Long-term risk of mortality associated with selective and combined elevation in office, home and ambulatory blood pressure. Hypertension. 2006;47:846–53.
47. Ohkubo T, Kikuya M, Metoki H, Asayama K, Obara T, Hashimoto J, Totsune K, Hoshi H, Satoh H, Imai Y. Prognosis of "masked" hypertension and "white-coat" hypertension detected by 24-hour ambulatory blood pressure monitoring. 10 year follow-up from the Ohasama study. J Am Coll Cardiol. 2005;46:508–15.
48. Miyajima E, Yamada Y, Yoshida Y, Matsukawa T, Shionoiri H, Tochikubo O, Ishii M. Muscle sympathetic nerve activity in renovascular hypertension and primary aldosteronism. Hypertension. 1991;17:1057–62.
49. Grassi G, Seravalle G, Turri C, Mancia G. Sympathetic nerve traffic responses to surgical removal of pheochromocytoma. Hypertension. 1999;34:461–5.
50. Converse RL Jr, Jacobsen TN, Toto RD, Jost CMT, Cosentino F, Fouad-Tarazi F, Victor R. Sympathetic overactivity in patients with chronic renal failure. N Engl J Med. 1992;327:1912–8.
51. Grassi G, Quarti-Trevano F, Seravalle G, Arenare F, Volpe M, Furiani S, Dell'Oro R, Mancia G. Early sympathetic activation in the initial clinical stages of chronic renal failure. Hypertension. 2011;57:846–51.
52. Hering D, Zdrojewski Z, Krol E, Kara T, Kucharska W, Somers V, Rutkowski B, Narkiewicz K. Tonic chemoreflex activation contributes to the elevated muscle sympathetic nerve activity in patients with chronic renal failure. J Hypertens. 2007;25:157–61.

53. Mancia G, Dell'Oro R, Quarti Trevano F, Scopelliti F, Grassi G. Angiotensin-sympathetic system intercations in cardiovascular and metabolic disease. J Hypertens. 2006;24:51–6.
54. Zoccali C. The endothelium as a target in renal diseases. J Nephrol. 2007;20:S39–44.
55. Schlaich MP, Sobotka PA, Krum H, Lambert E, Esler MD. Renal sympathetic nerve ablation for uncontrolled hypertension. N Engl J Med. 2009;361:932–4.
56. Grassi G, Seravalle G, Brambilla G, Pini C, Alimento M, Facchetti R, Spaziani D, Cuspidi C, Mancia G. Marked sympathetic activation and baroreflex dysfunction in true resistant hypertension. Int J Cardiol. 2014;177:1020–5.
57. Gaddam KK, Nishizaka MK, Pratt-Ubunama MN, Pimenta E, Aban I, Oparil S, Calhoun DA. Characterization of resistant hypertension: association between resistant hypertension, aldosterone, and persistent intravascular volume expansion. Arch Intern Med. 2008;168:1159–64.
58. Narkiewicz K, van de Borne PJ, Cooley RL, Dyken ME, Somers VK. Sympathetic activity in obese subjects with and without sleep apnea. Circulation. 1998;98:772–6.
59. Grassi G, Facchini A, Quarti Trevano F, Dell'Oro R, Arenare F, Tana F, Bolla G, Monzani A, Robuschi M, Mancia G. Obstructive sleep apnea-dependent and –independent adrenergic activation in obesity. Hypertension. 2005;46:321–5.

Index

L. Landsberg (ed.), *Pheochromocytomas, Paragangliomas and Disorders of the Sympathoadrenal System*, Contemporary Endocrinology,
https://doi.org/10.1007/978-3-319-77048-2

R

S